Pulmonary Arterial Hypertension and Interstitial Lung Diseases

Robert P. Baughman • Roberto G. Carbone
Giovanni Bottino
Editors

Pulmonary Arterial Hypertension and Interstitial Lung Diseases

A Clinical Guide

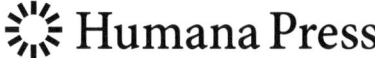 Humana Press

Editors
Robert P. Baughman
University of Cincinnati,
Department of Internal Medicine
Cincinnati, OH

Roberto G. Carbone
Regional Hospital
Department of Internal Medicine
Aosta, Italy

Giovanni Bottino
Regional Hospital
Department of Internal Medicine
Aosta, Italy

ISBN: 978-1-58829-695-5   e-ISBN: 978-1-60327-074-8
DOI: 10.1007/978-1-60327-074-8

Library of Congress Control Number: 2008937495

springer.com

wife Elise Lower,
in Memory of mother Attilia Innesti Carbone
wife Elena Bottino

Preface

Interstitial lung disease (ILD) is a broad category of lung diseases that includes more than 150 disorders characterized by scarring or fibrosis of the lungs. Even among the many types of the disease, ILD's progression can vary from person to person, and people respond differently to therapy. In the past, emphasis in treating ILDs has focused on the effect on gas exchange and loss of lung volume. This is a direct effect of the damage to the interstitium. However, an important indirect effect is on the pulmonary vasculature with resulting pulmonary hypertension. The association between interstitial lung disease and pulmonary hypertension has long been recognized, it was often associated with hypoxia and fibrosis alone. Recent studies that demonstrate response to pulmonary vasodilators stresses the vascular component of this process. In this book, we examine the various interstitial lung diseases. We also examine the incidence and outcome of pulmonary hypertension in the various interstitial diseases.

The book is divided into two main sections. The first discusses general issues. Drs. Carbone and Bottino introduce both ILD and associated pulmonary hypertension in the first two chapters of the book. The next chapter is by Drs. Meyer and Raghu, who discuss the evaluation of idiopathic interstitial lung diseases. They point out that this includes not only idiopathic pulmonary fibrosis, but other conditions such as nonspecific interstitial pneumonitis and cryptogenic organizing pneumonia. Drs. Moreira and Travis provide a detailed analysis of the pathology of the various ILDs. The pathologist often has the final say about what disease, although a comprehensive approach the clinician, radiologist, and pathologist gives a better definition of many cases. Finally, Drs. Carbone and Bottino summarize the evaluation of pulmonary hypertension. Although most of the information available is from patients with primary pulmonary hypertension, the observations can often be extended to patients with ILD.

The other section of the book deals with specific categories of disease. Dr. Lynch and colleagues discuss bronchiolitis, an increasingly recognized problem leading to airway obstruction and restriction. The use of inspiratory and expiratory high-resolution computed tomography scan has markedly enhanced the recognition of this process. Dr. Selman and his group then discuss hypersensitivity pneumonitis, a diffuse group of diseases bound together by common clinical and pathological features.

Drs. Brown and Strange discuss the collagen vascular diseases. Scleroderma has been one of the most widely studied lung diseases that can cause both interstitial lung process as well as pulmonary hypertension. In the past few years, large clinical trials have been published showing the benefits of some forms of therapy in these diseases. Dr. Martinez discusses the specific problem of pulmonary hypertension with idiopathic pulmonary fibrosis. Because idiopathic pulmonary fibrosis is associated with a high mortality, treatment for this complication may have major impact on the disease. Dr. Lee Newman examines the interstitial lung diseases associated with various occupational exposures. This divergent group can have a quite variable outcome. However, as a group it represents a major part of the differential diagnosis of all patients with interstitial lung diseases.

Dr. Baughman and colleagues discuss sarcoidosis. This multi organ disease affects the lungs in more than 90% of cases. Although most patients do well, there is a group with persistent pulmonary disease. Up to half of these patients will have pulmonary hypertension. Drs. Baughman, Lower, and Engel provide an evaluation for the disease and treatment strategies for the disease and associated pulmonary hypertension.

Finally, the editors would like to again to thank all the authors for their efforts in preparing this book. We would also like to thank Richard Lansing of Humana Press for his support.

Contents

Contributors

Robert P. Baughman, MD
Professor of Medicine, Interstitial Lung Disease and Sarcoidosis Clinic,
University of Cincinnati Medical Center, Department of Medicine,
Cincinnati, OH

Giovanni Bottino, MD
Professor of Medicine, Dept. of Internal Medicine, Docent of Respiratory
Diseases, DIMI-University of Genoa, Genoa, Italy

Alan N. Brown, MD
Associate Professor of Rheumatology and Immunology, Department of Medicine,
Medical University of South Carolina, Charleston, SC

Roberto G. Carbone, MD, FCCP
Department of Internal Medicine, Respiratory Unit, Regional Hospital,
Aosta, Italy; Consultant Physician of DIMI University of Genoa, Genoa, Italy,
for Interstitial Lung Disease, Consultant Physician of University of Turin,
Turin, Italy, for Asbestosis correlated with Mesothelioma, Aosta, Italy

Guillermo Carrillo, MD
Instituto Nacional de Enfermedades Respiratorias Ismael Cosío Villegas, México

Peter J. Engel, MD
Ohio Heart and Vascular Center, Cincinnati, OH

Michael C. Fishbein, MD
Department of Pathology and Laboratory Medicine, The David Geffen School
of Medicine at UCLA, Los Angeles, CA

Miguel Gaxiola, MD
Instituto Nacional de Enfermedades Respiratorias Ismael Cosío Villegas, México

Elyse E. Lower, MD
Professor of Medicine, Interstitial Lung Disease and Sarcoidosis Clinic,
University of Cincinnati Medical Center, Department of Medicine,
Cincinnati, OH

Joseph P. Lynch, III, MD
Division of Pulmonary, Critical Care Medicine and Hospitalists, Department
of Internal Medicine, The David Geffen School of Medicine at UCLA,
Los Angeles, CA.

Fernando J. Martinez, MD, MS
Department of Internal Medicine, Division of Pulmonary & Critical Care
Medicine, University of Michigan Health System, Ann Arbor, MI.

Keith C. Meyer, MD, MS, FACP, FCCP
Professor of Medicine, Medical Director of Lung Transplantation, Director,
Interstitial Lung Disease Clinic, Assoc. Director, Adult Cystic Fibrosis Clinic,
Section of Allergy, Pulmonary and Critical Care Medicine, Department
of Medicine, University of Wisconsin School of Medicine and Public Health.
Madison, WI.

Assaf Monselise, MD
Department of Internal Medicine, University of Tel Aviv, Tel Aviv, Israel

Fabio Montanaro, MB
Department of Epidemiology and Statistics University of Genoa, Genoa-Italy

Andre L. Moreira, MD, PhD
Department of Pathology, Memorial Sloan Kettering Cancer Center, NY, NY.

Carmen Navarro, MD
Instituto Nacional de Enfermedades Respiratorias Ismael Cosío Villegas, México

Lee S. Newman, MD, MA
Professor, Department of Preventive Medicine and Biometrics, Division
of Allergy and Clinical Immunology and Division of Pulmonary Sciences and
Critical Care Medicine, Department of Medicine, University of Colorado Denver,
School of Medicine, Denver, CO.

Ganesh Raghu, MD, FCCP, FACP
Professor of Medicine & Lab Medicine (Adjunct), Division of Pulmonary &
Critical Care Medicine, Director, Interstitial Lung Disease, Sarcoid and
Pulmonary Fibrosis Program, Medical Director Lung Transplant Program,
University of Washington. Seattle, WA.

Rajeev Saggar, MD
Division of Pulmonary, Critical Care Medicine, UC Irvine School of Medicine,
Irvine, CA

Moisés Selman, MD
Instituto Nacional de Enfermedades Respiratorias Ismael Cosío Villegas, México

Charlie Strange, MD
Professor of Pulmonary and Critical Care Medicine, Department of Medicine,
Medical University of South Carolina, Charleston, SC

Robert D. Suh, MD
Department of Radiology, The David Geffen School of Medicine at UCLA,
Los Angeles, CA

William D. Travis, MD
Department of Pathology, Memorial Sloan Kettering Cancer Center, NY, NY

Abbreviations

6MWT	six minute walk test
ACCESS	A Case Control Etiologic Study of Sarcoidosis
ACCP	American College of Chest Physicians
AIP	acute interstitial lung disease
ALK1	active/like kinase type/1
ANCA	antineutrophil cytoplasmic antibody
ANP	atrial natriuretic peptide
APC	antigen-presenting cells
AR	acute rejection
ASD	atrial septal defect
ATS	American Thoracic Society
AVP_1	vasopressin receptor
BAL	broncho alveolar lavage
BCG	bronchocentric granulomatosis
BeLPT	beryllium lymphocyte proliferation test
BIP	bronchiolitis interstitial pneumonia
BMPR2	bone morphogenetic protein receptor type-2
BNP	brain natriuretic peptide
BOOP	bronchiolitis obliterans organizing pneumonia
CCB's	calcium channel blockers
CFA	cryptogenic fibrosiing alveolitis (synonymous of IPF)
CMV	cytomegalovirus
COP	cryptogenic organizing pneumonia
CPI	composite physiologic index
CRP score	clinical radiological physiological score
CVD	collagen vascular disease
CXC	chemochine
DG	diacylglycerol
DIP	desquamitive interstitial pneumonia

DLco	diffusion capacity (of the lung) for carbon monoxide (CO)
DPI	Diphenyleniodonium
ERS	European Respiratory Society
ET	endothelin
ETA	endothelin receptor
EVE	endogenous vascular elastase
FVC	forced vital capacity
FEV1	Forced expiratory volume in one second
GIP	giant interstitial pneumonia
HHT	hereditary hemorrhagic teleangectasia
HPV	hypoxic pulmonary vasoconstriction
HSCT	HEMATOPOIETIC STEM CELL TRANSPLANTATION
IIP	idiopathic interstitial pneumonia
IL	interleukin
ILD	interstitial lung disease
IP	inositol phosphate
IP3	inositol triphosphate
IPAH	idiopathic pulmonary arterial hypertension
IPF	idiopathic pulmonary fibrosis
ISHLT	INTERNATIONAL SOCIETY OF HEART LUNG TRANSPLANTATION
LIP	lymphoid interstitial pneumonia
LIGHT	Lymph toxin-like Inducible protein that competes with Glycoprotein D for Herpes virus entry mediator on T lymphocytes
LTR	lung transplant recipients
NO	nitric oxide
NSIP	non-specific interstitial pneumonia
NYHA	New York Heart Association class
Octreoscan	^{111} In-DTPA-D-Phe1-Octreotide
ODTS	organic dust toxic syndrome
PAF	platelet activating factor
PAH	pulmonary arterial hypertension
PAP	pulmonary artery pressure
	PDE4, and PDE 5:phosphodiesterases
PAPm	mean pulmonary artery
PCW	pulmonary capillary wedge

PFT	pulmonary functional test
PGI2	prostaglandin I2
PH	pulmonary hypertension
PIP2	inositol polyphospholipids
P_{LA}	left atrial pressure
PLC	phospholypase C
PMF	progressive massive fibrosis
PPH	primary pulmonary hypertension
PVOD	pulmonary veno-occlusive disease
PVR	pulmonary vascular resistance
RA	right atrial
RB/ILD	respiratory bronchiolitis-associated with interstitial lung disease
RIPID	Italian registry for diffuse infiltrative lung disorders
RV	right ventricular/ ventricle
RVH	right ventricular hypertrophy
RVSP	right ventricular systolic pressure
S6c	peptide named sarafotoxin
SACE	serum angiotensing converting enzyme
SFTPC	surfactant protein C gene SFTPC
SLE	systemic lupus erythematous
SMC	smooth muscle cells
SOD	Super oxide Dismutase
SPAM cells	pulmonary artery smooth muscle cells
sPAP	systolic pulmonary arterial pressure
SPECT	Single Photon Emission Computed Tomography
SPH	secondary pulmonary hypertension
SSc	systemic scleroderma
TBB	transbronchial biopsy
TGF/β	transforming grown factor
TIE2	endothelial-specific receptor of angiopoietin-1
TNF	tumor necrosis factor
TR	tricuspid valve regurgitation
U.I.	uptake index
UIP	usual interstitial pneumonia
VEGT	Vascular endothelial growth factor
VF	ventricular fibrillation
V/Q	ventilation/perfusion

Part I
General Principles

Chapter 1
Interstitial Lung Disease: Introduction

Roberto G. Carbone, Fabio Montanaro, and Giovanni Bottino

Introduction

Interstitial lung diseases (ILDs) are a large group of heterogeneous inflammatory fibrosing disorders comprising more than 200 entities that predominantly affect the pulmonary interstitium rather than the airspaces [1]. Significant progress in the understanding of ILD was made since the 1960, with the recognition of collagen vascular diseases, drugs, and occupational exposures as potential causes. However, a wide spectrum of pathologies, presentations, and outcomes still remain unknown. Liebow and Carrington [2] were first to classify idiopathic interstitial pneumonia (IIP) into five histologic subgroups: usual interstitial pneumonia (UIP), bronchiolitis interstitial pneumonia, desquamative interstitial pneumonia, giant interstitial pneumonia, and lymphoid interstitial pneumonia. In 1998, the classification was modified by Katzenstein and Myers [3], with UIP corresponding to Hamman–Rich Syndrome [4], respiratory bronchiolitis associated with ILD, desquamative interstitial pneumonia, nonspecific interstitial pneumonia (NSIP), and acute interstitial lung disease. The modern classification, which was recognized by the American Thoracic Society and European Respiratory Society [5], included another entity: cryptogenic organizing pneumonia (Fig. 1.1). Different ancillary diagnostic procedures, such as chest x-ray, high-resolution computed tomography (HRCT), Gallium[67] scintigraphy, and bronchoalveolar lavage, are considered inaccurate and nonspecific in diagnosing this group of diseases, especially in the their early stages [6–11]. Imaging with radiolabeled indium-111 octreotide scintigraphy (Octreoscan, Mallinckrodt Medical, Inc., St. Louis, MO), which is used in the evaluation of patients with neuroendocrine tumours, meningiomas, astrocytomas as well as lymphomas and thymomas [12], has been proposed in the study of ILD by several clinicians and nuclear medicine specialists.

As for sarcoidosis, the use of Octreoscan was shown to be a sensitive diagnostic tool, particularly in the imaging of lymph nodes and spleen, and its use appears to enable the better identification of lung disease activity [13–15].

Recently, the authors of several studies [16–17] have proposed the use of echocardiography and cardiac catheterization as effective tools in the evaluation of pulmonary hypertension, which is a predictive factor of survival associated with

R.P. Baughman et al. (eds.), *Pulmonary Arterial Hypertension and Interstitial Lung Diseases,*
© Humana Press, a part of Springer Science + Business Media, LLC 2009

Classification of interstitial lung disease (ILD)

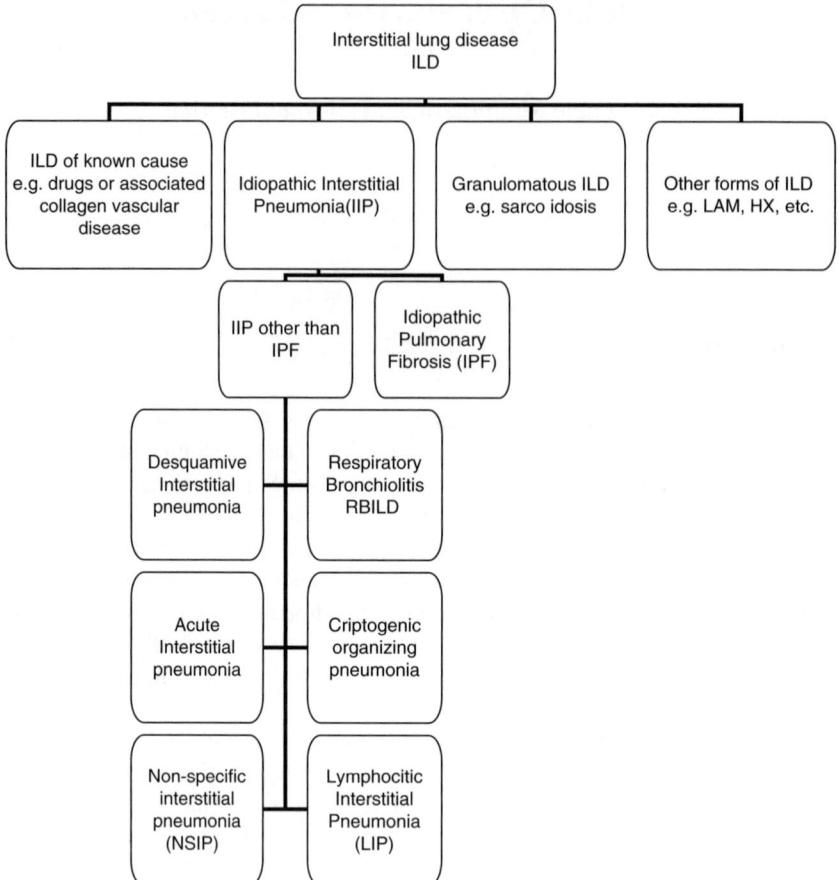

Fig. 1.1 Classification of ILD

systemic scleroderma. This hypothesis suggests a similar correlation between idiopathic pulmonary fibrosis (IPF) and pulmonary arterial hypertension [18].

Therapy for patients in the advanced stages of ILD has little or no benefit, which is why prompt diagnosis is important (especially with UIP or NSIP) and why lung biopsy considered the gold standard for the diagnosis. The importance of tissue morphology has been addressed in the American Thoracic Society/ European Respiratory Society / American College of Chest Physicians classification of IIP, where both histological and clinicoradiological findings with the use of HRCT are taken into account [19,20].

The difficulty in the clinical assessment and classification of ILD emphasizes the complexity of this group of diseases, which are still poorly understood and underdiagnosed. The scope of the following two chapters is to describe (1:) the epidemiology, the genetic factors of fibrotic lung diseases, the physiology, and the pathophysiology of the pulmonary circulation in correlation with ILD; (2) the role of imaging, such as HRCT, gallium-67, Octreoscan, and echocardiography in the development of new management strategies of ILD-associated pulmonary hypertension; and (3) the utility of different imaging techniques in the clinical medical practice.

Patients suspected of ILD must be referred to a specialist as soon as possible for the following reasons: (1) the earlier patients are referred to a pulmonologist, the greater the possibility of confirming the diagnosis; (2) an accurate diagnosis is crucial, because some ILDs are treatable; (3) early referral also may ensure that the patient is an eligible lung transplant candidate; (4) early diagnosis and intervention may improve outcomes and enable the patient to be enrolled in one of the many ongoing trials for potential new therapies; and (5) a prompt diagnosis of ILD should depend upon a multidisciplinary approach, in which clinical and radiological data assessed by physicians, pulmonologists, surgeons, cardiologists, pathologists, radiologists, and nuclear medicine specialists are integrated.

Epidemiology of ILD in Europe in Comparison With the USA

As mentioned previously, ILD is a group of approximately 200 different pathologies of heterogeneous origin, with different clinical aspects and prognosis. This implies that describing the "epidemiology of ILDs" involves the descriptions of each specific pathology included in this group.

Epidemiology of ILD

The first population-based registry of patients with ILD was established in Bernalillo County (NM, USA) in 1988 [21]. During the period of 1988–1993, 460 patients with ILD were enrolled in the patient registry: 56% were prevalent cases and 44% were incident cases diagnosed during the study period. The prevalence rates of ILD were estimated to be 80.9 per 100,000 among men and 67.2 per 100,000 among women and incidence rates of 31.5 per 100,000 and 26.1 per 100,000, respectively. This study had some limitations: first, only 7% of the cases had the diagnosis confirmed by open lung biopsy; second, the autopsy population—which was used to estimate the occurrence of preclinical and undiagnosed ILD in the general population—was much younger than the control group (average ages: 42 years versus 70 years, respectively); finally, concerns regarding possible overdiagnosis or underdiagnosis in the investigated community, possible overdiagnosis because of the activity of the registry itself, and the estimated pool of patients that could be undiagnosed were expressed by the authors but not investigated.

During the period of 1992–1996, in Flanders, a prospective registry collected information about 362 prevalent and incident cases of ILD. Cases came from 20 respiratory centers who responded to a standardized questionnaire. An incidence of 1.0 per 100,000/year was estimated [22].

In Germany, a prospective incidence registry of newly diagnosed cases of ILD started its activity in January 1995. Up to early 2000, 1,184 cases have been registered [23]. In Spain, an ILD registration was conducted on 23 pulmonary medicine centres during 1 year (Oct. 2000 to Sept. 2001). In the study period, 511 cases were registered, allowing researchers to estimate an incidence rate of 7.6 per 100,000/ year [24].

In Italy, two different registries were created. The first aimed to retrospectively survey the occurrence of different ILD through a questionnaire sent to 34 respiratory centres (17 respondents). Finally, 4,169 patients were registered and validated [25]. The second Italian registry, namely the Italian registry for diffuse infiltrative lung disorders (RIPID, i.e., Registro Italiano Pneumopatie Infiltrative Diffuse), was established in 1998 with the aim of creating a national database of these disorders, providing the background for epidemiological and clinical studies of adequate sample size [26]. During the period of 1998–2005, a total of 3,152 patients had been registered. Unfortunately, the prevalence and incidence rates could not be estimated because the size of the population covered by the participating centre was not exactly estimable, with the exception of Bolzano province, where 193 newly diagnosed cases of diffuse infiltrative lung diseases were enrolled in the registry and an incidence of 2.9 cases per 100,000 was estimated in the period 1990–2004. The most frequently reported interstitial lung disorders were sarcoidosis and IPF.

The RIPID did not include a series of 128 patients diagnosed with ILD of unknown etiology who were referred to Regional Hospital, Aosta (126,000 inhabitants) in the period 1995–2004. According to the recommendations of ATS Criteria, the diagnosis was made on clinical, radiological, and histological data:59 patients were diagnosed with UIP/IPF (46.1%), 19 with NSIP (14.8%), and the remaining 50 patients (39.1%) with other ILD (including:24 with sarcoidosis, 16 with Wegener granulomatosis, and 10 with extrinsic allergic alveolitis). All diagnosis of ILD were confirmed by biopsy:42 open pulmonary biopsies, 40 video-assisted thoracoscopies, 32 percutaneous biopsies, 12 mediastinoscopies, and 2 lymph node biopsies [27].

Because incidence/prevalence data were difficult to estimate or, where estimated, were susceptible to uncontrollable biases, the comparison of the occurrence in different areas could be not informative and likely biased. On the contrary, to compare the relative frequency of different ILD subgroups could be informative (Fig. 1.2). In all the registries, the most frequent diseases were IPF (more than 30% of cases except in Flanders) and sarcoidosis, ranging from 14.9% in Spain to 35.4% in Germany.

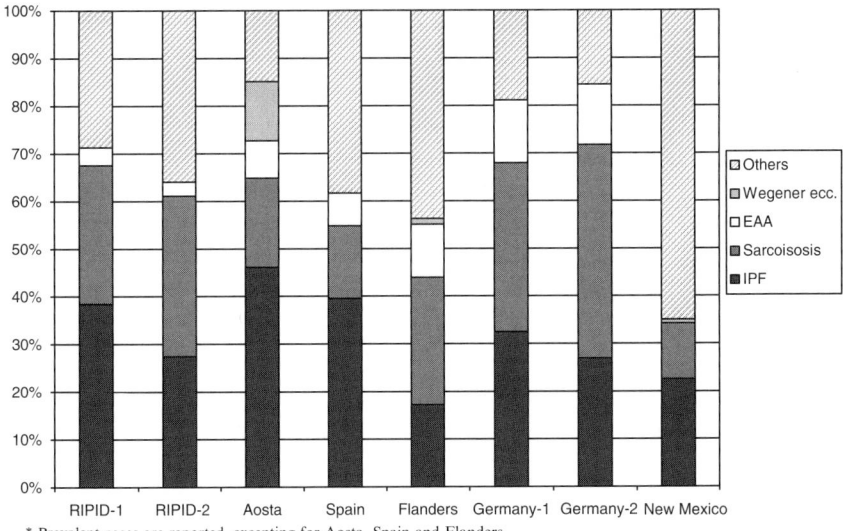

* Prevalent cases are reported, excepting for Aosta, Spain and Flanders.

Fig. 1.2   Relative frequency of ILD subgroups in different countries

Epidemiology of ILD Subgroups

Besides general ILD registries, epidemiological investigations on specific subgroup pathologies included in the large ILD disease also have been conducted.

IPF

IPF is not a rare disease. Approximately 80,000 cases of IPF have been identified in the USA, with an estimated 30,000 new cases developing each year. The descriptive epidemiology of IPF has not been deeply investigated, and estimates are quite limited. Moreover, criteria providing the basis for these estimates often are not precisely defined. In early 1990s, prevalence estimates of IPF in the general population varied from 3 to 6 cases per 100,000 [28,29], whereas the aforementioned New Mexico's ILD registry [21] revealed a prevalence of 20.2 and 13.2 per 100,000 among men and women, respectively, and an incidence of 10.7 per 100,000 per year among men and 7.4 among women. IPF is reported to occur more commonly in men than women [28,29].

Typically, patients present between the ages of 40 and 70 years, and approximately 66% of patients are older than 60 years of age at presentation. The mean age at diagnosis is 66 years, and the prevalence for people ages 35 to 44 years is 2.7 cases per 100,000 whereas the prevalence for people older than 75 years of age exceeds 175 cases per 100,000.

The incidence of IPF increases with age, as approximately two-thirds of patients with IPF are older than 60 years of age [28,30,31], and the incidence is 160 per 100,000 among 75 years of age and older [21]. There is no valid explanation as to why IPF is a disease that occurs predominately in older people.

Limited evidence exists that the geographical location and ethnicity are related to diagnosis. There is a slight male preponderance of disease, and the age-adjusted mortality rate for white patients exceeds that for black patients. Age-adjusted rates mortality rates from IPF appear to be greater among the white population and lower among the black population [31]. A geographic variation was observed that may reflect differences in occupational and environmental exposures.

Because IPF is a chronic disease that is almost uniformly fatal, the ratio of the prevalence to the incidence can provide a crude indication of the duration of survival after diagnosis [32]. Hubbard et al. [33] investigated the rate of mortality from IPF (i.e., cryptogenic fibrosing alveolitis) in England and Wales (UK), Australia, Canada, Scotland, Germany, USA, and New Zealand to determine whether mortality was increasing or decreasing compared with that observed in other seven countries. They observed that the greatest mortality rates for CFA were observed in UK, i.e., England and Wales, followed by Scotland, New Zealand, Australia, and Canada, whereas the USA and Germany had CFA mortality rates considerably lower than those for the other countries. Mortality from CFA had increased in England and Wales, Scotland, Canada, and Australia since 1979 whereas it decreased in the USA and it was low and stable in Germany.

Concerns regarding the accuracy of IPF diagnoses were raised. In the Italian RIPID, the diagnosis of IPF was based upon a surgical lung biopsy only in 20% of cases; this percentage of pathological diagnosis was slightly lower than that reported in the Spanish register (32%) [24], whereas in the Regional Hospital of Aosta, all diagnoses were biopsy-confirmed and 33% of all patients with IIP had open lung biopsies.

Sarcoidosis

Information on sarcoidosis can be traced from general ILD registries (Fig. 1.2) or from specific analytical studies; no specific registry of patients diagnosed with sarcoidosis have been established. Sarcoidosis represented 11.6% of prevalent cases registered by Coultas et al. [21] and 7.8 percent of incident ones in the same registry. Only approximately one-third of cases patients with sarcoidosis in the RIPID had a lung surgical biopsy.

A Case Control Etiologic Study of Sarcoidosis (ACCESS) generated a large database for a series of analytical epidemiological reports. In this study, in which the authors aimed to study the etiology of sarcoidosis, newly biopsy-confirmed patients with sarcoidosis from several US regions were examined with the use of a standardized evaluation [34–36].

In the first report, 736 patients were considered to be representative of sarcoidosis in the USA, even if some potential recruitment biases have been identified. In this report, organ involvement was investigated, revealing differences attributable to race, sex, and age [34]. Because of the considerable sample size of case and control relatives, Rybicki et al. [35] could demonstrate that sarcoidosis aggregates in family, confirming what was before based only on anecdotal reports. A third report based on ACCESS database was aimed to investigate the relationship between environmental and occupational factors and risk of sarcoidosis. The results of this study suggested that insecticides, agricultural environments, and exposure to microbial aerosol may be associated with sarcoidosis, whereas many other possible etiologic require further investigation [36].

Summary

The data of aforementioned registries confirmed that epidemiological registries can be useful tools to investigate rare or relatively rare disorders (e.g., sarcoidosis and IPF) to design multicentric clinical studies of adequate sample size, especially cohort and prospective studies, aimed at providing standardized diagnostic, management, and follow-up criteria with a particular regard to outcome measures such as survival and quality of life.

This consideration is a consequence of the fact that death certificates and state mortality data are neither sensitive nor accurate for describing the occurrence of ILD. Proof of that could be the apparently low mortality rates from IPF in USA when compared with other countries [37].

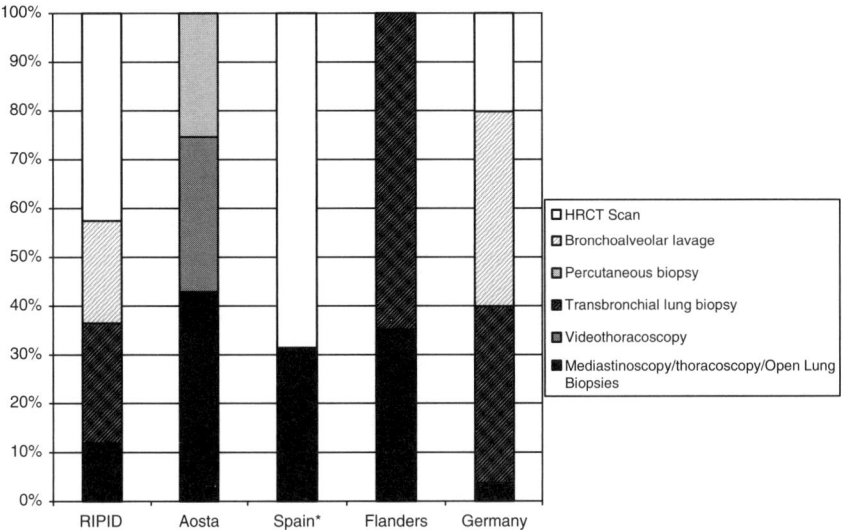

* IPF cases only. Both HRCT and open lung biopsies were used in combination with other diagnostic procedures.

Fig. 1.3 Diagnostic procedures in ILD in different countries

A limitation in the data of ILD registries is the limited use of biopsies. As reported in this chapter, only low percentages of cases had a histology confirmed diagnosis, whereas most diagnoses are based upon clinical observation and radiological and HRCT scan findings. Unfortunately, the accuracy of the HRCT scan is limited, as only approximately 50% of IPF diagnosis obtained in that way could be confirmed and the remaining should be inexorably wrong [7]. Therefore, the use of open lung biopsy should be the gold standard. Only Aosta Valley had all its cases histologically confirmed (Fig. 1.3). Comparability of registries included in Fig. 1.2 is limited, as RIPID included only 167 cases of 4,169 and Flanders only 71 out of 362. Finally, different diagnostic procedures for each patient have been registered in Spain.

References

1. Green FHY. Overview of pulmonary fibrosis. Chest 2002;122:334S–339S.
2. Liebow AA, Carrington CB. The interstitial pneumonia. In: Simon M, Potchen EJ, Le May M, editors. Frontiers of pulmonary radiology. New York: Grune & Sratton; 1969. p. 102–141.
3. Katzenstein ALA, Myers JL. Idiopathic pulmonary fibrosis. Clinical relevance of pathologic classification. Am J Respir Crit Care Med 1998;157:1301–1315.
4. Hamman L, Rich A. Acute diffuse interstitial fibrosis of the lung. Bull Johns Hopkins Hosp 1944;74:177–212.
5. American Thoracic Society and European Respiratory Society. American Thoracic Society/European Respiratory Society international multidisciplinary consensus classification of the idiopathic interstitial pneumonias. Am J Respir Crit Care Med 2002;165:277–304.
6. Turner-Warwick M, McAllister W, Lawrence R, et al. Corticosteroid treatment in pulmonary sarcoidosis: do serial lavage lymphocyte counts, serum angiotensin converting enzyme measurements and gallium-67 scan help management? Thorax 1986;41:903–913.
7. Gross TJ, Hunninghake GW. Idiopathic pulmonary fibrosis. N Eng J Med 2001;345:517–525.
8. Grijm K, Verberne HJ, Krowels FH, Weller FR, Jansen MH, Bresser P. Semiquantitative ^{67}Ga scintigraphy as an indicator of response to and prognosis after corticosteroid treatment in idiopathic interstitial pneumonia. J Nucl Med 2005;46:1421–1426.
9. Wells AU, Hansell DM, Rubens MB, Cullinan P, Haslam PL, Black CM, Du Bois RM. Fibrosing alveolitis in systemic sclerosis. Bronchoalveolar lavage findings in relation to computed tomographic appearance. Am J Respir Crit Care Med 1994;150:462–468.
10. Aqusti C, Xaubert A, Luburich P, Ayuso MC, Roca J, Rodriguez-Roisin R. Computed tomography-guided bronchoalveolar lavage in idiopathic pulmonary fibrosis. Thorax 1996;51:841–845.
11. Leung AN, Brainer MW, Caillat–Vigneron N. Sarcoidoisis activity: correlation of HRCT findings with those of ^{67}Ga scanning, bronchoalveolar lavage, and serum angiotensin-converting enzyme essay. J Comput Assist Tomogr 1998;22:229–234.
12. Musi M, Carbone RG, Bertocchi C, Cantalupi DP, Michetti G, Pugliese C, Virotta G. Bronchial carcinoid tumours: a study on clinicopathological features and role of octreotide scintigraphy. Lung Cancer 1998;22:97–102.
13. Lebthai R, Crestani B, Belmatoug N, Daou D, Genin R, Dombret MC, Palazzo E, Faraggi M, Aubier M, Le Guludec D. Somatostatin receptor scintigraphy and gallium scintigraphy in patients with sarcoidosis. J Nucl Med 2001;42:21–26.
14. Carbone R, Filiberti R, Grosso M, Paredi P, Peano L, Cantalupi D, Villa G, Monselise A, Bottino G, Shah P.. Octreoscan perspectives in sarcoidosis and idiopathic interstitial pneumonia. Eur Rev Med Pharmacol Sci 2003;7:97–105.

15. Carbone RG, Musi M, Cantalupi DP, et al. Somatostatin receptor versus Gallium-67 scintigraphy in interstitial lung diseases. Chest 1999;119:315S.
16. McGoon M, Gutterman D, Steen V, Barst R, McCrory DC, Fortin TA, Loyd JE; American College of Chest Physicians. Screening early detection, and diagnosis of pulmonary arterial hypertension. ACCP evidence-based clinical practice guidelines. Chest 2004;126:14S–34S.
17. Mc Laughlin VV, Presberg KW, Doyle RL, Abman SH, McCrory DC, Fortin T, Ahearn G; American College of Chest Physicians. Prognosis of pulmonary arterial hypertension. ACCP evidence-based clinical practice guidelines. Chest 2004;126:78S–92S.
18. Nadrous HF, Pellika PA, Krowka MJ, Swanson KL, Chaowalit N, Decker PA, Ryu JH. Pulmonary hypertension in patients with idiopathic pulmonary fibrosis. Chest 2005;128:2393–2399.
19. American Thoracic Society. Idiopathic pulmonary fibrosis: diagnosis and management. International Consensus Statement. Am J Respir Crit Care Med 2000;161:646–664.
20. Leslie KO. Historical perspective. A pathologic approach to the classification of idiopathic interstitial pneumonia. Chest 2005;128:513S–519S.
21. Coultas DB, Zumwalt RE, Black WC, Sobonya RE. The epidemiology of interstitial lung diseases. Am J Respir Crit Care Med 1994;150:967–972.
22. Roelandt M, Demedts M, Callebaut W, Coolen D, Slabbynck H, Bockaert J, Kips J, Brie J, Ulburghs M, De Boeck K, et al. Epidemiology of interstitial lung disease (ILD) in Flanders: registration by pneumologists in 1992–1994. Working group on ILD, VRGT. Vereniging voor Respiratoire Gezondheidszorg en Tuberculosebestrijding. Acta Clin Belg 1995;50:260–268.
23. Schweisfurth H. Report by the Scientific Working Group for Therapy of Lung Diseases: German Fibrosis Register with initial results [in German]. Pneumologie 1996;50:899–901.
24. Xaubet A, Ancochea J, Morell F, Rodriguez-Arias JM, Villena V, Blanquer R, Montero C, Sueiro A, Disdier C, Vendrell M; Spanish Group on Interstitial Lung Diseases, SEPAR.. Report on the incidence of interstitial lung diseases in Spain. Sarcoidosis Vasc Diffuse Lung Dis 2004;21:64–70.
25. Agostini C, Albera C, Bariffi F, De Palma M, Harari S, Lusuardi M, Pesci A, Poletti V, Richeldi L, Rizzato G, Rossi A, Schiavina M, Semenzato G, Tinelli C; Registro Italiano Pneumopatie Infiltrative Diffuse. First report of the Italian register for diffuse infiltrative lung disorders (RIPID). Monaldi Arch Chest Dis 2001;56:364–368.
26. Tinelli C, De Silvestri A, Richeldi L, Oggionni T. The Italian register for diffuse infiltrative lung disorders (RIPID): a four-year report. Sarcoidosis Vasc Diffuse Lung Dis 2005;22(Suppl 1):S4–S8.
27. Carbone R, Montanaro F, Bottino G. Outcome in interstitial lung disease. Eur Resp J 2005; 26:268.
28. Scott J, Johnston I, Britton J. What causes cryptogenic fibrosing alveolitis? A case-control study of environmental exposure to dust. BMJ. 1990;301:1015–1017.
29. Iwai K, Mori T, Yamada N, Yamaguchi M, Hosoda Y. Idiopathic pulmonary fibrosis. Epidemiologic approaches to occupational exposure. Am J Respir Crit Care Med 1994;150: 670–675.
30. Hubbard R, Lewis S, Richards K, Johnston I, Britton J. Occupational exposure to metal or wood dust and aetiology of cryptogenic fibrosing alveolitis. Lancet 1996;347:284–289.
31. Mannino DM, Etzel RA, Parrish RG. Pulmonary fibrosis deaths in the United States, 1979–1991. An analysis of multiple-cause mortality data. Am J Respir Crit Care Med 1996;153:1548–1552.
32. Weycker D, Oster G, Edelsberg J, et al. Economic costs of idiopathic pulmonary fibrosis. Paper presented at: CHEST 2002, November 2–7, 2002; San Diego, California.
33. Hubbard R, Johnston I, Coultas DB, Britton J. Mortality rates from cryptogenic fibrosing alveolitis in seven countries. Thorax 1996;51:711–716.
34. Baughman RP, Teirstein AS, Judson MA, Rossman MD, Yeager H Jr, Bresnitz EA, DePalo L, Hunninghake G, Iannuzzi MC, Johns CJ, McLennan G, Moller DR, Newman LS, Rabin DL, Rose C, Rybicki B, Weinberger SE, Terrin ML, Knatterud GL, Cherniak R; Case Control Etiologic Study of Sarcoidosis (ACCESS) research group. Clinical characteristics of patients in a case control study of sarcoidosis. Am J Respir Crit Care Med 2001;164:1885–1889.

35. Rybicki BA, Iannuzzi MC, Frederick MM, Thompson BW, Rossman MD, Bresnitz EA, Terrin ML, Moller DR, Barnard J, Baughman RP, DePalo L, Hunninghake G, Johns C, Judson MA, Knatterud GL, McLennan G, Newman LS, Rabin DL, Rose C, Teirstein AS, Weinberger SE, Yeager H, Cherniack R; ACCESS Research Group. A case-control etiologic study of sarcoidosis (ACCESS). Am J Respir Crit Care Med 2001;164:2085–2091.
36. Newman LS, Rose CS, Bresnitz EA, Rossman MD, Barnard J, Frederick M, Terrin ML, Weinberger SE, Moller DR, McLennan G, Hunninghake G, DePalo L, Baughman RP, Iannuzzi MC, Judson MA, Knatterud GL, Thompson BW, Teirstein AS, Yeager H Jr, Johns CJ, Rabin DL, Rybicki BA, Cherniack R; ACCESS Research Group. A case control etiologic study of sarcoidosis: environmental and occupational risk factors. Am J Respir Crit Care Med 2004;170:1324–1330.
37. Coultas DB, Hughes MP. Accuracy of mortality data for interstitial lung diseases in New Mexico, USA. Thorax 1996;51:717–720.

Chapter 2
Pulmonary Hypertension in Interstitial Lung Disease

Roberto G. Carbone, Assaf Monselise, and Giovanni Bottino

Genetic Factors Associated With Interstitial Lung Disease (ILD): View in Relation to Pulmonary Hypertension (PH)

The development of family registries and the banking of deoxyribonucleic acid has enabled researchers to search for a marker for familial PH on chromosome 2q 31/32. As a result, the bone morphogenetic protein factor receptor type 2 gene (BMPR2) on chromosome 2q 33, having 13 exons, was discovered. Mutations in familial PH have been reported in all exons except for 5 and 13. Humbert et al. [1] cited mutations of BMPR2 in PH associated with fenfluramine derivates. These data are concordant with the working hypothesis that gene–gene or gene–environmental interactions are required for PH. Conversely, Morse et al. [2] and Tew el al. [3], who studied patients with scleroderma and PH, did not find the presence of BMPR2 mutations.

Recently, Trembart et al. [4] have found a second PH gene in some patients with hereditary hemorrhagic teleangectasia lesions whose mutation in active/like kinase type/1 (ALK1) receptor confers a predisposition to PH and hereditary hemorrhagic teleangectasia lesions. Both BMPR2 and ALK1 genes are two receptors in the transforming grown factor (TGF)-β family. Multiple genetic causes associated with PH are summarised in Fig. 2.1.

Du et al. [5,6] have described the genetic mechanism of PH. According to their hypothesis, an unknown stimulus involved in the TGF-β receptor pathway increases angiopoietin-1 and its receptor TIE2, which decreases the BMPR1A receptor. The latter is required for the optimization of the BMPR2A receptor. Mutant forms of BMPR2A and mALK1 are associated with familial forms of PH, and both are involved in signaling through growth promoting proteins, which finally stimulate vascular smooth muscle remodelling. The study of genes associated with the risk of acquiring PH is complex from a statistical point of view. PH is probably the result of an interaction between the BMPR2 genes with environmental factors and will be continue to be a subject of future investigations.

R.P. Baughman et al. (eds.), *Pulmonary Arterial Hypertension and Interstitial Lung Diseases,*
© Humana Press, a part of Springer Science + Business Media, LLC 2009

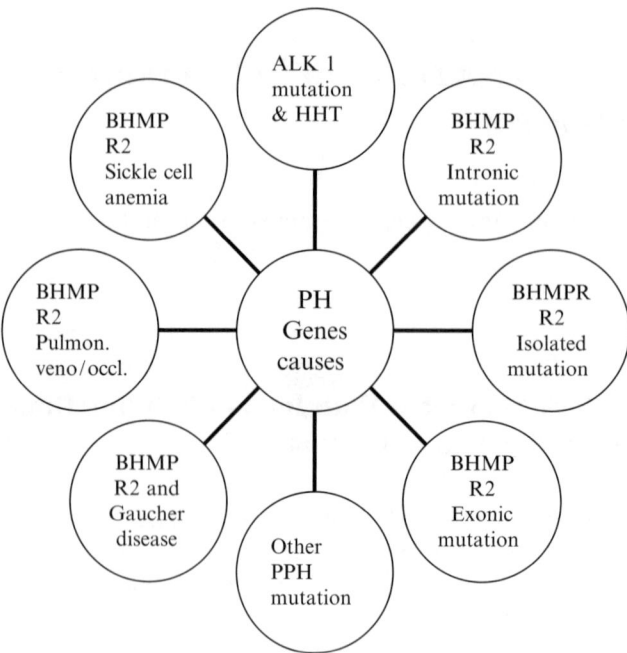

Fig. 2.1 PH genetic causes

View in Relation to ILD

Mutations of the surfactant protein C gene could be the cause of pathological forms of IPF, including nonspecific interstitial pneumonia (NSIP), desquamitive interstitial pneumonia (DIP), and usual interstitial pneumonia (UIP). Nogee et al. [7] showed that mature surfactant protein C is derived from the proteolysis of a 197 amino acid pro-protein. The surfactant protein C precursor protein is an integral membrane protein that is anchored to the membrane by a mature surfactant protein C. A deletion in the domain of the surfactant protein C precursor protein causes a disruption in the intracellular transport with a consequent degradation of this protein. A lack of mature surfactant protein C in lung tissue and bronchoalveolar lavage (BAL) fluid is an indication that the precursor protein has not being processed and secreted normally.

The absence of the surfactant protein/C (SP/C) or an abnormal production of the pro SP/C protein could both lead to severe ILD, as recently described by Amin et al. [8] in a family with ILD. In particular, the defective SP/C could be the cause of mechanical injury to the respiratory epithelial type II cells and thereby the alveoli, contributing to the pathogenesis of IPF. The clinical course of ILD as the result of surfactant protein C gene mutations appears could be quite long, ranging up to few decades. Evidence suggests a common viral respiratory infection as a trigger for the disease. Nineteen percent of patients who received a lung transplantation for IPF had a positive family history. Studying IPF in families may be the most effective method for understanding this disease. Several studies have provided evidence for the importance of TGF-β1 gene polymorphism in disease progression of IPF [9–13].

A study of the distribution, concentration, and profibrotic effects of a mutant TGF-β1 protein in lung tissue of patients with IPF is expected in the near future. A hypothesis that suggests a potential role for a genetic variant of TGF-β1 in disease progression of IPF must be confirmed in larger studies [14].

PH: Physiology in ILD

Pulmonary circulation is influenced by different physiologic conditions. Regional differences in blood flow occur during standing as the result of differences in the hydrostatic pressures between pulmonary artery, alveolar, and venous pressures. Blood flow does not depend on the pulmonary venous pressure but on a pressure gradient existing between pulmonary artery and alveolar pressure. For illustrative purposes, the lung can be divided in four zones: West zones I–IV in the standard position. In West zone I, the pulmonary artery pressure exceeds the alveolar pressure, and it is not present in human subjects under physiologic conditions because the pulmonary artery pressure always exceeds the alveolar pressure. The apex of the lung corresponds to West zone II. Blood flow in this zone follows the waterfall principle (Sterling resistance). The middle and lower portions of the lung correspond to West zones III and IV, respectively. Pulmonary vessels here are characterised by their capability to fully distend as a result of the augmented perfusion during physical activity.

In addition to this passive recruitment, an active vasodilation also could take place. The vasoconstrictive effect of hypoxia on pulmonary vessels is denominated hypoxic pulmonary vasoconstriction (HPV). HPV is mediated by cyclic AMP (cAMP) and cyclic GMP (cGMP) in smooth muscle cells of precapillary vessels. These two molecules regulate calcium concentration in the cytoplasm, thereby permitting the interaction of actin and myosin filaments. A cascade of events begins with the activation of G proteins by a series of ligands: caffeine, thromboxane A_2, noradrenaline, vasopressin (AVP_1 receptor), angiotensin II, and endothelin (ETA receptor), or by membrane depolarization, which blocks the potassium channels. Activated G proteins lead to PLC (phospholypase C)-mediated breakdown of inositol polyphospholipids PIP2 from membrane phospholipids, which give origin to inositol triphosphate IP3 and diacylglycerol DG. The interaction of the former with the sarcoplasmic reticulum causes an efflux of calcium ions into the cytoplasm.

Potassium channels also play an important role in the mechanism of HPV by influencing the membrane potential, which leads to the generation of cAMP and cGMP [15–17]. Cyclic GMP (cGMP) is activated by nitric oxide (NO), a potent vasoactive mediator, as well as by atrial natriuretic peptide (ANP) and brain natriuretic peptide. Cyclic AMP (cAMP) is actived by prostacyclin via the IP receptor and by catecholamines via B_2 adrenergic and D_1 dopaminergic receptors).

Phosphodiesterases (PDE4 and PDE5) inactivate cAMP and cGMP by cleavage of the two molecules, thereby permitting vasodilation.

Different subtypes of potassium channels have been identified in pulmonary vessels. Of particular interest is the K_{DR} subtype, which is important for the control of pulmonary vascular resistance. One of the K_{DR} channel components is present in scarce quantities in patients with PPH and is therefore thought to predispose them to the disease. Some subtypes of potassium channels are inhibited by appetite suppressants, such as dexfenfluramine. It seams that HPV is regulated by O_2 concentration, mechanism of which lies within pulmonary artery smooth muscle cells (SPAM cells). The mechanism is not well understood, but it appears to be related to an NADPH oxidase shown to exist also in oxygen-sensitive cells of the carotid body. During hypoxia, SPAM cells produce super oxide anions, which are converted by super oxide dismutase to hydrogen peroxide. The latter is degraded by a catalase to H_2O and O_2. It may be possible to block HPV by inhibiting the enzyme NADPH oxidase with diphenyleniodonium or by blocking the super oxide dismutase (Fig. 2.2) [18,19].

The final step in the chain of reactions bringing to HPV is dependent upon SPAM cell intracytoplasmatic concentration of calcium ions [20]. During hypoxia, the decrease in SPAM cells in the potassium concentration leads to membrane depolarisation, thereby permitting the influx of calcium ions into the cytoplasm, which leads to a cascade of events terminating in vasoconstriction.

Oxygen may be a direct activator of the potassium channels; otherwise, its effect could be mediated by intracellular changes in the redox potential with the formation of super oxide and peroxide anions, calcium ions. Indeed, it has been suggested that the NADPH oxidase is part of this oxygen-sensitive potassium channel. Recent studies have demonstrated that calcium channel antagonists, endothelin, and alpha-adrenergic antagonists block HPV. Some vasodilators, such as prostacyclin and NO, are able to counteract HPV [21].

Prostacyclin is an endothelium-derived antiaggregator molecule with vasodilating properties. Prostaglandin I_2 is a potent vasodilator with antiproliferative effects on smooth muscle fibres and fibroblasts [6]. It is an unstable molecule with a half-life of 2–3 min in the circulation, necessitating a continuous infusion while treating patients with PH.

Endothelin 1 (ET-1), a polypeptide synthesised by endothelial cells, is considered to be the most potent vasoconstrictor among the vasoactive peptides known.

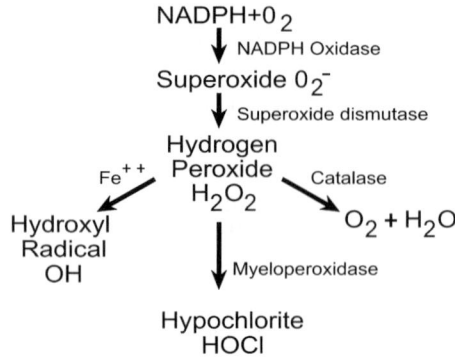

Fig. 2.2 Structure

The profibrotic, proinflammatory, proliferative, and vasoconstrictive effects of ET-1 are mediated through ET receptors [22,23]. Increased pulmonary vascular tone in PH is caused by a combination of factors: (1) enhanced ET-1 activity, a result of increased circulating ET-1 and increased expression of ET_A receptors, which mediates pulmonary vasoconstriction; (2) a decrease in vasodilators such as prostacyclin and NO; (3) vascular remodeling through the proliferation of pulmonary artery smooth muscle cells, resulting in medial hypertrophy and intimal hyperplasia; and (4) ET-1-induced platelet aggregation and hypoxia, which lead to an increase in endothelin secretion and stimulation of fibroblast proliferation. Stimulation of the ET-1R is a feature common to many disorders characterised by abnormal vasoconstriction, cell proliferation, and fibrosis, such as PH, pulmonary fibrosis, scleroderma, chronic heart failure, hypertension, and chronic renal failure (Table 2.1).

Two subtypes of ET-1 receptors are known: ET_A and ET_B [24,25]. The ET_A risoform is selective in that it binds ET-1 and ET-2 with a higher affinity than ET-3, whereas the ET_B R binds, in addition, a peptide named sarafotoxin S6c. Both subtypes are widely expressed on endothelial cells in lung and brain tissue. The expression ratio of the $ET_B R/ET_A R$ in the lung interstitium, alveolar epithelium, and large pulmonary vessels is in favor of the former. Furthermore, an increased

Table 2.1 Pathophysiology of PH

a) Factors contributing to hypoxemia

Endhotelin-1 (ET-1) and serotonin play an important role in pulmonary vasoconstriction in vivo:

ET-1 + serotonin →   high plasma levels
               ↓
Hypoxemia →   chronic hypoxaemia
         ↓
Pronounced vasoconstriction
         ↓
Remodeling of pulmonary arteries. Hypertrophy and proliferation of pulmonary vascular smooth muscle cells and increased number of platelets (the latter effected only by serotonin)
         ↓
High pulmonary vascular resistance
         ↓
Increased Pulmonary Hypertension
         ↓
Major detrimental impact on the quality of life
         ↓   ↓   ↓
Low exercise tolerance   overall morbidity   low prognosis and survival

b) Factors that antagonise the effects of hypoxaemia

1. O_2 therapy

2. Calcium antagonists

3. Inhaled nitric oxide

4. Prostaglandin infusion

5. Prostaglandin infusion in association with bosentan

6. Prostaglandin by aerosol

expression of ET-1 was shown to exist in the airway epithelium and type-II pnue-mocytes of patients with IPF [26,27], and the lungs of patients with scleroderma, as compared with subjects without [28]. In the rat model of bleomycin-induced pulmonary fibrosis, ET-1 was found to be increased in airway epithelial cells and inflammatory cells. An ET antagonist could attenuate the development of fibrosis, which could be the result of a decrease in the inflammatory process [29]. Further support for the role of ET-1 in pulmonary fibrosis comes from the observation that overexpression of ET-1 in the lung is associated with progressive pulmonary fibro-sis and recruitment of inflammatory cells, predominantly CD4 lymphocytes.

In this study by Hocher et al. [30], there was no significant development of PH. At present, there are a few studies in which the authors addressed the inflammatory and proliferative properties of ET[101–103]. Data regarding ET effects on angiogenesis related to pulmonary fibrosis are lacking. Indeed, the histopathological characteristics of IPF show features of dysregulated and abnormal repair with exaggerated angiogen-esis, fibroblast proliferation, and deposition of extra cellular matrix, leading to pro-gressive fibrosis and restrictive damage, as expressed in pulmonary function tests.

The first evidence of neovascularization in IPF was identified by Turner-Warwick et al. [31], who examined lungs of patients affected with interstitial lung diseases, and demonstrated neo vascularization leading to anastomoses between the systemic and pulmonary microvasculature.

Peao et al. [32] confirmed the evidence of neovascularization in the pathogenesis of bleomycin-induced pulmonary fibrosis after the perfusion of rat lungs with methacrylate resin. Using electron microscopy, Peao et al. [32] showed that the major vascular alterations that were located in the peribronchial regions consisted of the remodelling of the alveolar capillaries. The neovascularization was closely associated with regions of pulmonary fibrosis, similar to the findings in human lungs. However, further studies are necessary to investigate factors involved in angiogenetic regulation in pulmonary fibrosis.

In two reports, Kean et al. [33,34] demonstrated an imbalance of the CXC chemochine promoters of angiogenesis (CXCL5 and CXCL8) and inhibitors of angiogenesis (CXCL10) in IPF lung tissue. The chemochine imbalance, which promotes angiogenic activity in the lung tissue of patients with IPF, was reflected by increased levels of CXCL5 and CXCL8, in comparison with control patients. Lung epithelium was the source of CXCL5, whereas pulmonary fibroblasts were the predominant interstitial source of CHCL8. The increased angiogenic activity attributed to CXCL8 was accom-panied by a decrease in the angiostatic factor CXCL10.

Hyde et al. [35] proposed that interferon (IFN)-γ, a major inducer of CXCL10, could be an inhibitor of wound repair because of its angiostatic properties. However, at the same time, it has been shown to reduce fibrosis in bleomycin-induced pulmonary fibrosis. Kean et al. [36] confirmed that the imbalance of CXC chemok-ines was relevant to the process of pulmonary fibrosis: CHCL2 and CXCL10 were measured during bleomycine-induced pulmonary fibrosis in whole lung tissues and were found to be directly and indirectly correlated, respectively, with hydroxypro-line concentration, a measure of collagen deposition. Indeed, these findings give further support to the theory that CXC chemokine regulated angiogenesis, is an important factor in the process of pulmonary fibrosis.

It is important to mention the interactions between ET-1and ANP, an antagonist of the former. The importance of the vasoconstrictive effects of ET-1 are of particular concern in the phase of increased ANP levels. ANP suppresses ET-1 by a negative feedback mechanism, preventing endothelin-induced hypertension.

Pathophysiology

PH, which is characterised by vasoconstriction and structural changes in the small pulmonary muscular arteries and arterioles, is a devastating disease, with progressive elevation of pulmonary artery pressure (PAP) and pulmonary vascular resistance, ultimately producing right heart failure and death [37].

Two facts are accepted to be related with the disease: (1) PH and the subsequent development of cor pulmonale are recognised consequences of ILD and (2) the presence of PH in patients with ILD results from hypoxic vasoconstriction. New data suggest that the PH mechanism is much more complex than it seemed to be. The mechanism leading to the development of PH involves primarily the obliteration of lung microvasculature caused by pulmonary thromboembolism and mechanical stress, the result of heart defects. Second, any form of PH, which may be caused by inflammatory diseases of the lung, collagen vascular diseases, toxic oil syndromes, and hypoxic pulmonary vasoconstriction, occurs with hypoxia and alveolar hypoventilation. The different tyhpes of ethiopathogenesis cited lead to vasoconstriction and pulmonary vascular remodeling, aggravated by in situ thrombosis of the small pulmonary arteries.

PH is classified into three categories, based on the severity of the pulmonary hemodynamics: (1) latent PH, (2) manifest PH, and (3) severe or very severe PH. If one rules out the passive PH caused by an increase in left ventricular filling pressure, the possible causes of PH are (1) vasoconstriction, (2) loss of vascular cross-sectional area as the result of remodeling and the occlusion of small arteries, (3) the loss of parenchymal elasticity, and (4) a reduction in the active vasodilation mechanism.

Latent PH

In patients with PH, at rest, the mean PAP remains normal (<21 mmHg). During physical exercise, the PAP increases to 28–30 mmHg. Patients are asymptomatic or manifest dyspnoea during strenuous physical activity.

Manifest PH

In patients with manifest PH, PH is within normal range at rest. The majority of patients with a mean PAP between 21 and 30 mmHg exhibit lung diseases with secondary pulmonary hypertension (SPH). The maximum cardiac output shows a distinct limitation in the unadapted patient. The PAP increases to 30 mmHg or greater during exercise. Cardiac output is limited during physical exercise only in adapted patients. The patients suffers from dyspnoea.

Severe or Very Severe PH

In patients with severe or very severe PH, a mean PAP of 30–45 mmHg at rest correlates with decompesation and lung diseases. A mean PAP of 40–70 mmHg at rest correlates with decompensation and chronic pulmonary embolism. Finally, a mean PAP of between 65 and 120 mmHg at rest correlates with Eisenmenger's Syndrome. When patients are at rest, there is reduced cardiac output.

Right ventricular adaptation is one of the most important prognostic factors in pulmonary hypertension. Initially, right ventricular hypertrophy compensates for the increased after load. The chamber decompensates when the pressure increases more rapidly than the adaptation mechanism. A moderate increase of pulmonary resistances and a slow progression of disease are good conditions for the development of right ventricular adaptation. On the whole, the factors that influence right ventricular remodeling are largely unknown.

There is evidence that the local ACE system of the heart might be activated during PH [38]. Pulmonary arteries develop structural changes in parallel with the chronic vasoconstriction. In situ thrombosis develops, accelerating the remodeling of small cells. As a consequence, there is a reduction of the vascular cross-sectional area and a loss of compliance. Structural changes in pulmonary arteries differ between small and large vessels: the latter assume aneurismal forms, whereas the lumen of the former is progressively diminished as the result of the remodeling process.

The term remodelling is used to describe changes in small diameter pulmonary vessels [39,40]. Normal-appearing pulmonary arterial vessels have a continuous media down to a diameter of approximately 80 μm. Distally to this point, vessels are partially muscular and contain so-called intermediate cells, which range in their properties somewhere between pericytes and smooth muscle cells. In the most peripheral vascular areas, there are only few pericytes, and the remaining cell population consists of endothelial cells.

The process of vessel remodeling results in (1) intimal fibrosis, (2) hypertrophy of the media, and (3) the formation of myocytes ex novo. The smooth muscles of the media grow distally, initially in a longitudinal direction, providing a complete muscular layer to smaller pulmonary arterial vessels having a diameter down to 15 μm. The smooth muscle cells produce extracellular matrix proteins such as glycoprotein and elastin. At same time, there are changes in other vascular layers, such as the adventitia and intima. The adventitia shows a proliferation of fibroblasts with migration of these cells in the vessel wall. The intimal cells responsible for fibrosis are poorly characterised and are described as my fibroblasts secreting extracellular matrix proteins such as collagen type I and III. As for the intima, changes involve the glycocalyx layer of the endothelial cells, with a reduction of heparan sulphate, which can trigger smooth muscle proliferation.

It seems that endothelial cell mediators shift from an anticoagulatory to protrombotic profile. The internal elastic lamina is fragmented and allows cells to migrate into the intimal layer.

The plexogenetic arteriopathy is characterised by a formation of multiple endoluminal channels in small, thin-walled branches of pulmonary arteries that appear similar to glomeruli in the kidney. Tuder et al. [41] described the channels as multilayer endothelial cells. They named the process "misguided angiogenesis." According to their hypothesis, endothelial proliferation could be the result of a frustrated attempt to build new vessels. In contrast, Yi et al. [42] described the plexiform lesion as a subtype of intimal fibrosis, consisting of the same cells types. Plexiform lesions occur in PPH and SPH. The latter is also associated with congenital heart defects and liver cirrhosis. The cells in lesions of SPH were polyclonal, whereas monoclonal lesions were found in PPH and dexfenfluramine-induced PH. The presence of monoclonal lesions suggests that all the cells stem from a single cell and show properties of tumour-like proliferation.

Today, we know that two elements are involved in the pathogenesis of PPH and SPH: cellular calcium concentration and vessel remodelling. Although the former could be reversible within a short time, the latter, if reversible at all, would need a considerably longer period of time. PH leads to a vicious circle of disordered endothelial function: mechanical obstruction by thrombi corroborates vascular remodeling by the release of fibrin degradation products and thrombin which are potent growth factors. Vascular remodelling enhances mechanical obstruction. Furthermore, an alteration of gene expression in association with hypoxia and reduced endothelial concentration of NO synthase was documented in patients with severe PPH [43].

Arterial hypoxia is a cause of polycythemia, which occurs as a result of many reasons: high altitudes, lung disease, heart disease, chronic pulmonary embolism, and PH. The primary mechanism involves hypobaric hypoxia, hypoventilation, ventilation/perfusion mismatch, shunting of pulmonary blood flow and vessel, or structural heart defects. The increase in viscosity resulting from polycytemia increases the perfusion resistance and pulmonary pressure. Arterial supply of O_2 is increased as the result of a high concentration of haemoglobin and a decline in cardiac output.

The increased tension on blood vessels in PH depends upon different factors: static and hydrostatic forces, shear stress that is dependent on blood viscosity and the diameter of the vessel. Vessels that are exposed to hydrostatic strain are subjected to infiltration of different cells and secretion of matrix proteins and growth factors, which together act on the remodelling process. Vascular adaptations protect vessels from dilation and the interstitial space from extravasation of plasma, hereby increasing pulmonary resistance, which might culminate in PE. The concomitant presence of endothelin and prostacyclin maintains the vascular tone balanced, even though remodeling has taken place. Increased levels of plasminogen activator-inhibitor explain the tendency for the local development of thrombosis. Repeated distension of fibroblasts leads to their activation with an increase of fibrosis.

Pressure-induced endothelial injury leads to penetration of the vessel wall by serum factors, which induce the liberation of endogenous vascular elastase, followed by a cascade of events in which the glycoprotein tenascin, as well as fibronectin, plays an important role. It is yet unclear whether humoral mediators cause PH or whether PH induces these factors; however, it seems that the endothelium has an important role in this process. Three groups of mediators have been individualised. The first comprises Thromboxan A_2, angiotensin II, thrombin, and platelet activating factor, which interact with the vessel wall but do not have vasoconstrive effects. The second group of mediators have few or no vasoactive properties but contribute to the remodelling process of the vascular wall. Among the third group, NO, ANP, and prostaglandin I2 have antiproliferative and vasodilative properties.

Fibrosis in patients with ILD is a slow, progressive process, leading eventually to remodelling of the connective and vascular tissue and ending finally with PH. Many recent studies suggest that alveolar type II cell injury and apoptosis may be an important early feature in the pathogenesis of ILD.

Wang et al. [44] have suggested that fibroblasts in the lungs of patients with IPF produce angiotensin-related peptides that promote epithelial cell apoptosis. Kuwano et al. [45] showed that TGF-β promotes epithelial cell apoptosis. Hagimoto et al. [46] explained the mechanism in ILD as the result of the increased production of oxidants in the phase of glutathione deficiency. In addition, Wang et al. [47] described an increase of tumour necrosis factor (TNF)- α, which promotes the apoptosis of alveolar epithelial cells. These data suggests a potential role for TNF-α in the pathogenesis of ILD, especially in IPF. The use of anti-TNF-α agents could, therefore, be a possible therapeutic approach for ILD.

The studies reported herein propose a pathogenetic mechanism for ILD, which includes epithelial cell injury and the consequent accumulation of a variety of growth factors (keratocyte growth factor, TGF-α and β, insulin-like growth factor-1, platelet-derived grown factors, fibroblast growth factor), that promote epithelial cell proliferation. Many growth factors activate tyrosine kinase, which induces fibroblast proliferation and matrix production, a process culminating in epithelial cell regeneration with recruitment of fibroblast and myofibroblasts. Keane et al. [48] hypothised that the progressive fibrosis stems from an angiogenetic process attributed to an imbalance of pro- and anti–angiogenetic chemokines. Vascular endothelial growth factor, a potent inhibitor of endothelial cell apoptosis, has a role in promoting angiogenesis and fibrosis. In contrast, Renzoni et al. [49] and Koyama et al. [50] suggested a decreased concentration of vascular endothelial growth factor in ILD with less angiogenesis in IPF in comparison with the granulation tissue in organizing pneumonia. The early stages of IPF are characterised by enhanced angiogenesis, whereas the late stages are dominated by paucity of blood vessels.

The initiation and maintenance of pulmonary fibrosis may be perpetuated by a sequence of host cytokine responses. Initially, high concentrations of IFN-γ, a type 1 cytokine, cause the activation of phagocytes (i.e., neutrophils, monocytes, and macrophages) as well as the induction of MHC class II expression on antigen-presenting cells. Moreover, IFN-γ suppresses fibroblast proliferation and collagen deposition. Subsequently, type 2 cytokines (interleukin [IL]-4, IL-5, and IL-13) predominate, with activated fibroblasts and fibrosis.

The authors of numerous recent studies have demonstrated a role for IL-4 and IL-5 in fibroblast activation. Weller et al. [51] described a correlation between fibroblast activation and the production of eosinophils. The authors of several studies have showed an increase of eosinophils in association with pulmonary fibrosis. In fact, the evolution of chronic immune-mediated lung diseases depends first on an abortive type 1 (high IFN-γ) response and, second, on a shift to a type 2 response with high levels of IL-4 and IL-13, IgE antibodies, eosinophils, and Th2 cells. A persisting insulting agent activates a type 2 response with the production of fibroblasts resulting in matrix deposition to "wall-off" the agent from the host.

Summary

The pathophysiology of IPF is characterised by a shift towards the increased production of Th2 and the decreased production of Th1 cytokines as the result of an as-yet-unknown lung injury. Overexpression of the Th2 cytokine TGF-β leads to angiogenesis, activation of lung fibroblasts with fibrogenesis, and deposition of extracellular matrix, all hallmarks of IPF. The Th1 cytokine IFN-γ produces biological effects opposite from those of TGF-β. IFN-γ inhibits the proliferation of lung fibroblasts and, in the bleomycin-induced model of lung fibrosis, down-regulates the transcription of the gene for TGF-β [52,53]. Production of IFN-γ may be decreased in patients with IPF [54]. Therefore, IFN-γ may have a potential therapeutic role in the management of IPF.

Clinical Role of High-Resolution Computed Tomography (HRCT)

Numerous reports have shown that HRCT is significantly more accurate than chest x-ray in the diagnosis of ILD. The use of Thin-section or HRCT increases spatial resolution, facilitating visualization of the pulmonary parenchyma to the level of the lobule, thereby permitting the ability to discern the different anatomical patterns of ILD.

According to studies, HRCT is 10–20% more accurate in the diagnosis of ILD as compared with a chest x-ray [55,56]. A correct diagnosis was made in 65% of cases when chest x-rays are used versus 74% of cases when low-dose HCRT is used ($p<0.02$) and 80% when conventional HRCT is used ($p<0.05$) [57]. A high confidence level in diagnosis was obtained in 42% of chest x-rays, 61% of low-dose HRCT, and 63% of conventional-dose HRCT, which were correct in 92%, 90%, and 96% of the studies, respectively [57].

Despite the overall similarity in the results of different studies, important drawbacks, highlight the differences in the reported accuracies of HRCT, including scanning techniques, retrospective design, lack of clinical correlation, lack of correlation with disease stage, referral bias, inconsistent definition of degrees of confidence, and poor interobserver concordance. The radiological findings of pulmonary fibrosis on HRCT correlate strongly with fibrosis on histology ($p=0.0001$). Also, a ground-glass appearance correlates well with interstitial inflammation ($p=0.03$). The use of HRCT could play an important role in the selection of optimal sites for lung biopsy and to exclude patients with severe end-stage fibrosis, who may not benefit from biopsy [58]. In contrast, no significant correlation was found between the presence of pulmonary nodules as detected by HRCT and disease activity in the assessment of patients with sarcoidosis when the authors of several publications compared the efficacy of HRCT to pulmonary functional tests, histology, BAL, and serum angiotensin-converting enzyme in assessing disease.

Nevertheless, the presence of "ground glass" in HRCT studies proved to be of value as a predictor both of response to therapy as well as overall prognosis in patients with ILD [59]. Wells et al. [60] found that the presence of ground glass opacity was related to prognosis and likelihood of response to treatment. In this study, HRCT abnormalities were interpreted as predominantly ground glass (group 1), mixed ground glass and reticular pattern (group 2), or opacities that were predominantly reticular pattern (group 3). The 4-year survival rate was greatest in patients who had predominantly ground-glass opacity and greater in patients who had mixed opacities as opposed to those who had reticular abnormalities; these findings were independent of the duration of symptoms or severity of pulmonary function abnormalities ($p<0.001$). Similarly, the response rate to therapy in previously untreated patients was significantly greater in patients who had predominantly ground-glass opacity and greater in group 3. The study concludes that the evolution of disease is correlated with histology and independent of its extension. In fact, a patient with an 80% ground glass opacity pattern who is a responder to therapy has a 40% survival rate greater than a patient with a fibrotic or reticular pattern.

HRCT findings in group 1 patients, described by Wells et al. [60], bear a striking resemblance to HRCT findings in patients who had NSIP, raising the possibility that the improved survival in at least some of the patients in this group is related to variations in the underlying pathology. NSIP pathology is divided in two histological subsets: cellular (plasma cells and lymphocytes) and fibrotic findings [60]. The former, which is less common than the latter, has a better prognosis, with good survival in patients at 5 and 10 years. Imaging with HRCT of cellular NSIP shows that the thickening of alveolar septa is caused by inflammatory cells, whereas the fibrotic variant is characterised by homogenously thickened septae with scarce inflammatory cells.

IPF, a chronic progressive ILD that can be fatal within 3 years of diagnosis, probably is the most common IIP, accounting for 62% of the cases. When a peripheral reticular pattern consistent with fibrosis by histology is present, the results of HRCT are reported to be approximately 90% accurate in the diagnosis of patients who have suspected IPF.

A reticular pattern or honeycombing are always more prominent in the lower lung zones, but they may involve the whole lung in advanced disease. Honeycombing, described by Zerhouni et al. [61], when associated with an intermediate reticular pattern typical of an intralobular interstitial thickening, gives rise to the morphology of IPF (97%). Hunninghake et al. [62] reported that the positive predictive value of a diagnosis of IPF made with HRCT by experienced radiologists is 96%. McDonald et al. [63] suggested that a biopsy is not always necessary when HRCT can be used to visualised the typical features of UIP (reticular pattern with little or any ground glass abnormality). Daniil et al. [64] noted that patients with a typical HRCT pattern of IPF had reduced survival as compared with those who have an atypical HRCT pattern. Flaherty et al. [65] concluded that the survival of patients with a positive HRCT and histological features of UIP was significantly worse as compared with those with a histological pattern of UIP and an indeterminate HRCT. HRCT features correlated closely with the histological pattern of UIP, but an indeterminate HRCT could be correlated with UIP or NSIP. The greatest mortality was described among patients with typical features of UIP as visualised by HRCT [65].

Gay et al. [66] proposed an HRCT fibrosis score for predicting survival of patients with IPF. The authors determined scoring by considering the severity of ground glass and fibrosis patterns by evaluating the correlation between HRCT, histology, and survival. Thirty-eight patients with IPF were recruited; all were treated with steroids for at least 3 months. The major importance of this study was in proposing predictive factors of outcome that may be important in selecting a subset of patients for lung transplantation. There was a good correlation between the histologic and HRCT fibrosis scores, which validates the use of HRCT scoring in the assessment of patients with IPF. The major drawback of this study was the small group of patients observed. In two prospective studies, King et al. [67,68] examined factors influencing survival in IPF patients: A clinical radiological physiological score was calculated.

The strength of these studies are supported by many factors: a histologic support, the numbers of cases, duration of follow-up, and an accurate statistical analysis. The major drawbacks were the absence of HRCT imaging and that all patients completed maximum exercise testing and DL_{CO}. For the authors, the HRCT results would likely strengthen the clinical radiological physiological score,because the assessment score and detection of PH with the use of a chest x-ray is subjective. Wells et al. [69] developed a composite physiologic index, where patients with IPF were evaluated with HRCT and pulmonary functional tests (i.e., forced vital capacity, forced expiratory volume in 1 second, and diffusion capacity of the lung for carbon monoxide [DLco]). The strength of the composite physiologic index lies in the fact that it does not require a complete exercise test nor the presence of experienced radiologists for the interpretation of HRCT. This index could be a useful clinical guide for staging disease severity and predicting outcome in patients with ILD.

The importance of HRCT was further emphasised by Mogulkoc et al. [70], who demonstrated that the HRCT fibrosis score was an independent predictor factor of survival in IPF. The Joint Statement of American Thoracic Society (ATS) and European Respiratory Society has approved that, in the absence of an open lung biopsy, HRCT should be one of the four major criteria necessary for the diagnosis of IPF, that is, after excluding other causes of ILD established by history, transbronchial biopsy, BAL, and abnormal pulmonary functional tests. The additional presence of at least three of four minor criteria (age >50 years, insidious onset of dyspnoea, duration of disease greater than 3 months, bibasilar crackles) is necessary [71].

Because features of NSIP on HRCT may significantly overlap with IPF/UIP, DIP, and cryptogenic organizing pneumonia (COP), NSIP is commonly misdiagnosed on HRCT. Cellular and fibrotic NSIP subtypes appear differently. The former exhibits a prominent ground-glass appearance (70–100%), whereas the latter has a fine reticular fibrosis, thickened septal lines, and honeycombing. The pattern is very similar to that of IPF (Fig. 2.3). Radiological and clinical features can be used to differentiate between fibrotic NSIP and IPF; the former shows an improvement in patients after steroid therapy. The Joint Statement of ATS and European Respiratory Society suggests that NSIP should be considered at first a provisional clinical diagnosis (Fig. 2.4). NSIP could be regarded as idiopathic only after excluding possible associations with collagen vascular diseases, drugs, and extrinsic allergic alveolitis.

On HRCT, the features of respiratory bronchiolitis/ILD and DIP (Fig. 2.5) typically overlap. The use of HRCT reveals areas of dense ground glass in association with mild reticulations in the upper zone of the lung with centrilobular emphysema. Mild bronchiol ectasias and centrilobular nodules are present in particular in the upper zones of the lungs. Honeycombing is uncommon. Both types of ILD have a good response to the use of steroids and the cessation of smoking.

The features of COP on HRCT typically show a mixed consolidation area of ground glass distributed in different patterns: triangular, patchy, and peripheral (Fig. 2.6). Approximately 85% of patients have a rapid response to steroid therapy, but in the remaining 10–15%, the disease is progressive. The relationship between UIP and COP has not been fully studied, but a reticular HRCT pattern in COP, similar to that of UIP, portends poor prognosis.

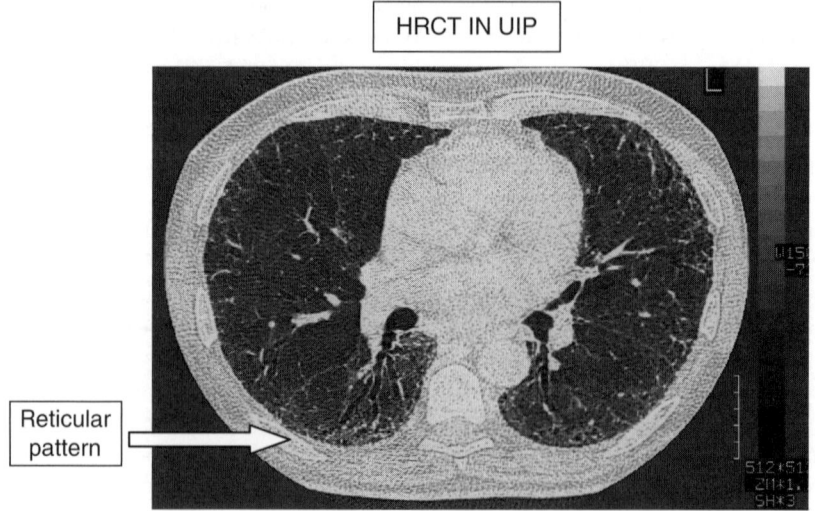

HRCT IN UIP

Reticular pattern

Fig. 2.3 UIP

HRCT IN NSIP

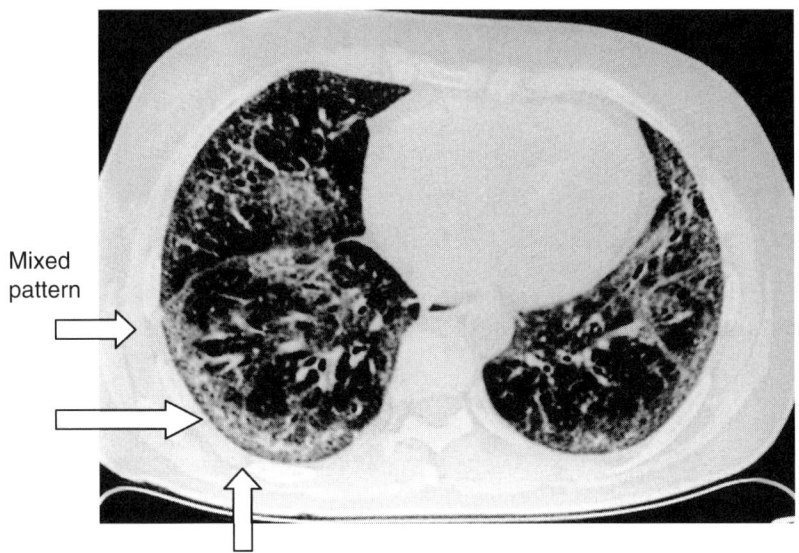

Mixed
pattern

Fig. 2.4 NSIP

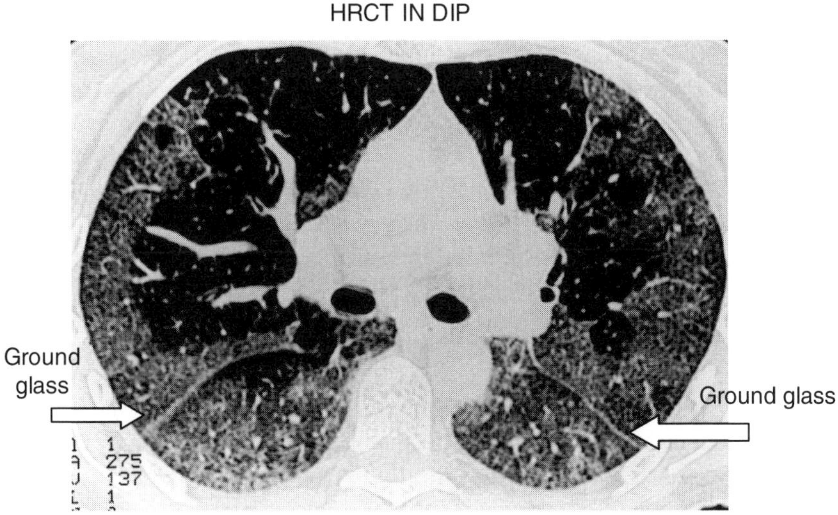

HRCT IN DIP

Ground
glass

Ground glass

Fig. 2.5 DIP

The features of acute interstitial lung disease on HRCTare characterised by
ground glass extended a random (100%), and partially consolidated (overall 60%).
Honeycombing is uncommon. Acute interstitial lung disease has a mortality rate of
approximately 60%; the remainder of patients experience long-term survival. LIP

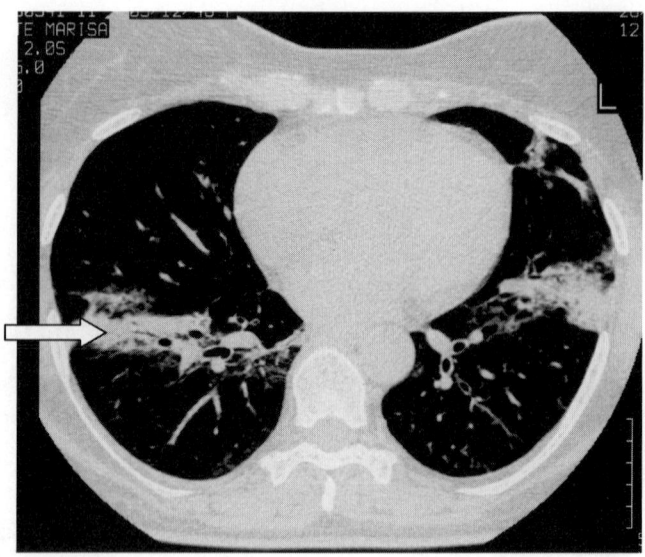

Fig. 2.6 COP

on HRCT appears as ground glass and numerous parenchymal fine nodules with a centrilobular distribution.

The features of UIP/IPF on HRCT may mimic UIP secondary to collagen vascular diseases asbestosis and limited bibasilar fibrosis resulting from recurrent aspiration. A granulomatous appearance on HRCT is typical of sarcoidosis (small hard nodules) and hypersensitivity pneumonia (soft centrilobular nodules). Moreover, hypersensitivity pneumonia may exhibit a patchy consolidation and therefore could be confused with respiratory bronchiolitis/ILD or COP. Finally, neoplastic ILD (lymphangitic metastasis) may appear as a reticular and ground glass pattern.

When considering the differential diagnosis of ILD, one should take into account other HRCT findings, such as a dilated esophagus in patients with systemic scleroderma, pleural plaques in asbestosis, lymph nodes in sarcoidosis and, in lymphangitic metastasis, hepatomegaly in amiodaron-induced lung disease. A score capable of predicting survival could be a useful tool for evaluating ILD. Other means currently available for the follow-up of patients with ILD are not accurate: DL_{CO} lacks standardization; the HRCT fibrosis score is a semiquantitative visual score. A CT score combining the ground glass severity scale, fibrosis, and periaxial score at different sections could be solution.

Some cases of ILD may present on HRCT with increased periaxial deposition of connective tissue. The evaluation in these cases is based on scoring of different CT sections where the ratio of airway wall thickness (T) to bronchial diameter (D) [T/D] is considered. We have studied the correlation of HRCT periaxial with pulmonary function tests, DL_{CO}, the 6-minute walk test (6MWT), dyspnea, and PH. In CT, periaxial score T/D, the normal value of which is 0.23, was not different in small and large airways [72].

Our evaluation of the 0 score is $\chi = 0.15$–0.23 and pathological values have been calculated, by defining the extent of the disease by means of the ratio between the areas A and A_0 of the cross sections of the sick and the normal bronchi, respectively. In this way, we have obtained the following formula:

$$T/D = 0.50 - \chi \sqrt{(A/A_0)}$$

The results of this work concluded that the HRCT periaxial score in patients with ILD had a good correlation to a restrictive pattern of pulmonary function tests, a normal DL_{CO} and PH, a negative 6MWT, and mild dyspnea.

Indeed, HRCT is a useful and noninvasive tool for the diagnosis and evaluation of ILD. It is important to bear in mind that a normal HRCT does not always exclude early and clinically significant ILD, especially in the phase of abnormal physiological tests.

Summary

A HRCT scan with a basal pattern of honeycombing (reticular pattern) and traction bronchiectasis is highly suggestive of IPF and carries with it a poor prognosis. In this setting, an open-lung biopsy is not necessary, although some clinicians perform bronchoscopy to exclude other diseases. On the other hand, the absence of a reticular pattern or fibrosis and the predominance of a ground glass pattern suggest NSIP. Here, the prognosis and response to treatment are better, and open lung biopsy is often performed. The HRCT fibrosis score is still a semiquantitative visual score. Therefore, we suggest that calculating a CT score based on a ground glass severity scale and CT fibrosis and periaxial score, at different sections, would be more accurate.

Clinical Role of BAL in ILD

BAL in combination with HRCT imaging and the clinical setting can play an important role in the differential diagnosis of ILD. A recently published study on a large cohort of patients ($n = 3{,}118$), showed the importance of the predictive value of BAL in the diagnosis of ILD. BAL cell counts were most useful for the diagnosis of relatively common entities, such as sarcoidosis, in contrast to rare forms of ILD. The ratio of T lymphocytes CD4+:CD8+ BAL is usually is increased in patients with clinically active pulmonary sarcoidosis. However, although older age may be a contributing factor for a high ratio, many patients do not have an increased ratio. Thus, the sensitivity of an increased CD4+:CD8+ ratio for sarcoidosis is relatively low. A decreased CD4+:CD8+ ratio has been reported in patients with hypersensitivity pneumonitis (HP), drug-induced lung disease, COP, eosinophilic pneumonia (EP), and IPF. A BAL lymphocyte differential count greater than 25% could be indicative of an ILD associated with granuloma formation, (e.g., sarcoidosis and hypersensitivity pneumonitis), or drug toxicity, that is, after excluding other diseases such as mycobacterial or fungal infection.

An exposure history to an antigen known to cause HP, when combined with BAL rich in lymphocytes (especially with differential counts equal or greater than 50%), is strongly suggestive of this disease. An eosinophil count equal or greater than 25% could be caused by an eosinophilic lung disease, especially EP, if the presentation is acute. In contrast, an extreme increase in the BAL content of neutrophils is likely caused by infection or an acute and diffuse lung injury. Because infection can cause the subacute onset of diffuse lung infiltrates or coexist with noninfectious ILD, BAL should be examined and screened for mycobacterial or fungal infection when performed to evaluate diffuse infiltrates.

Increased numbers of mast cells have been associated with HP, drug reactions, sarcoidosis, ILD associated with collagen vascular disease, IPF, COP, EP, or malignancy. Plasma cells have been observed in BAL in HP, drug reactions, EP, malignancy, or infection. Alveolar macrophages may also display morphological changes, such as a foamy appearance in HP, markedly vacuolated cytoplasm positively staining for fat in chronic aspiration pneumonitis, cytoplasmic inclusions associated with viral infection (e.g., cytomegalovirus pneumonia), ingested red blood cells with diffuse alveolar haemorrhage, or ingested asbestos bodies. Bloody lavage fluid is characteristic of diffuse alveolar haemorrhage. BAL fluid that has a milky or light brown to whitish color suggests the diagnosis of pulmonary alveolar proteinosis. A BAL with CD1a-positive cells in the right clinical setting and imaging can support a diagnosis of pulmonary Langerhans cell histiocytosis.

Acute-onset ILD is defined as an illness of less than 4 weeks' duration, with symptoms of shortness of breath, hypoxaemia, and diffuse radiographic infiltrates. The patient should have no history of previous lung disease, and no obvious risk factors for acute respiratory distress syndrome, such as sepsis or trauma. Diagnostic considerations in acute-onset ILD include infection and noninfectious ILD (i.e., acute interstitial pneumonia, acute EP, diffuse alveolar haemorrhage, acute HP, acute COP, drug toxicity, or acute exacerbation of previously undiagnosed IPF). Bronchoscopy with BAL at the time of acute presentation may facilitate the diagnosis and avoid the need for a surgical lung biopsy.

Recent advances in ILD assessment have demonstrated that the BAL procedure is an excellent tool in the clinical diagnosis of IPF when surgical lung biopsy is not performed. To make a diagnosis of IPF without a surgical lung biopsy, all four major criteria (exclusion of other known causes of ILD, a restrictive ventilatory defect and impaired gas exchange on pulmonary function testing, bibasilar reticular abnormalities with little or no ground-glass opacities on HRCT, and transbronchial biopsy or BAL showing no features to support an alternative diagnosis) and at least three of the four minor criteria (age > 50 years, the insidious onset of otherwise-unexplained dyspnea on exertion, duration of illness ≥ 3 months, and chest auscultation showing bibasilar inspiratory crackles) must be present [73].

Some experts suggest, however, that when lower lung honeycombing occurs and upper lung zone reticular lines are present, the positive predictive value of these HRCT findings for a diagnosis of IPF/UIP is at least 85%, and a confident diagnosis of UIP can be made when these findings are present [73].

We suggest that, in cases of atypical HRCT, nondiagnostic patterns, or in elderly patients with extensive honeycombing and advanced disease, that the IPF diagnosis be made with the use of a minimally invasive approach such as BAL or indium-111 octreotide scanning (Octreoscan, Mallinckrodt Medical, Inc., St. Louis, MO). The latter seems to show a close correlation with IPF (UIP histological features).

Furthermore, clinicians should be aware that radiographic imaging, including HRCT, may not show pathologic changes, particularly when certain forms of ILD (e.g., non-IPF interstitial pneumonias or HP) are present. If BAL is performed on a symptomatic patient who has undergone radiographic imaging that is not suspicious of ILD, an abnormal cell profile consistent with the presence of an alveolitis can indicate the need for additional investigation including lung tissue biopsy [73].

Summary

The role of the BAL procedure in the diagnosis and staging of ILD has been subject to intense study and will continue to increase in importance. The ATS and guidelines for BAL in ILD are currently being completed. The algorithm described below describes an updated approach to BAL in the diagnosis of ILD (Fig. 2.7).

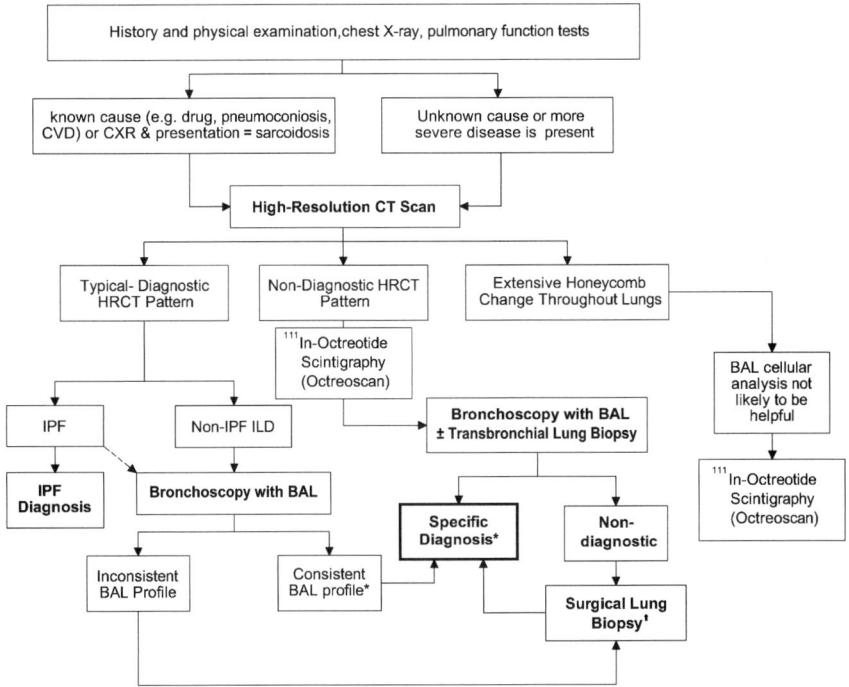

*Infection malignancy, and hemorrhage must be excluded as required by clinical features
'Surgical lung biopsy should sample at least two different lung regions and be guided by the HRCT image.

Fig. 2.7 Flowchart

Clinical Role of the Scintigraphy (i.e., Gallium-67 and Indium-111 Octreotide Scan [Octreoscan])

The evaluation of patients with sarcoidosis (unlike those affected with IPF) requires a combination of clinical, radiographic, scintigraphic, or bronchoscopic data. Given the contradictory results of these studies, it is apparent that a definitive conclusion regarding the role of HRCT in diagnosis and assessment of disease activity in patients with sarcoidosis remains to be determinated. Leung et al. [74] demonstrated a poor correlation between the extent of nodular involvement on HRCT and the intensity of lung gallium uptake ($r=46$; $p<0.02$), BAL lymphocytes ($r=50$; $p<0.01$), and serum angiotensin-converting enzyme levels ($r=38$, $p<0.05$).

Gallium-67 scintigraphy routinely was used for the study of ILD, especially sarcoidosis [75,76]. This test, whose sensitivity is now known to be suboptimal, was used in the past for its prognostic value [77]. Today, it is known that gallium imaging has no proven value for evaluation of IPF [77]. It is an expensive ancillary test, is associated with radiation exposure, and requires two hospital visits by the patient, the first for injecting the contrast and the second for scanning. The interpretation of gallium scans is difficult, and a negative scan does not exclude disease. Confounding factors such as steroid treatment must be considered, and patients should be instructed to stop therapy 1 week before the procedure [78,79].

Turner-Warwick et al. [80] had suggested that if no symptoms caused by extrapulmonary disease are present, then the evaluation of disease extent in sarcoidosis can be limited to clinical history, chest-X-ray, and pulmonary function tests. Although HRCT is more sensitive than chest-X-ray for detecting ILD, it is of limited value because worsening of symptoms and a decrease in lung function tests are not correlated with CT imaging [81].

In the face of a lack in imaging techniques capable of providing adequate information on the disease extent and predict its severity disease, the use of somatostatin receptor imaging could be promising. Octreotide is a somatostatin derivate that binds to granuloma somatostatin T lymphocyte receptors, especially CD4-T cells, thereby demonstrating active granulomatous disease in sarcoidosis. Somatostatin receptors (subtype 2) are also present in epithelioid cells and giant cells [78,82]. Somatostatin receptor whole-body scintigraphy was obtained at 4 and 24 h after the administration of 5mCi of [111] In-DTPA-D-Phe1-octreotide (Octreoscan). Thoracic imaging was obtained with single-photon emission computed tomography. The Octreoscan uptake index (UI) was defined as the ratio between normal and pathologic accumulation of the tracer in lung tissue. Octreoscan UI was scored by the use of a similar procedure described in literature used for gallium-67 and compared with the data of a group of healthy individuals. Normal values at 4 and 24 h were considered for UI$\leq$10.

As for patients with sarcoidosis, the use of Octreoscan was shown to be a more sensitive diagnostic tool than gallium-67 scintigraphy, particularly when lymph nodes and spleen were imaged. Octreoscan is useful for the identification of disease activity and extension of lung disease (Fig. 2.8) [78,79,83]. Lebthay et al. [78]

confirmed that the use of Octreoscan also was more accurate than gallium-67 scintigraphy for evaluating the extent of sarcoidosis in patients receiving steroid therapy. Finally, the increased costs associated with Octreoscan, are outweighed by the accuracy of this test.

Summary

The Octreoscan UI is strongly correlated with the degree of dyspnea in patients with sarcoidosis and can effectively quantify pulmonary involvement (Fig. 2.8). Further studies are warranted to evaluate Octreoscan as an early test in the prediction of disease.

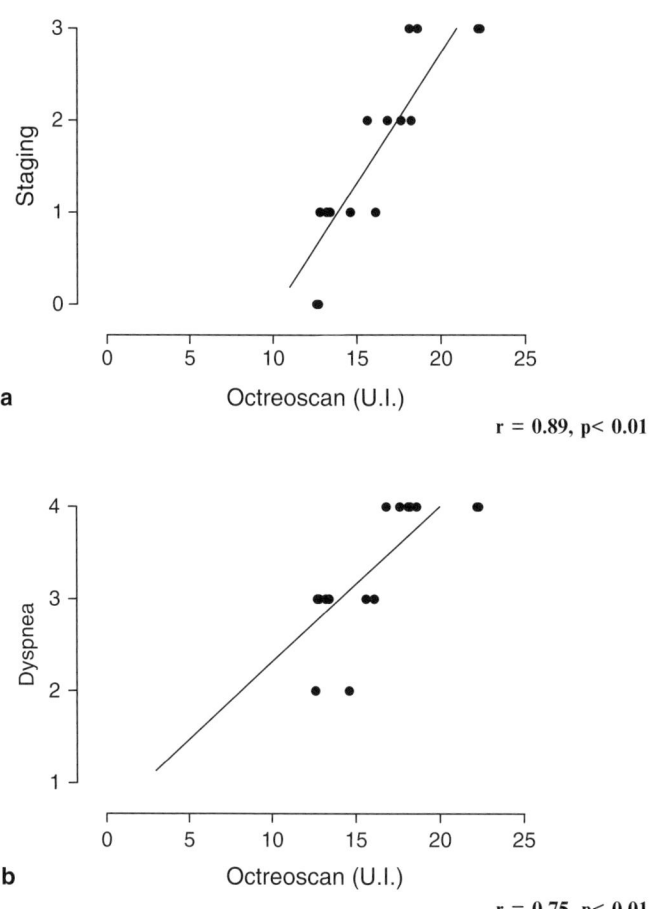

Fig. 2.8 Octreoscan in sarcoidosis. Correlation with staging (**a**) and degree of dyspnea (**b**)

The Octreoscan UI could be particularly useful in monitoring extrathoracic sarcoidosis and NSIP, probably because these two conditions are characterised by a
preponderant inflammatory infiltrate (particularly lymphocytes) and less fibrosis
(Fig. 2.9a). As for UIP, HRCT is still the most prevalent imaging technique for

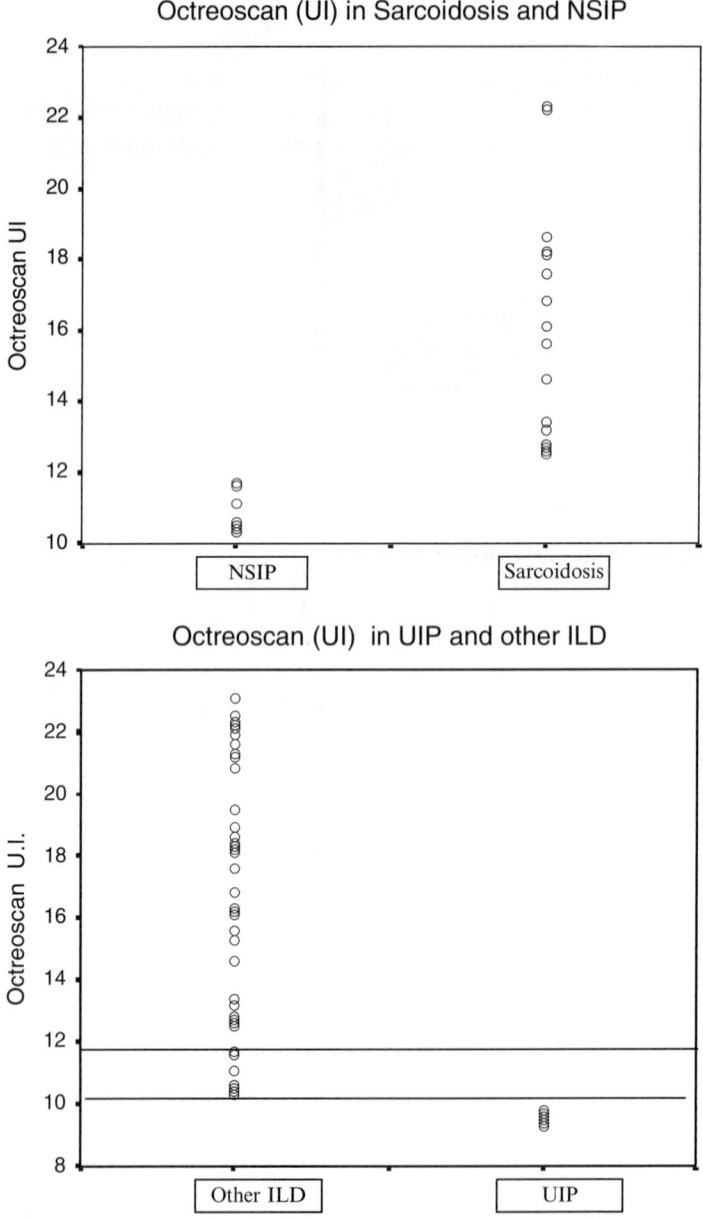

Fig. 2.9 a Octreoscan in sarcoidosis and NSIP. **b** Octreoscan (IU) in UIP and other ILD

assessing the extension of disease. Larger studies are necessary to evaluate the substitution of HRCT by Octreoscan in the assessment of UIP (Fig. 2.9b. Figs. 2.10–2.18, Octreoscan imaging).

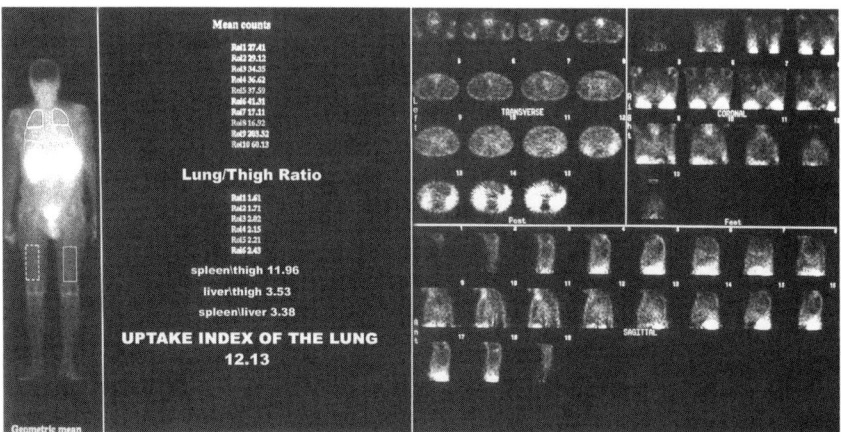

Fig. 2.10 Octreoscan of NSIP

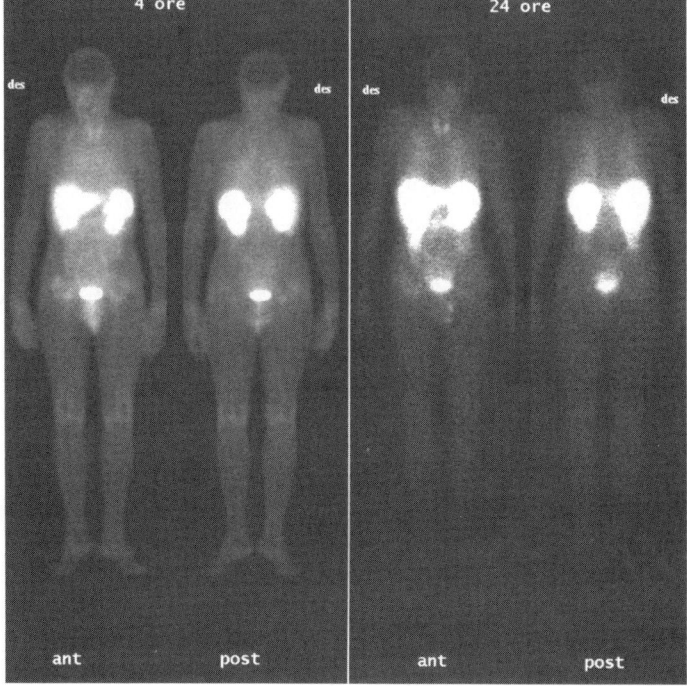

Fig. 2.11 Anterior and posterior Octreoscan scans of NSIP

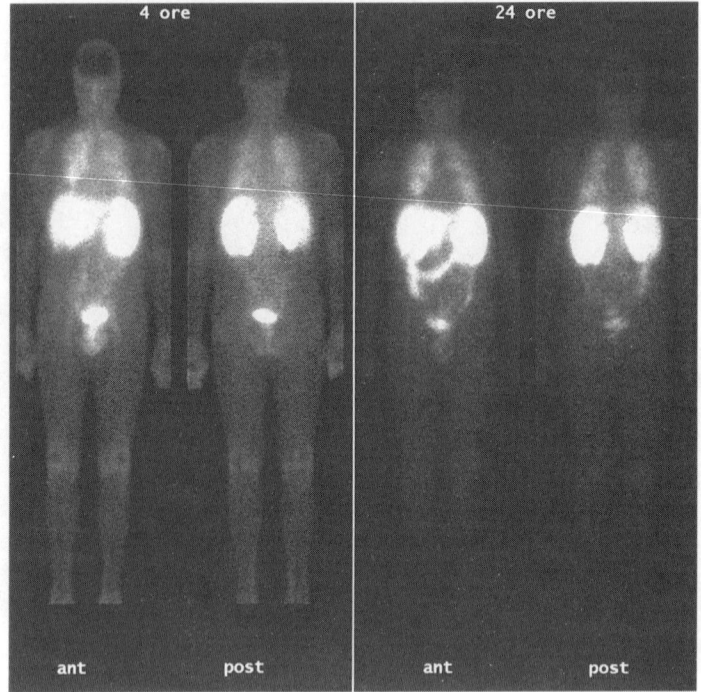

Fig. 2.12 Octreoscan of sarcoidosis

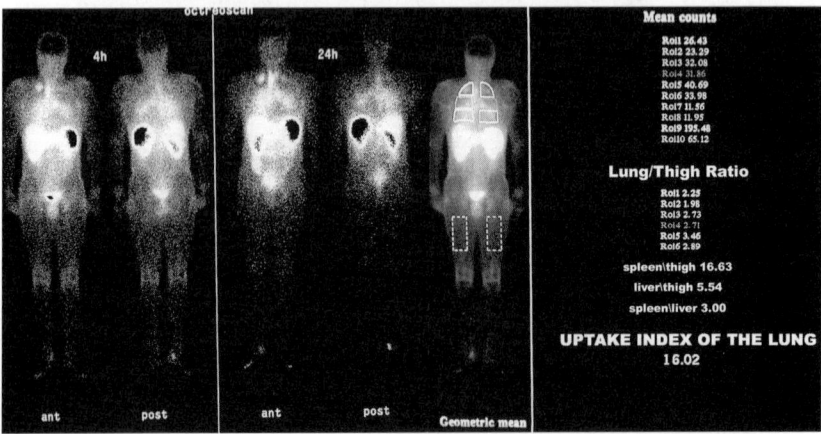

Fig. 2.13 Anterior and posterior Octreoscan scans of sarcoidosis

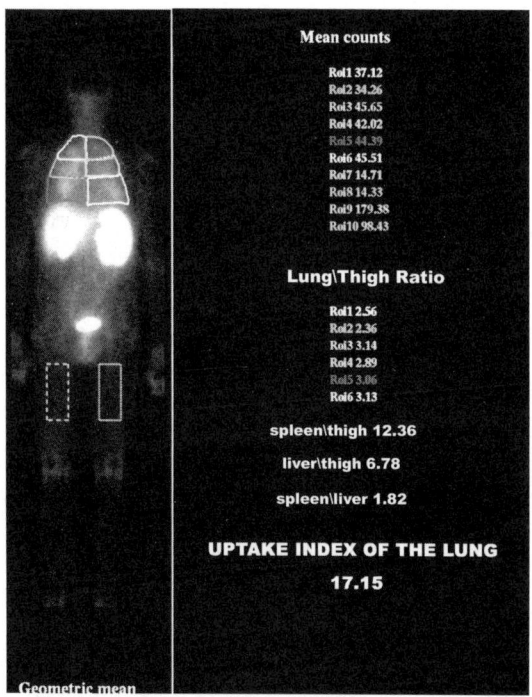

Fig. 2.14 Octreoscan of sarcoidosis

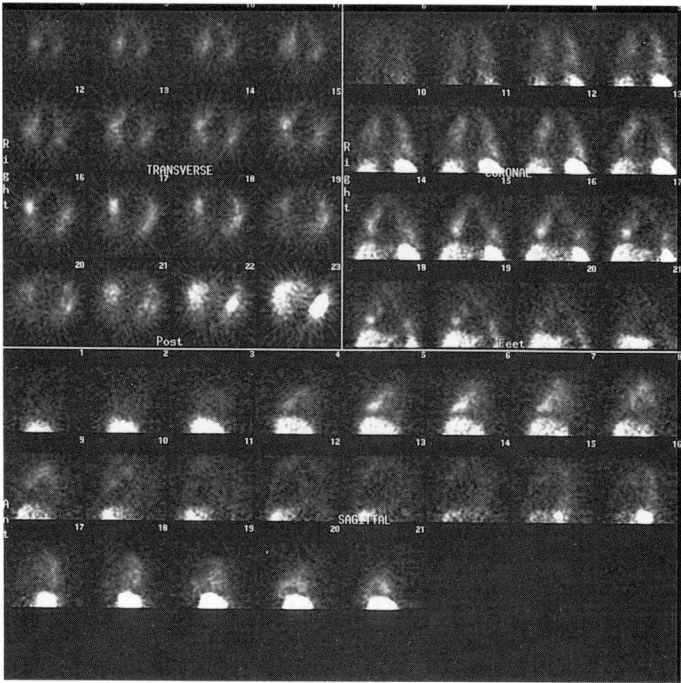

Fig. 2.15 Sarcoidosis on single-emission photon computed tomography

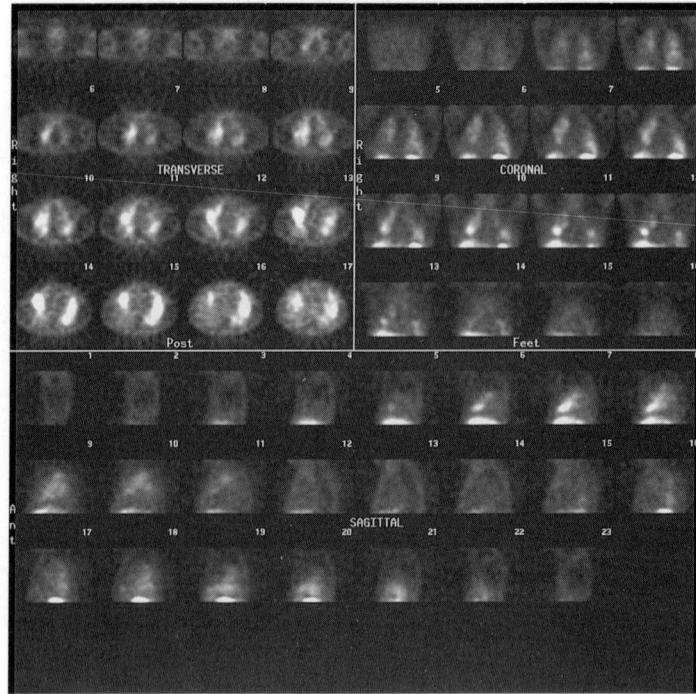

Fig. 2.16 Sarcoidosis on single-emission photon computed tomography

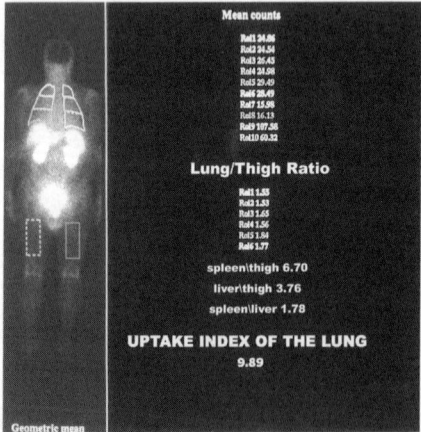

Fig. 2.17 Octreoscan of UIP

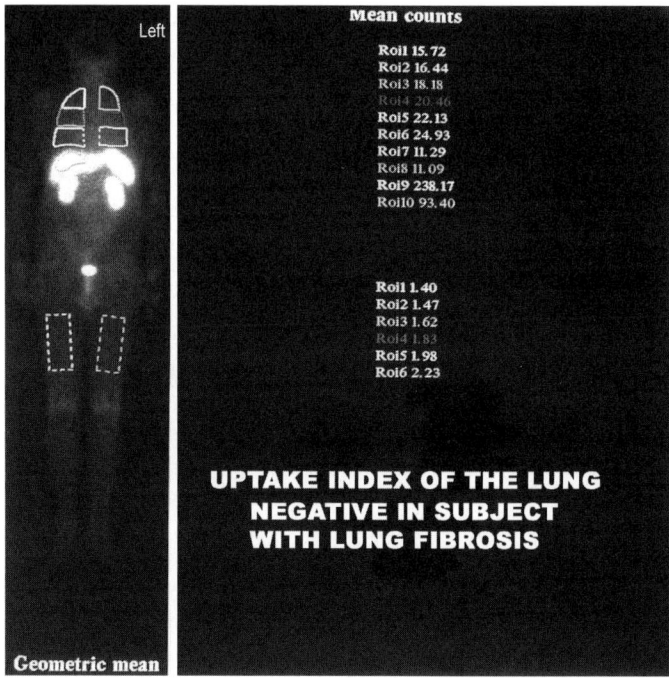

Fig. 2.18 UIP on single-emission photon computed tomography

Correlation Between Heart and Lung in ILD: Cardiological Procedures

Pulmonary arterial hypertension has been observed in all connective tissue diseases, but most frequently in systemic scleroderma (SSc). A good correlation between HRCT and pulmonary arterial hypertension could improve the clinical assessment, therapy, and survival prediction of patients with ILD. The development of pulmonary hypertension is a marker of poor prognosis. Up to 80% of patients affected with IPF and up to 50% of those with SSc develop secondary pulmonary artery hypertension, which begins with extravascular inflammation.

In the latter, echocardiography is a good screening test for early PH; it has a high sensitivity and specificity [84]. Echocardiography, as an adjunct to clinical evaluation, is currently the optimal screening approach for evaluating patients with SSc-related pulmonary arterial hypertension, which carry a worse prognosis than those with idiopathic pulmonary hypertension [85]. Burdt et al. [86] found that PH secondary to mixed connective tissue diseases, in particular overlap of scleroderma, systemic lupus erythematous, and myositis, was the most common cause of death, occurring in 38% of patients. Increased pulmonary arterial pressure occurred less frequently in patients with systemic lupus erythematous, polymyositis, and rheumatoid arthritis. PH was associated with Raynaud's phenomenon in each of the cases, suggesting a similar pathogenesis of these vasculopathies.

When PH is suspected clinically, Doppler echocardiography should be performed as soon as possible. Systolic pulmonary arterial pressure (sPAP), which is considered equal to right ventricular systolic pressure in the absence of pulmonary valve stenosis or outflow tract obstruction, can be evaluated by Doppler echocardiography with a sensitivity and specificity that ranges from 0.79 to 1, and 0.6 to 0.98, respectively.

McQuillan et al. [87] assessed the clinical correlates of sPAP on a large echocardiographic database of 102.818 patients: the mean sPAP was 28.3 ± 4.9 mmHg (95% confidence interval 18.7–37.9 mmHg). The author concluded that the evolution of Doppler techniques during the last decade has permitted the detection of minimal tricuspid valve regurgitation (TR) and thereby has made the estimation of sPAP more accurate.

The percentage of normal echocardiographic tests in which less-than-moderate TR was detected has increased from 48% in 1990 to 80% in 1999. Barst et al. [88] defined PH for values sPAP>35 mmHg. According to this author a Doppler examination by an experienced sonographer yields quantifiable TR in 74% of cases. Other studies reported absent or non quantifiable TR in 39% of patients, but pulmonary diastolic pressure also can be estimated by the use of Doppler echocardiography and correlates well with invasive measurements ($r=0.92$) [89]. The authors of many studies use correlation coefficients as measures of accuracy, for example, comparing echo estimate and the value measured by right-catheterization.

Screening examinations depend not only on the sensitivity and specificity of the test used, but also on the prevalence of disease in the study population. False-positive results will be more frequent when the prevalence of disease is low. Consequentially Doppler echocardiography may underestimate the sPAP in patients with severe PH and overestimate sPAP in populations comprising mostly subjects with normal pressures.

The debate between experts about the efficiency of echocardiography as an accurate examination for the diagnosis of PH resides in the fact that the use of this examination results in an underestimation of the disease. According to Baughman et al. [90], the use of echocardiography could be a useful tool in ruling out significant PH in patients with sarcoidosis only if a TR jet is clearly visualised. This group confirmed the presence of PH in more than half of sarcoidosis patients with persistent dyspnea. Sulica et al. [91] reported the detection of PH by echocardiography in 40% of patients with sarcoidosis.

Arcasoy et al. [92] studied a group of 374 patients with advanced lung disease who underwent echocardiography and right heart ventricular catheterization within 72 h of each other: the use of echocardiography had a sensitivity of 85% in diagnosing PH, the specificity was lower, and a large percentage of patients were misclassified as having PH, especially when the estimated right ventricular systolic pressure was close to the cut-off point of 40 mmHg. Furthermore, Nadrous et al. [93] described a subgroup of patients in which PH could not be estimated because of a lack of TR. This patient group did not survive for a long time. The authors of a study that evaluated mortality in association with PH found that subjects with IPF had a very poor survival rate, especially those with concomitant left ventricular dysfunction. The preservation of cardiac output can be an important factor in IPF associated PH as well as in idiopathic pulmonary hypertension.

Doppler echocardiography should be performed as a noninvasive effective tool that can detect, in some cases, an interstitial lung disease developed after cardiac surgery. It is known that cardiopulmonary surgery is associated with an acute inflammatory process that leads to lung damage caused by ischemia/reperfusion injury [94–96]. The latter is not limited to cardiomyocytes but also extends to the entire organism and especially in the alveolar/capillary unit and the interstitial lung tissue. Our clinical investigations hypothesised an injury of the capillaries and, most generally, of the interstitium of the lung with an inflammatory response 2 months after beginning cardiac surgery and often remaining at chronic clinical levels without treatment, probably leading to progressive fibrosis with definitive damage of pulmonary interstitium.

In the early inflammatory cellular phase after cardiac surgery, an interstitial lung process was shown: (1) BAL fluid containgin a decrease of T-helper CD4 lymphocytes and an increase in T-suppressor CD8 lymphocytes, (2) pulmonary function tests with a restrictive pattern often involving the small airways and DLco (77.9%±SD16), (3) a moderately increased mean sPAP (44±SD 10 mmHg), and (4) a significant response after treatment with steroids.

Therefore, a Doppler echocardiography accurate study must be conducted to diagnose and exclude left cardiac failure and/or diastolic dysfunction. In fact, the vascular/alveolar units are vulnerable to injury as a result of disorders affecting the heart, releasing endotoxin, secretion of metabolic markers, and generation of oxygen-derived free radicals by polymorph nuclear neutrophils. At the anatomic level, the interstitium is defined as the alveolar walls, including epithelial cells and capillaries, septae, and perivascular, perilymphatic, and peribronchiolar connective tissues. This structure is characterised from a wall extremely thin of alveolar–interstitial–capillary–plasma–erythrocyte and at same time immensely strong to withstand the stresses caused from the changes of the internal and external pressure.

The stress leads to multiple events of injury/inflammation of the alveolar–capillary constituents compromising the normal basement membrane integrity. In response to injury, an intraalveolar exudative process takes place with infiltration of macrophages, fibroblasts, and other inflammatory cells. The resistance to stress is guaranteed from collagen IV of basement membranes enmeshed in an extracellular matrix that defends the alveolar–capillary barrier. Nevertheless, the physiologic and pathophysiologic phenomena can lead to chronic inflammation with remodeling of the extracellular matrix structure, progressing inevitably to end-stage pulmonary fibrosis.

Remodeling about the stress related to the larger pulmonary arterial and venous system is known, vice versa it's also needed to demonstrate the pathophysiological mechanism of injures related to capillary section. Another potential mechanism of disrepair seems to be the result of injuries caused from exchanges of capillary pressures and regulated from a modified gene for various procollagen formations and for the development the other grown factors. [97,98].

The 6MWT is a submaximal exercise test used to assess functional capacity in congestive heart failure. It is also useful for evaluating patients with PH for the following reasons: (1) the ease of reproducibility, (2) the good correlation with maximal exercise testing, and (3) the fact that most patients reach the end point of the test [99]. The 6MWT correlates with cardiovascular mortality and morbidity and helps a clinician to predict survival in patients with idiopathic pulmonary arterial hypertension.

The New York Heart Association (NYHA) classification is a simple method for classifying patients with congestive heart failure. NYHA has been used as a predictor of survival in several studies of patients with PH; however, its significance was proved in only three studies of SSc and idiopathic pulmonary hypertension. Little is known about the correlation between the NYHA classification and ILD associated PH. Carbone et al. [100] reported that NYHA could estimate survival and be used as a substitute for PAP in ILD (Figs. 2.19–2.23). Future prospective studies with mortality as an end point could shed more light on the utility of this classification.

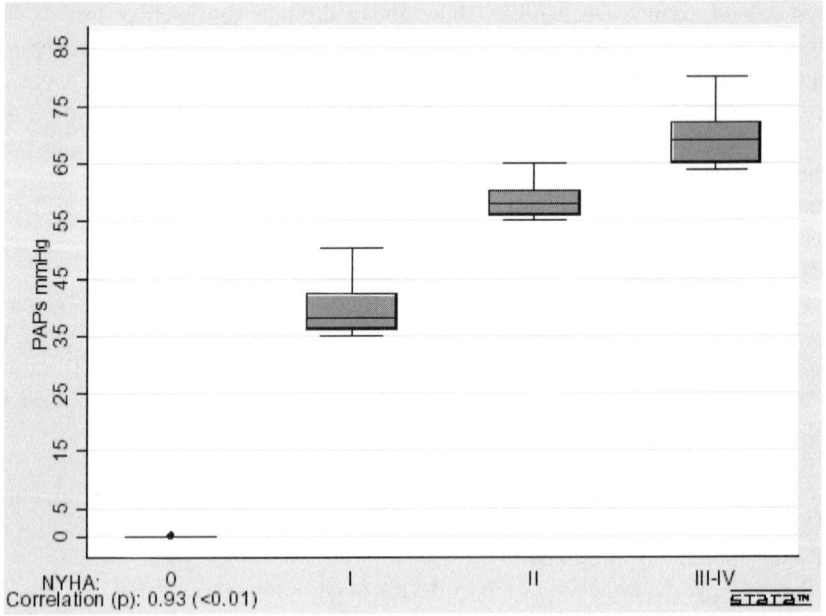

Fig. 2.19 Correlation PAPs: NYHA in ILD (94 patients)

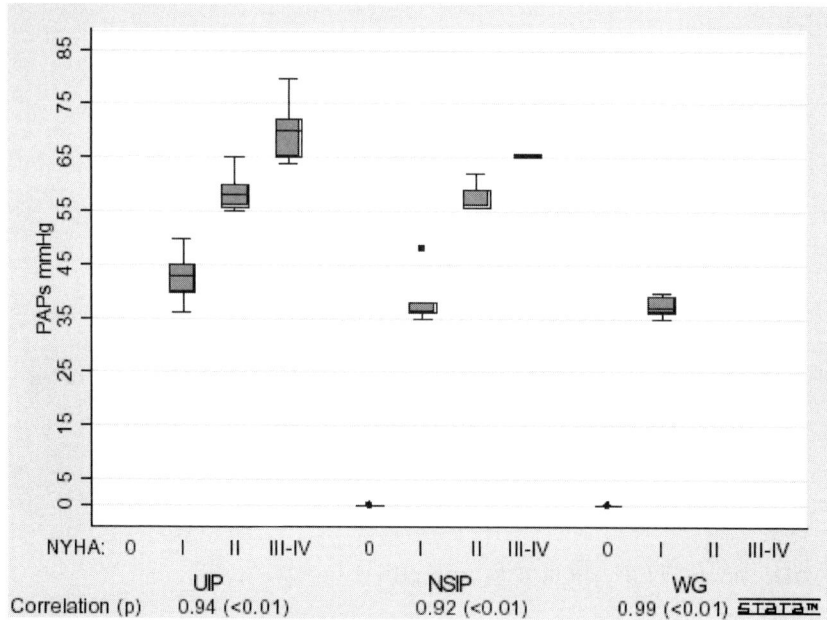

Fig. 2.20 Correlation PAPs: NYHA by diagnosis

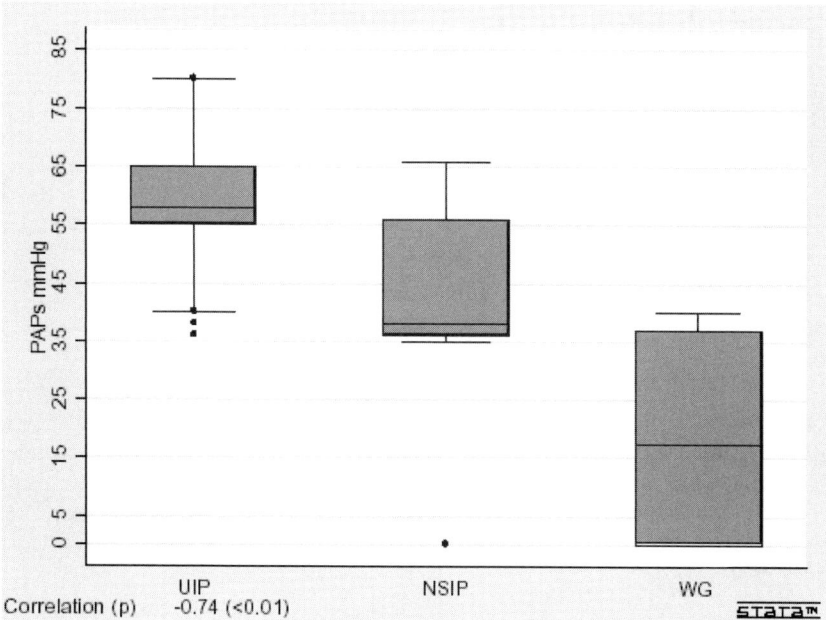

Fig. 2.21 PAPs by diagnosis

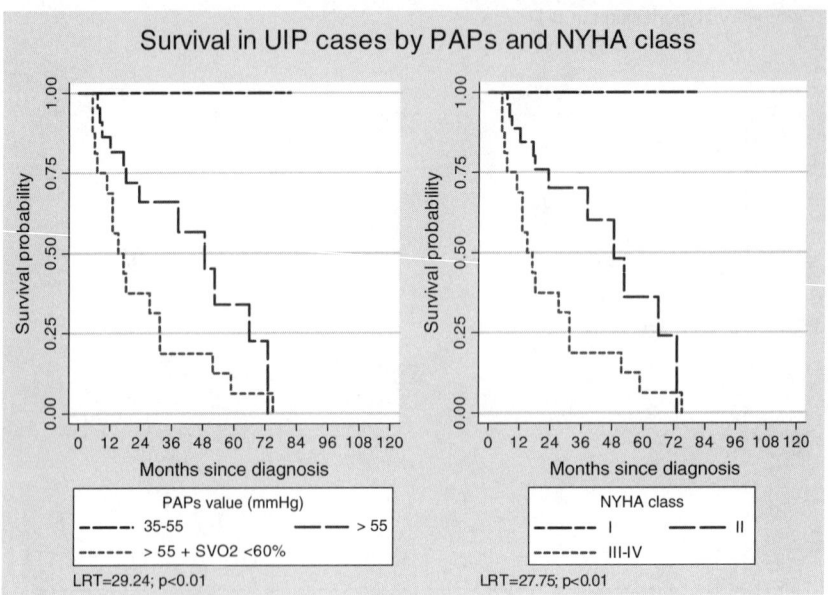

Fig. 2.22 Survival in UIP cases by PAPs and NYHA class

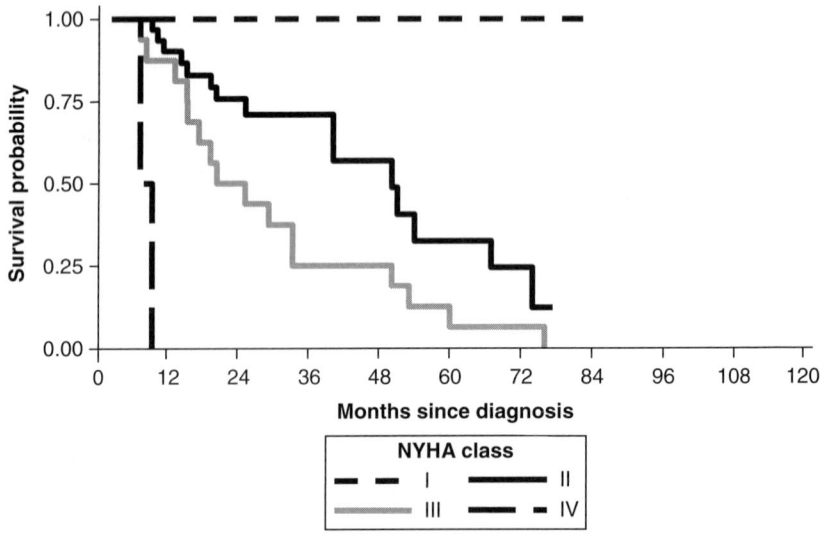

Fig. 2.23 Kaplan Meyer survival estimates in 104 patients with interstitial lung disease according to NYHA functional class

Summary

This section reviews the approach to diagnosis of PH in correlation with ILD diagnostic tests (Fig. 2.24). Cardiac parameters used for screening patients with suspected ILD

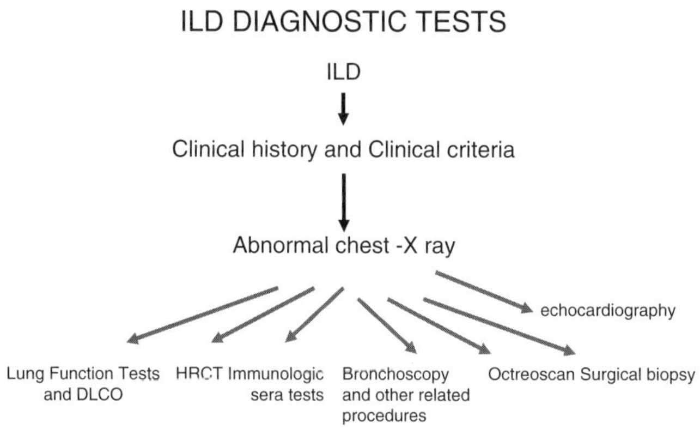

ILD DIAGNOSTIC TESTS

ILD

↓

Clinical history and Clinical criteria

↓

Abnormal chest -X ray

echocardiography

Lung Function Tests
and DLCO

HRCT Immunologic
sera tests

Bronchoscopy
and other related
procedures

Octreoscan Surgical biopsy

Fig. 2.24 Diagnostic tests for ILD

are discussed. Echocardiography, when a TR jet is visible, is an important tool both in terms of diagnosis and prognosis. Patients with suspected PH in whom a TR jet is not visible, could be considered for right ventricular catheterization. The 6MWT is a useful quantitative test for evaluating the prognosis of patients with ILD-associated PH. The utility of the NYHA classification as a prognostic factor of survival and mortality in ILD should be further evaluated in larger studies.

References

1. Humbert M, Deng Z, Simmoneau G, et al. BMPR2 germline mutations in pulmonary hypertension associated with fenfluramine derivates. Eur Respir J 2002;20:518–523.
2. Morse J, Barst R, Horn E, et al. Pulmonary hypertension in scleroderma spectrum of disease lack of bone morphogenetic protein receptor-2 mutations. J Rheumatol 2002;29:2379–2381.
3. Tew MB, Arnett PC, Reveille JD, et al. Mutation of bone morphogenetic protein receptor type 2 are not found in patients with pulmonary hypertension and underlying connective tissue diseases. Arthritis Rheum 2002;46:2829–2830.
4. Trembart JRC, Thomson JR, Machado RD, et al. Clinical and molecular genetic features of pulmonary hypertension in patients with hereditary hemorrhagic telangiectasis. N Engl J Med 2001;345:325–334.
5. Du I, Sullivan CC, Chu D, et al. Signaling molecules in non familial pulmonary hypertension. N Eng J Med 2003;92:984–991.
6. Farber HW, Loscalzo J. Pulmonary arterial hypertension. N Eng J Med 2004;351:1655–1665.
7. Nogee LM, Dunbar, III, AE, Wert SE, et al. A mutation in the surfactant protein C gene associated with familial interstitial lung disease. N Eng J Med 2001;344;573–579.
8. Amin RS, Wert SE, Baughman RP, et al. Surfactant protein deficiency in familial interstitial lung disease. J Pediatr 2001;139:85–92.
9. Khalil N, Parekh TV, O'Connor R, et al. Regulation of the effect of TGF-beta 1 by activation of latent of TGF-beta 1 and differential expression of TGF-beta receptors /T-beta R-1 and T beta R-2) in idiopathic pulmonary fibrosis. Thorax 2001;56:907–915.
10. Sime PJ, Xing Z, Graham FL. Adenovector-mediated gene transfer of active transforming grown factor-beta 1 induces prolonged severe fibrosis in rat lung. J Clin Invest 1997;100:768–777.

11. Whyte M, Hubbard R, Meliconi R, et al. Increased risk of fibrosing alveolitis associated with interleukin-1 receptor antagonist and tumor necrosis factor-a gene polymorphisms. Am J Respir Crit Care Med 2000;162:755–758.

12. Zorzetto M, Ferrarotti I, Trisolini R, et al. Complement receptor 1 gene polymorphisms are associated with idiopathic pulmonary fibrosis. Am J Respir Crit Care Med 2003;168:330–334.

13. Pantelidis P, Fanning GC, Wells AU, et al. Analysis of tumor necrosis factor-α, lymphotoxin-α, tumor necrosis factor receptor II, and interleukin-6 polymorphisms in patients with idiopathic pulmonary fibrosis. Am J Respir Crit Care Med 2001;163:1432–1436.

14. Xaubert A, Marin-Arguedas A, Lario S, et al. Transforming growth factor-β_1 gene polymorphisms are associated with disease progression in idiopathic pulmonary fibrosis. Am J Respir Crit Care Med 2003;168:431–435.

15. Reeve HL, Archer SL, Weir EK. Ion channels in the pulmonary vasculature. Pulm Pharmacol Ther 1997;10:243–252.

16. Weir EK, Reeve HL, Talorova S, et al. Oxygen sensing in the pulmonary vasculature. In: Lopez-Barneo J, Weir EK, editors. Oxygen regulation of ion channels and gene expression. Armonk, NY: Futura Publishing Company, Inc.; 1998. p. 193–206.

17. Yuan JX, Aldinger AM, Juhaszova M, et al. Dysfunctional voltage- gated K^+ channels in pulmonary artery smooth muscle cells of patients with primary pulmonary hypertension. Circulation 1998;14:1400–1406.

18. Marshall RB, Mamary CAJ, Verhoeven AJ, et al. Pulmonary artery NADPH-oxidase is activated in hypoxic pulmonary vasoconstriction. Am J Respir Cell Mol Biol 1996;15:633–644.

19. Weissmann N, Tadic A, Winterhalder S, et al. Inhibition of hypoxic pulmonary vasoconstriction by superoxide dismutase inhibitors in isolated rabbit lungs. Am J Respir Crit Care Med 1999;159:A 569.

20. Robertson TP, Hague D, Aaronson PI, et al. Voltage-independent calcium entry in hypoxic pulmonary vasoconstriction of intrapulmonary arteries of the rat. J Physiol 2000;525:669–680.

21. Yuan JX, Tod M, Rubin L, et al. Deoxyglucose and reduced glutathione mimic effects of H, hypoxia on K^+ and Ca^{++} conductances in pulmonary artery cells. Am J Physiol 1994;267:L52–L63.

22. Yanagisawa M, Kurihara H, Kimura S, et al. A novel potent vasoconstrictor peptide produced by vascular endothelial cells. Nature 1988;332:411–415.

23. Giaid A, Yanagisawa M, Langleben SD, et al. Expression of endothelin-1 in the lungs of patients with pulmonary hypertension. N Eng J Med 1993;328:1732–1739.

24. Arai S, Hori S, Aramori I, et al. Cloning and expression of a cDNA encoding an endothelin receptor. Nature (Lond) 1990;348:730–732.

25. Sakurai T, Yanagisawa M, Takuwa Y, et al. Cloning of a cDNA encoding a non-isopeptide–selective subtype of the endothelin receptor. Nature (Lond) 1990;348:732–735.

26. Giaid A, Michel RP, Stewart DJ, et al. Expression of endothelin-1 in patients with cryptogenic fibrosing alveolitis. Lancet 1993;341:1550–1554.

27. Ugucccioni M, Pulsatelli L, Grigolo B et al. Endothelin-1 in idiopathic pulmonary fibrosis. J Clin Pathol 1995;48:330–334.

28. Abraham DJ, Vancheenswaran R, Dashwood MR, et al. Increased levels of endothelin-1 and differential endothelin type A and B receptor expression in scleroderma-associated fibrotic lung disease. Am J Pathol 1997;151:831–841.

29. Park SH, Saleh D, Giaid A, et al. Increased endothelin-1 in bleomycin-induced pulmonary fibrosis and the effect of an endothelin receptor antagonist. Am J Respir Crit Care Med 1997; 156:831–841.

30. Hocher B, Schwartz A, Fagan KA, et al. Pulmonary fibrosis and chronic lung inflammation in ET-1 transgenic mice. Am J Respir Cell Mol Biol 2000;23:19–26.

31. Turner-Warwick M. Precapillary systemic-pulmonary anastomoses. Thorax 1963;18:225–237.

32. Peao MND, Aguas AP, DeSa CM, et al. Neoformation of blood vessels in association with a rat lung fibrosis induced by bleomycin. Anat Rec 1994;238:57–67.

33. Keane MP, Arenberg DA, Lynch JP 3rd, et al. The CXC chemokines, IL-8 and IP-10, regulate angiogenic activity in idiopathic pulmonary fibrosis. J Immunol 1997;159:1437–1453.

34. Keane MP, Belperio JA, Burdick M, et al. ENA-78 is an important angiogenic factor in idiopathic pulmonary fibrosis. Am J Respir Crit Care Med 2001;164:2239–2242.
35. Hyde DM, Henderson TS, Giri SN, et al. Effect of murine gamma interferon on the cellular responses to bleomycin in mice. Exp Lung Res 1988;14:687–704.
36. Keane MP, Belperio JA, Arenberg DA, et al. IFN-gamma-inducible protein-10 attenuates bleomycin-induced pulmonary fibrosis via inhibition of angiogenesis. J Immunol 1999; 163:5686–5692.
37. Rich S, editor. Primary pulmonary hypertension. Executive summary from the World Symposium: Primary Pulmonary Hypertension 1998. htpp://www.who.int/ncd/cvd/pph.html. Accessed 14 Aug 2008.
38. Morell NW, Morris KG, Stenmark KR. Role of angiotensin-converting enzyme activity and expression is increased during hypoxic pulmonary hypertension. Cardiovasc Res 1997;34: 393–403.
39. Davis P, Burke G, Reid I. The structure of the wall of the rat interacinar pulmonary artery: an electron microscopic study of microdissected preparations. Microvasc Res 1986;32:50–63.
40. Jones RC. Role of interstitial fibroblasts and intermediate cells in microvascular remodelling in pulmonary hypertension. Eur Respir Rev 1993;3:569–575.
41. Tuder RM, Groves B, Badesch DB, et al. Exuberant endothelial cell growth and elements of inflammation are present in plexiform lesions of pulmonary hypertension. Am J Pathol 1994; 144: 275–285.
42. Yi ES, Kim H, Ahn H, et al. Distribution of obstructive intimal lesions and their cellular phe-notypes in chronic pulmonary hypertension. A morphometric and immunohistochemical study. Am J Respir Crit Care Med 2000;162:1577–1586.
43. Giaid A, Saleh D. Reduced expression of endothelial nitric oxide synthase in the lungs of patients with pulmonary hypertension. N Eng J Med 1993;328:1732–1739.
44. Wang R, Ibarra-Sunga O, Verlinski L, et al. Abrogation of bleomycin- induced epithelial apoptosis and lung fibrosis by captopril or by a caspase inhibitor. Am J Physiol Lung Cell Mol Physiol 2000;279:L143–L151.
45. Kuwano K, Kunitake R, Maeyama T, et al. Attenuation of bleomycin-induced pneumopathy in mice by a caspase inhibitor. Am J Physiol Lung Cell Mol Physiol 2001;280:L316–L325.
46. Hagimoto N, Kuwano K, Inoshima M, et al. TGF-beta 1 as an enhancer of Fas-mediated apoptosis of lung epithelial cells. J Immunol 2002;168:6470–6478.
47. Wang R, Alam G, Zagariya A, et al. Apoptosis of lung epithelial cells in response to TNF-alpha requires angiotensin II generation de novo. J Cell Physiol 2000;185:253–259.
48. Keane MP, Arenberg DA, Lynch JP Lynch JP 3rd, et al. The CXC chemokines, IL-8 and IP-10, regulate angiogenic activity in idiopathic pulmonary fibrosis. J Immunol 1997;159: 1437–1443.
49. Renzoni EA, Walsh DA, Salmon M, et al. Interstitial vascularity in fibrosing alveolitis. Am J Respir Crit Care Med 2003;167:438–443.
50. Koyama S, Sato E, Haniuda H, et al. Decreased level of vascular endothelial grown factor. Am Respir J Crit Care Med 2002;166:382–385.
51. Weller PA. Eosinophils and fibroblasts: the medium in the mesenchyme. Am J Respir Cell Mol Biol 1989:1:267–268.
52. Elias JA, Freundlich B, Kern JA, Rosenbloom J. Cytokine networks in the regulation of inflammation and fibrosis in the lung. Chest 1990;97:1439–1445.
53. Gurujeyalakshmi G, Giri SN. Molecular mechanisms of antifibrotic effect of interferon gamma in bleomycin-mouse model of lung fibrosis: down regulation of TGF-β and procol-lagen I and III gene expression. Exp Lung Res 1995;21:791–808.
54. Prior C, Haslam PL. In vivo levels and in vitro production of interferon-gamma in fibrosing interstitial lung diseases. Clin Exp Immunol 1992;88:280–287.
55. Gaensler EA, Carrington CB. Open biopsy for chronic diffuse infiltrative lung disease: clini-cal, roentgenographic, and physiologic correlation in 502 patients. Ann Thorac Surg 1980; 30:411–426.

56. Padley SPG, Hansell DM, Flower CDR, et al. Comparative accuracy of high resolution computed tomography and chest radiography in the diagnosis of chronic diffuse infiltrative lung disease. Clin Radiol 1991;44:222–226.
57. Lee KS, Primack SL, Staples CA, et al. Chronic infiltrative lung disease: comparison of diagnostic accuracies of radiography and low- and conventional-dose thin-section CT Radiology 1994;191:669–673.
58. Kazerooni EF, Martinez F, Flint D, et al. Thin-section CT obtained at 10 mm increments versus three-level thin-section CT for idiopathic pulmonary fibrosis: correlation with pathologic scoring. AJR Am J Roentgenol 1997;169:977–983.
59. Webb RW, Muller NL, Naidich DP. Clinical utility of high-resolution computed tomography. In: Webb RW, Muller NL, Naidich DP editors. High-resolution CT of the lun.g Philadelphia PA: Lippincott William & Wilkins; 2001. p. 569–597.
60. Wells AU, Hansell DM, Rubens MB, et al. The predictive value of appearances of thin-section computed tomography in fibrosing alveolitis. Am Respir Dis 1993;148:1076–1082.
61. Zerhouni EA, Naidich DP, Stitik FP. et al. Computed tomography of the pulmonary parenchyma: part 2. Interstitial disease. J Thorac Imaging 1985;1:54–64.
62. Hunninghake GW, Zimmerman MB, Schwarz DA, et al. Utility of a lung biopsy for the diagnosis of idiopathic pulmonary fibrosis. Am J Respir Crit Care Med 2001;164:193–196.
63. McDonald SL, Rubens MB, Hansell DM, et al. Nonspecific interstitial pneumonia and usual interstitial pneumonia: comparative appearances at and diagnostic accuracy of thin-section CT. Radiology 2001;221:600–605.
64. Daniil ZD, Giltchrist FC, Nicholson AG, et al. A histologic pattern of nonspecific interstitial pneumonia is associated with a better prognosis than usual interstitial pneumonia in patients with cryptogenic fibrosing alveolitis. Am J Respir Crit Care Med 1999;160:899–905.
65. Flaherty KR, Twaite EL, Kazerooni EA, et al. Radiological versus histological diagnosis in UIP and NSIP: survival implications. Thorax 2003;58:143–148.
66. Gay SE, Kazerooni EA, Toews GB, et al. Idiopathic pulmonary fibrosis: predicting response to therapy and survival. Am J Respir Crit Care Med 1998;157:1063–1072.
67. King TE Jr, Schwarz MI, Brown K, et al. Idiopathic pulmonary fibrosis: relationship between histopathologic features and mortality. Am J Respir Crit Care Med 2001;164:1025–1032.
68. King TE Jr, Tooze JA, Schwarz MI, et al. Predicting survival in idiopathic pulmonary fibrosis: scoring system and survival model. Am J Respir Crit Care Med 2001;164:1171–1181.
69. Wells AU, Desai SR, Rubens MB, et al. Idiopathic pulmonary fibrosis: a composite physiologic index derived from disease extent observed by computed tomography. Am J Respir Crit Care Med 2003;167:962–969.
70. Mogulkoc N, Brutsche MH, Bishop PW, et al. Pulmonary function in idiopathic pulmonary fibrosis and referral for lung transplantation Am J Respir Crit Care Med 2001;164:103–108.
71. American Thoracic Society. Idiopathic pulmonary fibrosis: diagnosis and management. International Consensus Statement. Am J Respir Crit Care Med 2000;161:646–664.
72. Awadh N, Muller NL, Park CS, et al. Airway wall thickness in patients with near fatal asthma and control groups: assessment with high resolution tomographic scanning. Thorax 1998; 53:248–253.
73. Meyer KC. Bronchoalveolar lavage as a diagnostic tool. Semin Respir Crit Care Med 2007; 28:546–560.
74. Leung AN, Brainer MW, Caillat-Vigneron N. Sarcoidoisis activity: correlation of HRCT findings with those of ^{67}Ga scanning, bronchoalveolar lavage, and serum angiotensin-converting enzyme essay. J Comput Assist Tomogr 1998;22:229–234.
75. Sulavik SB, Spencer RP, Palestro CJ, et al. Specificity and sensitivity of distinctive chest radiographic and /or ^{67}Ga images in the noninvasive diagnosis of sarcoidosis. Chest 1993;103:403–409.
76. Alavi A, Palevsky HI. Gallium-67 citrate scanning in the assessment of disease activity in sarcoidosis. J Nuc Med 1992;33:751–755.
77. Grijm K, Verberne, Krowels FH, et al. Semiquantitative ^{67}Ga scintigraphy as an indicator of response to and prognosis after corticosteroid treatment in idiopathic interstitial pneumonia. J Nucl Med 2005;46:1421–1426.

78. Lebthai R, Crestani B, Belmatoug N, et al. Somatostatin receptor scintigraphy and gallium scintigraphy in patients with sarcoidosis. J Nucl Med 2001;42:21–26.
79. Carbone R, Filiberti R, Grosso M, et al. Octreoscan perspectives in sarcoidosis and idiopathic interstitial pneumonia. Eur Rev for Med and Pharmacol Sci 2003;7:97–105.
80. Turner-Warwick M, McAllister W, Lawrence R, et al. Corticosteroid treatement in pulmonary sarcoidosis: do serial lavage lymphocyte counts, serum angiotensin converting enzyme measurements and gallium-67 scan help management? Thorax 1986;41:903–913.
81. Clarke D, Mitchell AWM, Dick R, et al. The radiology of sarcoidosis. Sarcoidosis 1994;11:90–99.
82. Kwekkeboom DJ, Krenning EP, Kho GS, et al. Somatostatin receptor imaging in patients with sarcoidosis. Eur J Nucl Med 1998;25:1284–1292.
83. Carbone RG, Musi M, Cantalupi DP, et al. Somatostain receptor versus gallium-67 scintigraphy in interstitial lung diseases. Chest 1999;119:315S.
84. McGoon M, Gutterman D, Steen V, et al. Screening early detection, and diagnosis of pulmonary arterial hypertension. ACCP evidence-based clinical practice guidelines. Chest 2004;126:14S–34S.
85. Mukerjee D, St George D, Knight C, et al. Echocardiography and pulmonary function as screening tests for pulmonary arterial hypertension in systemic sclerosis. Rheumatology 2004;43:461–466.
86. Burdt MA, Hoffman RW, Deutscher SL, et al. Long term outcome in mixed connective tissue disease: longitudinal clinical and serologic findings. Arthritis Rheum 1999;42:899–990.
87. Mc Quillan BM, Picard MP, Leavitt M, et al. Clinical correlates and reference intervals for pulmonary artery systolic pressure among echocardiographically normal subjects. Circulation 2001;104:2797.
88. Barst RJ, McGoon M, Torbicki A, et al. Diagnosis and differential assessment of pulmonary hypertension. J Am Coll Cardiol 2004;43:40S–47S.
89. Stephen B, Dalal P, Berger M, et al. Noninvasive estimation of pulmonary artery diastolic pressure in patients with tricuspid regurgitation by Doppler echocardiography. Chest 1999;116:73–77.
90. Baughman R, Lower EE, Engel P. Echocardiography to detect pulmonary hypertension in sarcoidosis. Sarcoidosis Vasc Diffuse Lung Dis 2005;22:244–245.
91. Sulica R, Teirstein AS, Kakarda S, et al. Distinctive clinical, radiological, and functional characteristics of patients with sarcoidosis-related pulmonary hypertension. Chest 2005;128:1483–1489.
92. Arcasoy SM, Christie JD, Ferrari VA, et al. Echocardiography assessment of pulmonary hypertension in patients with advanced lung disease. Am Respir J Crit Care 2003;167:735–740.
93. Nadrous HF, Pellika PA, Krowka MJ, et al. Pulmonary hypertension in patients with idiopathic pulmonary fibrosis. Chest 2005;128:2393–2399.
94. Bourbon A, Vionnet M, Leprince P, et al. The effect of methylprednisolone treatment on the cardiopulmonary bypass-induced systemic inflammatory response. Eur Cardiothorac Surg 2005;27:729–730.
95. Gothard J. Lung injury after thoracic surgery and one-lung ventilation. Curr Opin Anaesthesiol 2006;19:5–10.
96. Ng CS, Wang S, Arifi AA, et al. Inflammatory response to pulmonary ischemia–reperfusion injury. Surg Today 2006;36:205–214.
97. Berg JT, Fu Z, Breen EC, et al. High lung inflation increases mRNA levels of ECM components and grown factors in lung parenchyma. J Appl Physiol 1997;83;120–128.
98. Berg JT, Breen EC, Fu Z, et al. Alveolar hypoxia increases gene expression of extra cellular matrix protein and platelet-derived growth factor-B in lung parenchyma. Am Respir Crit Care Med 1998;138:1920–1928.
99. Carbone R, Bossone E, Bottino G, et al. Secondary pulmonary hypertension- diagnosis and management. Eur Rev for Med Pharmacol Sci 2005;9:331–342.
100. Carbone R, Montanaro F, Bottino G. Outcome in interstitial lung disease. Eur Respir J 2005;26:268S.

101. Garbin U, Fratta Pasini A, Stranieri C, et al. Effects of nebivolol on endothelial gene expression during oxidative stress in human umbilical vein endothelial cells. Mediators Inflamm. 2008; 2008:367590.
102. Lee SH, Channick RN, Endothelin antogonism in pulmonary arterial hypertension. Semin Respir Crit Care Med. 2005 Aug;26(4):402–8. Review.
103. Ishaque A, Dunn MJ, Sorokin A, Cyclooxygenase-2 inhibits tumor necrosis factor alpha-mediated apoptosis in renal glomerular mesangial cells. J Biol Chem. 2003 Mar 21;278(12):10629–40.

Chapter 3
Idiopathic Pulmonary Fibrosis and Associated Pulmonary Hypertension: Genetics, Pathobiology, Diagnosis, and Management

Keith C. Meyer and Ganesh Raghu

Introduction

Idiopathic pulmonary fibrosis (IPF) accounts for the majority of cases of idiopathic interstitial pneumonia (IIP) and carries a poor prognosis for the patient. Although the term, IPF, was once used for a number of forms of IIP, IPF is now defined as a specific disease entity. IPF is characterized by radiological and/or histopathological patterns of usual interstitial pneumonia (UIP) on surgical lung biopsy or a constellation of clinical criteria that predict a confident diagnosis of IPF in the absence of a surgical lung biopsy [1,2]. When the diagnosis of IPF is made, it infers that patients lack other explanations for the presence of a UIP lesion, such as an associated connective tissue disorder or an iatrogenic/environmental exposure that can cause pulmonary fibrosis with a histopathological pattern suggestive of UIP.

The diagnosis of IPF is often made relatively late in the course of the disease, when patients have fairly impaired lung function. IPF has proven to be generally refractory to immunosuppressive therapies [3], and the authors of less-recent studies who suggested that a beneficial response to immunosuppressive therapy may occur were likely to have included some patients with non-IPF forms of IIP. Other forms of IIP, such as nonspecific interstitial pneumonia (NSIP) or cryptogenic organizing pneumonia (COP), can respond to immunosuppressive pharmacologic agents (e.g., corticosteroids, cytotoxic drugs). Pulmonary hypertension (PH) has been increasingly recognized as a complication of IPF and portends a much poorer prognosis for survival.

Epidemiology of IPF

A relative lack of studies based on population screening combined with a lack of uniform diagnostic criteria have made it difficult to establish a reasonably accurate estimate of the incidence and prevalence of IPF because most of the available studies were performed before the current definition of IPF was adopted. Despite these problems, IPF has not been shown to have a biased expression on the basis of race or ethnic

R.P. Baughman et al. (eds.), *Pulmonary Arterial Hypertension and Interstitial Lung Diseases,*
© Humana Press, a part of Springer Science + Business Media, LLC 2009

background, although men more frequently are affected than are women. Coultas et al. [4] reported the incidence and prevalence of IPF in the desert southwestern region of the USA as 11 and 20 per 100,000 per year, respectively, for men and 7 and 13 per 100,000 per year for women. A study from the UK in which the authors examined data from a longitudinal computerized general practice database estimated the incidence of IPF at 4.6 per 100,000 person-years and observed a progressive increase in the incidence for the periods of 1991–1995 to 2000–2003 [5].

A more recent study by Raghu et al. [6], using relatively narrow criteria (diagnostic code for IPF plus procedure code for lung biopsy, transbronchial biopsy, or thoracic computed tomography [CT] scan), found the incidence and prevalence of IPF in the USA as 6.8 and 14 per 100,000/year. If broader diagnostic criteria were used (diagnostic code only), the incidence and prevalence were 16.3 and 42.7 per 100,000/year. Both Coultas et al. [4] and Raghu et al. [6] found a dramatic increase in the incidence and prevalence of IPF with advancing age. Coultas et al. reported that the incidence and prevalence of IPF in persons ages 75 and older were 102 and 175 for men and 57 and 73 per 100,000 for women. Similarly, Raghu et al. estimated an incidence and prevalence of 71 and 271 per 100,000/year for elderly men and 67 and 266 per 100,000/yr for elderly women. In comparison, the incidence of IPF approaches that of primary lung cancer in the elderly [7], and the incidence of colorectal cancer is estimated at 15–18 per 100,000/year [8]. Increased death rates also have been reported recently throughout the USA [9].

A number of epidemiological studies have established risk factors for IPF. Individuals at increased risk include workers who are exposed to metal or wood dust, fumes, or livestock; men are more likely to have these types of exposures [10,11]. Cigarette smoking appears to be an independent risk factor in both sporadic and familial IPF [12], and viral infections, particularly Epstein–Barr virus infection, also have been linked to IPF pathogenesis [13]. Additionally gastro-esophageal reflux disease has been strongly linked to IPF, with a prevalence of approximately 90% in patients with IPF [14,15].

Genetics and Pathobiology of IPF

Pulmonary fibrosis is a manifestation of the disease state in various genetic disorders (Table 3.1), and numerous specific gene mutations and polymorphisms have been associated with IPF [16,17]. These associations indicate that genetic factors undoubtedly play a role in disease susceptibility, although gene–gene interactions, gene–environment interactions, and epigenetic factors undoubtedly influence susceptibility to pulmonary fibrosis, and multiple genetic polymorphisms may simultaneously play a role in the pathogenesis of IPF. Other observations that support a genetic predisposition to IPF include the differential responses that inbred mouse strains display to fibrogenic agents and the considerable variation in susceptibility to developing pneumoconioses that has been observed in humans exposed to fibrogenic dusts, such as asbestosis or silica, in the workplace. Additionally, factors that are inherent to advancing age may come into play

Table 3.1 Genetic abnormalities linked to pulmonary fibrosis

- Clinical disorders associated with pulmonary fibrosis
  - Tuberous sclerosis
  - Neurofibromatosis
  - Niemann-Pick disease
  - Gaucher disease
  - Hermansky-Pudlak syndrome
  - Familial hypocalciuric hypercalcemia
  - Familial IPF
    - Surfactant protein C
    - ELMOD-2
- Gene polymorphisms associated with pulmonary fibrosis
  - IL-1 receptor antagonist
  - TNF-α
  - Complement receptor-1
  - Surfactant associated proteins (SP-A, SP-B)
  - ACE
  - TGF-β1
  - Plasminogen activator inhibitor-1

and explain the greatly increased susceptibility of older individuals to pulmonary fibrosis. These factors include age-associated reduction in telomerase activity in human somatic cells [18], which can decrease the inhibitory effect of telomerase on the differentiation of fibroblasts into myofibroblasts [19], or altered expression of plasminogen activator inhibitor-1, which has been associated with fibrosis, by senescent fibroblasts [20].

Because the vast majority of patients develop pulmonary fibrosis in their sixth decade of life or beyond, telomerase mutations that are associated with adult-onset pulmonary fibrosis may be of particular interest. Telomerase antagonizes or reverses telomere shortening, and cultured cells exhibit replicative senescence as telomeres shorten. Additionally, telomeres are shorter in older versus younger individuals, and telomere shortening has been linked to human aging. Mutations in the reverse transcriptase protein component (hTERT) of the telomerase ribonucleoprotein complex have been linked to dyskeratosis congenita and sporadic bone marrow failure [21], and hTERT mutations have recently been linked to familial pulmonary fibrosis [22,23]. Cultured fibroblasts and other cell types from patients with IPF associated with telomerase complex gene mutations display reduced telomere lengths. However, hTERT mutations and telomere shortening occur in family members without pulmonary fibrosis, indicating that other factors (e.g., environmental effects, other genes) modulate clinical expression of disease.

Lung histopathology in UIP demonstrates areas of seemingly normal lung interspersed with fibrotic lesions that are characterised by temporal heterogeneity. Architectural distortion of the lung parenchyma typically is present, and other histopathologic findings that are characteristic of UIP include the presence of fibroblast foci (discrete collections of fibroblasts, myofibroblasts, and newly formed

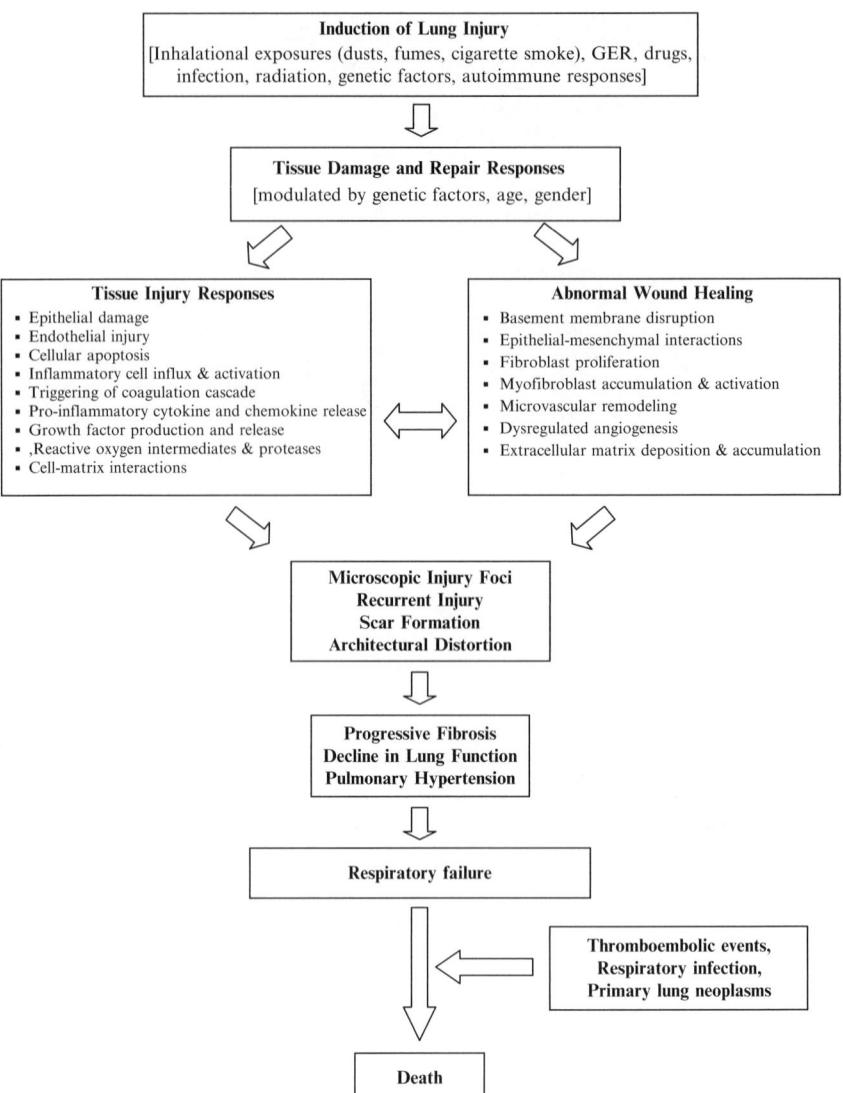

Fig. 3.1 Pathobiology and natural history of IPF

collagen), smooth muscle hyperplasia, and honeycomb cysts (dilated airspaces lined with bronchiolar epithelium and usually filled with inspissated mucus and inflammatory cells). Interestingly, when native lung explants were examined from patients with a pretransplant diagnosis of IPF, areas consistent with changes of NSIP as well as desquamative interstitial pneumonia were identified in nearly all explants [24]. Flaherty et al. [25] found that surgical lung biopsies from different lung regions in a given patient often show discordant histopathology, with one biopsy showing UIP but another showing NSIP. Survival was much better for patients with concordant NSIP/NSIP and worst for those with concordant UIP/UIP, while that for patients with UIP/NSIP was similar to that for UIP/UIP.

The pathogenesis of IPF involves features of wound healing and tissue remodeling, and abnormal wound healing may account for the progressive nature of the lung lesions and the inability to restore the lung to normal structure and function (Fig. 3.1). Increased levels of proinflammatory cytokines and chemokines that promote inflammation and fibroproliferation [26] support a role for inflammation and polarization of the immune response, even though conventional anti-inflammatory/immunosuppressive therapies appear to have little effect on disease progression. Key cytokines implicated in promoting fibrosis include tumour necrosis factor (TGF)-β, interleukin-13, and CC chemokines [26]. Other abnormalities that have been identified include epithelial injury associated with apoptosis and loss of type I alveolar cells accompanied by a proliferation of type II cells and basement membrane disruption, and reactive oxygen intermediates are released as inflammatory cells are recruited to the lungs.

Another aspect of damage and remodeling of the lung parenchyma consists of microvascular changes that include evidence of endothelial cell death accompanied by recruitment of endothelial cells and fibroblasts, activation of the coagulation cascade, and deposition of excessive extracellular matrix. Turner-Warwick [27] described extensive microvascular remodeling that was characterised by neovascular changes in areas of fibrosis and in areas where anastomoses between systemic and pulmonary microvasculature were identified. Aberrant vascular remodeling has also been described in animal models of pulmonary fibrosis [28], and communications between the systemic and pulmonary microvasculature may promote right-to-left shunting and hypoxaemia in patients, especially during physical exertion. Additionally, more extensive microvascular changes may predispose patients to develop secondary PH and further exacerbate gas exchange in patients who develop this complication. Vascular remodeling in IPF has been associated with an imbalance of angiogenic and angiostatic CXC chemokines with net augmentation of angiogenic activity [29], but a relative lack of the potent angiogenic factor, vascular endothelial growth factor [30], as well as enhanced expression of angiostatic factors such as pigment epithelial-derived factor have also been described in IPF [31]. One interesting distinction between granulation tissue seen in organizing pneumonia and the fibroblast foci of UIP is a relative paucity of proangiogenic cytokines in the fibroblast foci of UIP [32].

Diagnosis of IPF

Most patients present with progressive dyspnea, and many have cough. Most patients are in their sixth to eighth decade of life and tend to have relatively advanced disease and high-resolution computed tomography (HRCT) findings that are typical for IPF. Because UIP can be associated with certain exposures or various rheumatologic disorders, a detailed clinical history should be taken to help exclude environmental exposures associated with pulmonary fibrosis, to identify medications that can induce a pneumotaxic reaction, and to detect the presence of a collagen–vascular disorder. Physical examination usually reveals bilateral rales at the lung bases on chest auscultation, and many patients have digital clubbing. Patients typically have evidence of a restrictive ventilatory defect on pulmonary function testing and a reduction in the diffusion capacity for carbon monoxide (DL_{CO}). Arterial hypoxaemia is usually present with advanced disease, and oxyhemoglobin desaturation can often be brought out by exertion when milder disease is present by performing cardiopulmonary exercise testing or a 6-minute walk test (6MWT).

Chest radiographs typically reveal bilateral interstitial opacities that are most prominent at the lung bases and in peripheral subpleural locations, but such changes can be seen with other forms of ILD, such as other forms of IIP, asbes-

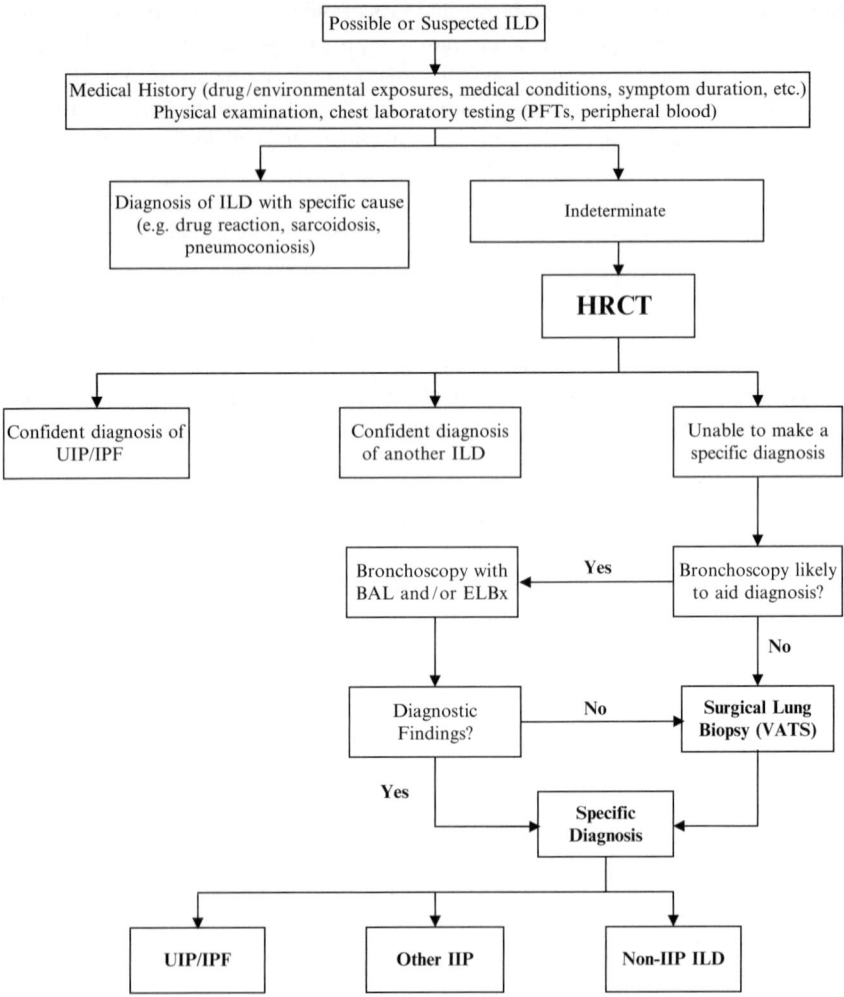

Fig. 3.2 Diagnostic approach to suspected ILD. VATS, video-assisted thorascopic surgery

tosis, or hypersensitivity pneumonitis. Occasionally, the routine chest radiograph may not reveal any significant abnormalities, and the disease is detected only when HRCT is performed. HRCT is a key tool for evaluating patients with diffuse parenchymal lung disease, and typical HRCT changes in UIP include a predilection for basilar and peripheral lung zones with patchy involvement and relative sparing of more central areas [33]. Linear opacities, which represent thickened intralobular and interlobular septae, are observed, and more advanced disease is characterised by honeycomb cysts (representing bronchiolectasis) and traction bronchiectasis. Ground-glass opacities should be minimal or absent, and the finding of prominent ground-glass opacities on HRCT would suggest an alternative diagnosis such as NSIP or COP.

Although bronchoscopy with bronchoalveolar lavage (BAL) and transbronchial lung biopsy can provide useful information that establishes a diagnosis of a specific form of ILD or at least substantially narrows the differential diagnosis (Fig. 3.2), adequate sampling from two or more segments/lobes via a surgical lung biopsy (SLB) is required to characterise the histological pattern as UIP and thus make a definitive diagnosis of IPF in patients who have other features suggesting an alternative diagnosis for the ILD/IIP. BAL typically reveals a differential cell count that shows a modest increase in neutrophils and/or eosinophils in IPF [34]. The presence of a BAL cell lymphocytosis pattern or the finding of a marked increase in eosinophils would suggest an alternative diagnosis. Although transbronchial lung biopsies may occasionally show changes consistent with IPF [35], the likelihood of retrieving adequate alveolar tissue and the ability to characterise the histological pattern of UIP in transbronchial lung biopsy specimens seems very low.

However, bronchoscopy was incorporated into the 2000 expert consensus statement on making a clinical diagnosis of IPF (Table 3.2) in the absence of a surgical lung biopsy [2]. With increasing awareness of typical clinical features and of a classic HRCT pattern of UIP, the trend in accepting a diagnosis of IPF without the need for subjecting patients to bronchoscopy and/or confirmation of the UIP pattern via the SLB has become evident. However, in the presence of atypical clinical and/or HRCT features, especially in new-onset ILD, the diagnosis of IPF can only be ascertained by recognition of UIP pattern in the SLB [1]. When lung biopsies are performed, the likelihood of the accuracy of the diagnosis of IPF is greater

Table 3.2 Criteria for the clinical diagnosis of IPF (Reference 2)

Major (all 4 required)
- Typical HRCT appearance
- Exclude other diseases
- PFTs showing parenchymal restriction and impaired gas exchange
- BAL or transbronchial lung biopsy not showing alternative diagnosis

Minor (3 of 4 required)
- Bibasilar velcro like crackles
- Age>50
- Duration of illness > 3 months
- Insidious onset

when the clinician interacts with an experienced pathologist and radiologist familiar with ILD/IIP [36].

Clinical Course of IPF

Median survival in IPF has been shown by various investigators to range between 2 and 5 years [37], and the survival of patients with IPF is clearly worse than that for patients with other forms of IIP such as cellular NSIP. However, survival varies according to various factors, such as age, extent of fibrosis, the presence of secondary hypertension, or other specific features of the clinical presentation. Flaherty et al. [38] found that patients who had an indeterminate HRCT combined with a surgical lung biopsy that showed UIP had a median survival of 5.8 years, whereas those with typical HRCT findings had a median survival of 2.1 years. One explanation for this considerable difference in survival may be that individuals with indeterminate HRCT findings were diagnosed earlier in the course of their disease. Interestingly, survival with collagen-vascular disease-associated UIP has been observed to be better than that for patients with idiopathic UIP/IPF [39].

Various clinical findings and measures of lung function have been linked to disease progression and survival (Table 3.3), but the clinical course of IPF can be quite variable. Some patients can have sustained and relatively rapid decline in lung function that leads to respiratory failure, whereas others can have fairly stable and relatively gradual decline in lung function over long periods of time. The triggers for acute and/or rapid decline in respiratory status are unknown, and acute exacerbations can occur in patients who are otherwise stable and result in a precipitous decline and death [40,41]. Although the exact incidence and prevalence of acute exacerbation in IPF is unknown, it is apparent that such rapid decline may manifest in approximately 5–15% of patients with IPF. A recent perspective by experts implicates occult infection, gastroesophageal reflux and microvascular coagulation as potential risks and/or causative factors [42].

Some of the most useful measures that correlate with disease severity/progression are subjective dyspnea, change in forced vital capacity over time, baseline DL_{CO} and change over time, and degree of oxyhemoglobin desaturation or change in walk distance during a 6MWT [43–47] or a modified 6MWT [48]. Individuals who have severe reduction in resting DL_{CO} are more likely to have secondary PH as a complication of their disease [49].

Although most patients succumb to respiratory complications of their disease, some die of causes other than respiratory failure, such as cardiac events or malignancy [50]. Pulmonary malignancy can occur, and patients with IPF are at increased risk of developing primary lung cancer, even when smoking is not a factor [51]. Patients with IPF are also at risk for pulmonary infection, venous thromboembolism, and adverse drug reactions.

Table 3.3 Clinical correlates of disease progression and survival

Clinical Assessment	Predictive characteristics
Dyspnea score	Changes over time correlate well with stability/progression
Respiratory event	Hospitalization for a respiratory complication increases the likelihood of more rapid progression
FVC	• Changes over time on serial testing correlate well with disease progression and mortality risk • >10% decline in serial values correlates with progressive disease
DLCO% predicted	• Worse survival if <35% predicted • ≈40% = breakpoint for advanced disease and increased risk of PH • 15% decline in serial value correlates with progressive disease
6-MWT	• Desaturation to ≤88% correlates with increased mortality risk (both IPF and NSIP) • Walk distance is more reproducible than SpO2 desaturation and correlates with mortality risk • Decline of walk distance (≥200 ft) on serial testing correlates with progressive disease
HRCT	• Extent of reticulation and honeycombing correlates with mortality • Worsening (↑honeycomb change) detected over longer time periods (≥2 yrs) correlates with decline in clinical status
Lung histopathology	• Extent of fibrosis (e.g. number of fibroblast foci) correlates with disease progression and mortality
Pulmonary artery pressure - Echocardiogram - Right heart catheterization	• Pulmonary hypertension (e.g. mean pulmonary artery pressure ≥35 mm Hg) correlates with increased risk of progression and mortality • Echocardiographic estimates of pulmonary arterial pressure are less reliable than right heart catheterization and may be misleading

Abbreviations Used: DLCO=diffusion capacity for carbon monoxide; 6-MWT=6-minute walk test; FVC=forced vital capacity; PH=pulmonary hypertension

Pulmonary Hypertension Complicating/Associated With IPF

It is clear that PH has an adverse effect on outcomes in chronic lung disease, and PH occurring as a complication of sarcoidosis has been identified as a marker for early death [52]. PH has also been identified as a frequent complication of IPF. Lettieri et al. [49] identified PH (defined as mean pulmonary artery pressure >25 mmHg) in 31.6% of patients undergoing pretransplant evaluation with cardiac catheterization. Greater pressures correlated with increased risk of death, and patients with PH had a lower DL_{CO}, lower walk distance, and greater oxyhemoglobin desaturation on a 6MWT, and were more likely to require supplemental oxygen therapy.

Nadrous et al. [53] found that echocardiographically estimated systolic pulmonary artery pressure [sPAP] correlated inversely with DL_{CO}, and patients with sPAP greater than 50 mmHg had a significantly worse survival than patients with milder PH. When a cohort of lung transplant candidates with IPF were re-evaluated with right heart catheterization just before undergoing lung transplant, the prevalence of PH increased from 33% to 85% of patients [54], suggesting that the risk of developing secondary PH gradually increases as lung function becomes progressively impaired. Additionally, examination of the United Network for Organ Sharing database identified PH in 46.1% of patients with IPF who had undergone right heart catheterization [55], and 6MWT distance was significantly lower in recently listed patients with IPF who had PH versus those who did not have PH [56]. Whelan et al. [57] identified increasing PAP as a risk factor for increased mortality after single lung transplant for IPF. Although it is conceivable that some patients may have occult PH at the time of onset/diagnosis, the incidence of this presentation is unknown.

Pathologic changes that affect the arteries, arterioles, capillary beds, and venules have been observed in IPF [27,58,59], and in situ thrombosis has been reported in small muscular pulmonary arteries [60]. Fibroblast and myofibroblast proliferation combined with deposition of extracellular matrix causes adventitial perivascular thickening, and pulmonary arterioles become muscularised and smooth muscle cell hypertrophy and proliferation combined with elastin and collagen accumulation occur in the media of small muscular arteries and distal pulmonary arterioles. Intimal hyperplasia combined with fibrosis and reduplication of the inner elastic laminae also occurs in small muscular arteries. Vascular regression appears to occur in areas of dense fibrosis and within fibroblast foci while increased capillary density combined with angiogenesis appears to occur in areas of seemingly normal lung flanking regions of dense fibrosis.

Altered expression of various pro- and anti-angiogenic cytokines and chemokines has been detected in lung tissue from patients with IPF [26], but it is unclear how these contribute to vascular remodeling and the development of PH. Vascular endothelial growth factor, which is highly expressed in the normal lung and likely plays an important role in maintenance of normal microvasculature by preventing endothelial cell apoptosis, is greatly reduced in the lung affected by UIP [30,31] and may contribute to depressed endothelial cell proliferation in response to injury (wound repair responses) and play a role in the destruction of capillary beds. Overall vessel density appears to be reduced in association with net vascular ablation [61], although an overall proangiogenic environment seems to exist with increased expression of angiogenic chemokines, such as CXCL5 and CXCL8, as opposed to angiostatic chemokines, such as CXCL10 [29,62,63]. Other mediators, such as endothelin-1 (ET-1), platelet-derived growth factor (PDGF), transforming growth factor (TGF-β), fibroblast growth factor, and serotonin display increased expression and may modulate changes in the media of pulmonary arteries. ET-1, a potent pulmonary vasoconstrictor and mitogen for smooth muscle cells, and other cytokines such as PDGF have been implicated in the pathogenesis of idiopathic pulmonary arterial hypertension, and mechanistic pathways that cause PH may be similar in patients with idiopathic pulmonary hypertension (IPAH) and those with IPF who develop PH.

Symptoms of PH, such as dyspnea and palpitations, may be difficult to differentiate from symptoms of progressive parenchymal fibrosis. Patients may have a loud pulmonic valve closure sound (P_2) on cardiac auscultation, or they may have a fixed, split S_2, or a holosystolic murmur attributable to tricuspid regurgitation. An early diastolic murmur may occur when pulmonic valve insufficiency is present, and a right ventricular heave or jugular venous distension may be present. An electrocardiogram may show a pattern of right ventricular strain, and chest radiography may show right ventricular enlargement, pulmonary artery dilation, and cardiomegaly. A very low DL_{CO} and requirement for supplemental oxygen should increase suspicion that PH may be present. However, further diagnostic testing is generally needed.

Transthoracic echocardiography (TTE) can be useful as a screening modality to detect PH, but its reliability is somewhat problematic, and PAPs can be underestimated or overestimated with TTE. Furthermore, Arcasoy et al. [64] found that technical difficulties often limit the ability to estimate right heart pressures. Right ventricular systolic pressure (RVSP) measurements were within 10 mmHg of sPAP from right heart catheterization (RHC) in only 37% of subjects, 40% of patients identified as having increased RVSP by TTE did not have PH by RHC (sPAP >45 mmHg), and 56% of patients identified as having normal RVSP were found to have PH by RHC. Finally, more than 25% of patients with normal RV morphology on TTE had PH when RHC was performed. Because of the limitations of TTE in accurately detecting and quantitating PH, a circulating biomarker that is predictive of PH would be clinically useful. Leuchte et al. [65] found plasma brain natriuretic peptide levels to be greater in patients with pulmonary fibrosis with mean PAP (mPAP) values >35 mmHg as compared with those with mPAP <35 mmHg.

Because of the shortcomings of clinical findings on physical examination and various measurements that reflect physiology and gas exchange (DL_{CO}, resting oxyhemoglobin saturation, supplemental oxygen requirements, 6MWT desaturation or distance), direct measurement of right heart and pulmonary artery pressures are required for accurate diagnosis and quantitation of severity of PH. Unfortunately, TTE lacks the accuracy of RHC, and the role of brain natriuretic peptide measurement as a screening tool remains unclear, leaving RHC as the best diagnostic procedure currently available for detecting and quantitating PH in patients with IPF.

Pulmonary vascular remodeling and the resultant PH as a complication of IPF clearly have a negative impact on the clinical status and survival of patients with IPF. A lower quality of life and a greater degree of exercise limitation characterise patients with IPF-associated PH, and circulatory impairment associated with PH appears to be independent of ventilatory compromise and have a greater impact on gas exchange and exercise limitation than ventilatory impairment [56,66]. Numerous studies have demonstrated an increased risk of death in patients with PH, and patients with PH who were listed for lung transplantation and had a normal pulmonary capillary wedge pressure

(≤15 mmHg) were found to have a 3-fold increased risk of death that was independent of age, race, percent predicted forced vital capacity, or 6MWT distance [56].

Treatment of IPF and IPF-Associated PH

It has become clear that anti-inflammatory and immunosuppressive pharmacologic therapies have had relatively little efficacy in the treatment of the majority of patients with IPF, as acknowledged by a National Institutes of Health expert panel [3] as well as the international consensus statement on IPF [1]. Various targets have been identified for the pharmacologic treatment of IPF (Table 3.4), and recent clinical trials have focused on antifibrotic therapies (e.g. interferon-γ, pirfenidone, bosentan, and etanercept) as potential treatments for IPF. A recent prospective, randomised, placebo-controlled, 2-year multicenter trial in which researchers examined recombinant human interferon-γ, which has been shown experimentally to down-regulate TGF-β production, was prematurely terminated because of a lack of efficacy. A post-hoc, subgroup analysis of a previous Phase III trial of 1-year duration had suggested that patients with less severe derangement in lung function may benefit from treatment with interferon-γ [67], but this observation was not supported by the subsequent 2-year trial. Phase II trials with etanercept, bosentan, and pirfenidone have been completed, and Phase III trials with pirfenidone and bosentan are currently in progress. Although immunomodulatory therapies have shown little benefit for clinically stable patients with IPF, corticosteroids may have a role in the treatment and stabilization of patients who develop an acute exacerbation of IPF.

Various mediators that appear to play a significant role in IPAH or experimental PH have been implicated or may play an important role in IPF-associated PH as well as in IPF lung fibrogenesis. These mediators include inflammatory cell-derived profibrotic leukotrienes generated by 5-lipoxygenase, which is up-regulated in pulmonary arteries of patients with IPAH [68,69], and ET-1, which promotes growth of pulmonary arterial smooth muscle as well as pulmonary arterial vasoconstriction [70]. Other mediators that can promote fibrogenesis and/or pulmonary vascular remodeling include TNF-α, PDGF, and fibroblast growth factor. Decreased prostaglandin E2 (PGE2) production can promote increased levels of TNF-α and TGF-β, and PGE2 levels are decreased in BAL fluids as well as alveolar macrophage-conditioned media from patients with IPF [68], and PGE2 and prostacyclin synthases have been shown to be depressed in vascular tissue of patients with IPAH [71].

There are relatively few studies that have examined the treatment of PH associated with IPF. However, a number of different pharmacologic agents have been approved for the treatment of IPAH. Agents used to treat IPAH target calcium-channels, ET-1 receptors, prostaglandin-mediated vasodilatation and phosphodiesterase-5 (PDE5) inhibition, although calcium-channel blockade has been useful for treating only a very small subset of patients with IPAH. Prostacyclin (PGI2), which is endogenously produced, induces vasodilation and also inhibits platelet aggregation and smooth muscle proliferation, and PGI2 analogs such as epoprostenol have

Table 3.4 Therapeutic targets for pharmacologic therapy

Target	Agent(s)	Rationale
TGF-β	• Pirfenidone • Anti-TGF-β	Down-regulation of TGF-β-stimulated collagen synthesis and extracellular matrix accumulation
Endothelin-I	Bosentan	Suppress TGF-β production and fibroblast/ myofibroblast stimulation via Endothelin-I antagonism
TNF-α	Etanercept	Antagonize the mitogenic effects of TNF-α on fibroblasts and suppress collagen synthesis
ROI (oxidant-antioxidant imbalance)	N-acetylcysteine	Replenish pulmonary glutathione stores and thereby antagonize signaling and tissue damaging effects of oxygen radicals (e.g. stimulatory effects of ROI on myofibroblasts)
Protein kinases	Imatinib mesylate	Inhibition of protein kinase-mediated fibroblast proliferation
CTGF	Anti-CTGF	Suppress fibroblast stimulation by CTGF
Inflammation	• Corticosteroids • Azathioprine • Cyclophosphamide • Mycophenolate	Suppression of any inflammatory component responsive to immunosuppressive therapy
Fibroblast activity & proliferation	Tetrathiomolybdate	Inhibit fibroblast activity via copper chelation
Leukotriene pathway	Zileuton	Suppress fibroblast stimulation by CTGF
Vasoconstriction	• Sildenafil • Inhaled epoprostenol	Relieve pulmonary hypertension

Abbreviations: TGF-β=Transforming growth factor; TNF-α=Tumor necrosis factor-α; ROI=Reactive oxygen intermediates; CTGF=connective tissue growth factor.

been shown to improve exercise capacity and hemodynamic indices as well as outcomes in IPAH [72]. ET-1 receptor antagonists [73,74] and the PDE5 inhibitor, sildenafil [75], have also been shown to benefit patients with IPAH.

Although epoprostenol may have benefit for IPF-associated PH and can decrease mPAP and increase cardiac index when given intravenously, it can significantly increase shunt [76]. However, in contrast to intravenous epoprostenol, inhaled epoprostenol can decrease mPAP without increasing shunt fraction [76]. A randomised clinical trial of inhaled epoprostenol has been completed, but results are not yet available.

Lung tissue from patients with IPF has increased expression of ET-1 [77,78], and ET-1 levels have been shown to correlate with PAP but correlate inversely with arterial oxygen levels [79]. ET-1 antagonism could potentially benefit patients with IPF-associated PH, and blockade of the profibrotic properties of ET-1 make ET-1 receptor antagonists an especially attractive treatment modality. Although the ET-1 antagonist, bosentan, has been examined for the treatment of IPF [80], only patients who lacked echocardiographic and clinical evidence of significant PH were enrolled in this trial, and no clinical trials of ET-1 antagonists have specifically targeted patients with IPF-associated PH.

The use of sildenafil has been shown to decrease vascular remodeling in animal models of hypoxic PH [81,82], and PDE5 inhibitors can block smooth muscle proliferation and promote vasodilatation by increasing cyclic guanosine monophosphate levels in the lung [75,83]. Ghofrani et al. [84] demonstrated decreased mPAP and shunt flow and increased arterial oxygen tension with a single dose of sildenafil. Collard et al. [85] subsequently performed a pilot study in 14 patients with IPF-associated PH and demonstrated improvement in 6-MWT distance. However, no randomised clinical trial has been performed to date to evaluate the efficacy of PDE5 inhibition for this patient population.

In situ thrombosis has been identified as playing a role in IPAH pathogenesis, and a nonrandomised epidemiologic study associated anticoagulation with improved outcome [86]. In situ thrombosis has also been suggested to contribute to PH in patients with pulmonary fibrosis [87], and a randomised clinical trial in patients with IPF suggested that anticoagulation may improve outcome [88]. However, this study had many problems, including the lack of a placebo arm that substantially limit any conclusions that can be drawn from this study, and a significant impact of anticoagulation therapies on IPF or IPF-associated PH remains to be identified.

Interventions other than immunomodulatory or antifibrotic pharmacologic therapies may benefit patients with IPF. Lung transplantation is an option for those who meet criteria for listing at a transplant center, and survival after listing for lung transplantation is decreased for waitlisted patients who do not undergo lung transplantation in comparison to those who receive transplants. In addition to survival, quality of life can improve considerably for those who undergo successful lung transplantation. Because the diagnosis of IPF confers a relatively poor prognosis, an expert panel convened under the auspices of the International Society for Heart and Lung Transplantation recommended referral of eligible patients to a transplant center at the time that a radiographic or histologic diagnosis of IPF is made [89]. Patients who undergo lung transplantation must comply with a complex medical treatment plan and have frequent monitoring to detect graft rejection or infection, and 5-year survival for single lung transplant (Kaplan-Meier) is only 43%. Other interventions, including those that target co-morbidities, may improve quality of life and relieve symptoms of the disease. Supplemental oxygen is generally given when evidence of resting hypoxaemia or significant exercise-induced or nocturnal hypoxaemia is detected.

Summary and Conclusions

IPF is a distinct form of IIP that is characterised by radiological and /or histopathologic changes of UIP in the lungs of adults in whom there is no clinical condition (e.g., rheumatologic disorder) or exposure associated with pulmonary fibrosis. IPF appears to be increasingly diagnosed today in comparison to past decades and portends a poor prognosis, especially if complicated by the development of PA hypertension. Extensive vascular remodeling occurs in IPF in association with progressive parenchymal scar formation, and many patients develop pulmonary hypertension as a complication of pulmonary fibrosis. No therapies have been able to make an impact on survival in IPF, and clinical studies/trials to determine effective pharmacologic therapies for PA hypertension complicating IPF are needed. Lung transplantation is currently considered the most effective therapy for IPF, and pharmacologic agents that prevent or modulate progressive lung fibrosis in IPF are currently underway.

References

1. American Thoracic Society. Idiopathic pulmonary fibrosis: diagnosis and treatment. International consensus statement. American Thoracic Society (ATS), and the European Respiratory Society (ERS). Am J Respir Crit Care Med 2000;161:646–664.
2. ATS/ERS. International Multidisciplinary consensus classification of the idiopathic interstitial pneumonias. Am J Respir and Crit Care Med 2002; 165:277–304.
3. Mason RJ, Schwartz MI, Hunninghake GW, Musson RA. NHLBI Workshop Summary. Pharmacological therapy for idiopathic pulmonary fibrosis. Past, present, and future. Am J Respir Crit Care Med 1999;160:1771–1777.
4. Coultas DB, Zumwalt RE, Black WC, Sobonya RE. The epidemiology of interstitial lung diseases. Am J Respir Crit Care Med 1994;150:967–972.
5. Gribbin J, Hubbard RB, Le Jeune I, Smith CJP, West J, Tata LJ. Incidence and mortality of idiopathic pulmonary fibrosis and sarcoidosis in the UK. Thorax 2006;61:980–985.
6. Raghu G, Weycker D, Edelsberg J, Bradford WZ, Oster G. Incidence and prevalence of idiopathic pulmonary fibrosis. Am J Respir Crit Care Med 2006;174:810–816.
7. Alberg AJ, Samet JM. Epidemiology of lung cancer. Chest 2003:123;21S–49s.
8. Jermal A, Murrray T, Samuels A, Ghafoor A, Ward E, Thun MJ. Cancer statistics 2003. CA Cancer J Clin 2003;53:5–26.
9. Olson AL, Swigris JJ, Lezotte DC, Norris JM, Wilson CG, Brown KK. Mortality from pulmonary fibrosis increased in the United States from 1992 to 2003. Am J Respir Crit Care Med 2007;176:277–284.
10. Hubbard R, Lewis S, Richards K, Johnston I, Britton J. Occupational exposure to metal or wood dust and aetiology of cryptogenic fibrosing alveolitis. Lancet 1996;347:284–289.
11. Baumgartner KB, Samet JM, Coultas DB, Stidley CA, Hunt WC, Colby TV, Waldron JA. Occupational and environmental risk factors for idiopathic pulmonary fibrosis: a multicenter case-control study. Collaborating Centers. Am J Epidemiol 2000;152:307–315.
12. Baumgartner KB, Samet JM, Stidley Ca, Colby TV, Waldron JA. Cigarette smoking: a risk factor for idiopathic pulmonary fibrosis. Am J Respir Crit Care Med 1997;155:242–248.
13. Tang YW, Johnson JE, Browning PJ, Cruz-Gervis RA, Davis A, Graham BS, Brigham KL, Oates JA Jr, Loyd JE, Stecenko AA. Herpesvirus DNA is consistently detected in lungs of patients with idiopathic pulmonary fibrosis. J Clin Microbiol 2003;41:2633–2640.
14. Tobin RW, Pope CE II, Pellegrini CA, Emond MJ, Sillery J, Raghu G. Increased prevalence of gastroesophageal reflux in patients with idiopathic pulmonary fibrosis. Am J Respir Crit Care Med 1998;158:1804–1808.
15. Raghu G, Freudenberger TD, Yang S, Curtis JR, Spada C, Hayes J, Sillery JK, Pope CE 2nd, Pellegrini CA. High prevalence of abnormal acid gastro-oesophageal reflux in idiopathic pulmonary fibrosis. Eur Respir J 2006;27:136–142.
16. Garcia CK, Raghu,G. Inherited interstitial Lung Disease. Clin Chest Med 2004;25:421–433.
17. Lawson WE, Loyd JE. The genetic approach in pulmonary fibrosis: can it provide clues to this complex disease? Proc Am Thorac Soc 2006;3:345–349.

18. Collins K, Mitchell JR. Telomerase in the human organism. Oncogene 2002;21:564–579.
19. Liu T, Hu B, Chung MJ, Ullenbruch M, Jin H, Phan SH. Telomerase regulation of myofibroblast differentiation. Am J Respir Cell Mol Biol 2006;34:625–633.
20. Mu XC, Staiano-Coico L, Higgine PJ. Increased transcription and modified growth state-dependent expression of the plasminogen activator inhibitor type-1 gene characterize the senescent phenotype in human diploid fibroblasts. J Cell Physiol 1998;174:90–98.
21. Garcia CK, Wright WE, Shay JW. Human diseases of telomerase dysfunction: insights into tissue aging. Nucl Acids Res 2007;1–11.
22. Armanios MY, Chen JJ, Cogan JD, Alder JK, Ingersoll RG, Markin C, Lawson WE, Xie M, Vulto I, Phillips JA 3rd, Lansdorp PM, Greider CW, Loyd JE. Telomerase mutations in families with idiopathic pulmonary fibrosis. N Engl J Med 2007;356:1317–1326.
23. Tsakiri K, Cronkhite JT, Kuan PJ, Xing C, Raghu G, Weissler JC, Rosenblatt RL, Shay JW, Garcia CK. Adult-onset pulmonary fibrosis caused by mutations in telomerase. Proc Natl Acad Sci U S A 2007;104:7552–7557.
24. Katzenstein AL, Zisman DA, Litzky LA, Nguyen BT, Kotloff RM. Usual interstitial pneumonia: histologic study of biopsy and explant specimens. Am J Surg Pathol 2002;26:1567–1577.
25. Flaherty KR, Travis WD, Colby TV, Toews GB, Kazerooni EA, Gross BH, Jain A, Strawderman RL, Flint A, Lynch JP, Martinez FJ. Histopathologic variability in usual and nonspecific interstitial pneumonias. Am J Respir Crit Care Med 2001;164:1722–1727.
26. Keane MP, Strieter RM, Lynch JP III, Belperio JA. Inflammation and angiogenesis in fibrotic lung disease. Semin Respir Crit Care Med 2006;27:589–599.
27. Turner-Warwick M. Precapillary systemic pulmonary anastomoses. Thorax 1963;18:225–237.
28. Peao MNDA, Aguas AP, DeSa CM, Grande NR. Neoformation of blood vessels in association with rat lung fibrosis induced by bleomycin. Anat Rec 1994;238:57–67.
29. Keane MP, Arenberg DA, Lynch JP III, Whyte RI, Iannettoni MD, Burdick MD, Wilke CA, Morris SB, Glass MC, DiGiovine B, Kunkel SL, Strieter RM. The CXC chemokines, IL-8 and IP-10, regulate angiogenic activity in idiopathic pulmonary fibrosis. J Immunol 1997;159:1437–1443.
30. Meyer KC, Cardoni A, Xiang Z. Vascular endothelial growth factor in bronchoalveolar lavage from normal subjects and patients with diffuse parenchymal lung disease. J Lab Clin Med 2000;135:332–338.
31. Cosgrove GP, Brown KK, Schliemann WP, Serls AE, Parr JE, Geraci MW, Schwarz MI, Cool CD, Worther GS. Pigment epithelial-derived factor in idiopathic pulmonary fibrosis. Am J Respir Crit Care Med 2004;170:242–251.
32. Lappi-Blanco E, Soini Y, Kinnula V, Pääkkö P. VEGF and bFGF are highly expressed in intraluminal fibromyxoid lesions in bronchiolitis obliterans organizing pneumonia. J Pathol 2002;196:220–227.
33. Wells A. Clinical usefulness of high resolution computed tomography in cryptogenic fibrosing alveolitis. Thorax 1998;53:1080–1087.
34. Meyer KC. The role of bronchoalveolar lavage in interstitial lung disease. Clin Chest Med 2004;25;637–649.
35. Barbescu EA, Katzenstein AL, Snow JL, Zisman DA. Transbronchial biopsy in usual interstitial pneumonia. Chest 2006;1129:1126–1131.
36. Flaherty KR, King TE Jr, Raghu G, Lynch JP 3rd, Colby TV, Travis WD, Gross BH, Kazerooni EA, Toews GB, Long Q, Murray S, Lama VN, Gay SE, Martinez FJ. Idiopathic interstitial pneumonia: what is the effect of a multidisciplinary approach to diagnosis? Am J Respir Crit Care Med 2004;170:904–910.
37. Collard HR, King TE Jr. Demystifying idiopathic interstitial pneumonia. Arch Intern Med 2003;163:17–29.
38. Flaherty KR, Thwaite EL, Kazerooni EA, Gross BH, Toews GB, Colby TV, Travis WD, Mumford JA, Murray S, Flint A, Lynch JP 3rd, Martinez FJ. Radiological versus histological diagnosis in UIP and NSIP: survival implications. Thorax 2003;58:143–148.
39. Park JH, Kim DS, Part I-N, Jang SJ, Kitaichi M, Nicholson AG, Colby TV. Prognosis of fibrotic interstitial pneumonia: idiopathic versus collagen vascular disease-related subtypes. Am J Respir Crit Care Med 2007;175:705–711.

40. Martinez FJ, Safrin S, Weycker D, Starko KM, Bradford WZ, King TE Jr, Flaherty KR, Schwartz DA, Noble PW, Raghu G, Brown KK; IPF Study Group. The clinical course of patients with idiopathic pulmonary fibrosis. Ann Intern Med 2005;142:963–967.
41. Brown KK, Raghu G. Medical treatment for pulmonary fibrosis: current trends, concepts, and prospects. Clin Chest Med 2004;25:759–772.
42. Collard HR, Moore BB, Flaherty KR, Brown KK, Kaner RJ, King TE Jr, Lasky JA, Loyd JE, Noth I, Olman MA, Raghu G, Roman J, Ryu JH, Zisman DA, Hunninghake GW, Colby TV, Egan JJ, Hansell DM, Johkoh T, Kaminski N, Kim DS, Kondoh Y, Lynch DA, Müller-Quernheim J, Myers JL, Nicholson AG, Selman M, Toews GB, Wells AU, Martinez FJ; Idiopathic Pulmonary Fibrosis Clinical Research Network Investigators. Acute exacerbations of idiopathic pulmonary fibrosis. Am J Respir Crit Care Med 2007;176:636–643.
43. Collard HR, King TE Jr, Bartelson BB, Vourlekis JS, Schwarz MI, Brown KK. Changes in clinical and physiologic variables predict survival in idiopathic pulmonary fibrosis. Am J Respir Crit Care Med 2003;168:538–542.
44. King TE Jr, Safrin S, Starko KM, Brown KK, Noble PW, Raghu G, Schwartz DA. Analyses of efficacy end points in a controlled trial of interferon-gamma1b for idiopathic pulmonary fibrosis. Chest 2005;127:171–177.
45. Wells AU, Desai SR, Rubens MB, Goh NS, Cramer D, Nicholson AG, Colby TV, du Bois RM, Hansell DM. Idiopathic pulmonary fibrosis: a composite physiologic index derived from disease extent observed by computed tomography. Am J Respir Crit Care Med 2003;167:962–969.
46. Lama RN, Flaherty KR, Toews GB, Colby TV, Travis WD, Long Q, Murray S, Kazerooni EA, Gross BH, Lynch JP 3rd, Martinez FJ. Prognostic value of desaturation during a 6-minute walk test in idiopathic interstitial pneumonia. Am J Respir Crit Care Med 2005;168:1084–1090.
47. Flaherty KR, Adin-Cristian A, Murray S, Fraley C, Colby TV, Travis WD, Lama V, Kazerooni EA, Gross BH, Toews GB, Martinez FJ. Idiopathic pulmonary fibrosis: prognostic value of changes in physiology and six-minute-walk test. Am J Respir Crit Care Med 2006;174:803–809.
48. Hallstrand TS, Boitano LJ, Johnson WC, Spada CA, Hayes JG, Raghu G. The timed walk test as a measure of severity and survival in idiopathic pulmonary fibrosis. Eur Respir J 2005;25:96–103.
49. Lettieri CJ, Nathan SD, Barnett SD, Ahmad S, Shorr AF. Prevalence and outcomes of pulmonary arterial hypertension in advanced idiopathic pulmonary fibrosis. Chest 2006;129:746–752.
50. Panos RJ, Mortenson RL, Niccoli SA, King TE, Jr. Clinical deterioration in patients with idiopathic pulmonary fibrosis: causes and assessment. Am J Med 1990;88:396–404.
51. Hubbard R, Venn A, Lewis S, Britton J. Lung cancer and cryptogenic fibrosing alveolitis: a population-based cohort study. Am J Respir Crit Care Med 2000;161:5–8.
52. Shorr AF, Helman DL, Davies DB, Nathan SD. Pulmonary hypertension in advanced sarcoidosis: epidemiology and clinical characteristics. Eur Respir J 2005;25:783–788.
53. Nadrous HF, Pellikka PA, Krowka MUJ, Swanson KL, Chaowalit N, Decker PA, Ryu JH. Pulmonary hypertension in patients with idiopathic pulmonary fibrosis. Chest 2005;128:2393–2399.
54. Nathan SD, Ahmad S, Koch J, Barnett S, Ad N, Burton N. Serial measures of pulmonary artery pressures in patients with idiopathic pulmonary fibrosis. Chest 2005;128:168S.
55. Shorr AF, Wainright JL, Cors CS, Lettieri CJ, Nathan SD. Pulmonary hypertension in patients with pulmonary fibrosis awaiting lung transplant. Eur Respir J 2007;30:715–721.
56. Lederer DJ, Caplan-Shaw CE, O'Shea MK, Wilt JS, Basner RC, Bartels MN, Sonett JR, Arcasoy SM, Kawut SM. Racial and ethnic disparities in survival in lung transplant candidates with idiopathic pulmonary fibrosis. Am J Transplant 2006;6:398–403.
57. Whelan TP, Dunitz JM, Kelly RF, Edwards LB, Herrington CS, Hertz MI, Dahlberg PS. J Heart Lung Transplant 2005;24:1269–1274.
58. Heath D, Gillund TD, Kay JM, Hawkins CF. Pulmonary vascular disease in honeycomb lung. J Pathol Bacteriol 1968;95:423–430.
59. Colombat M, Mal H, Groussard O, Capron F, Thabut G, Jebrak G, Brugière O, Dauriat G, Castier Y, Lesèche G, Fournier M. Pulmonary vascular lesions in end-stage idiopathic pulmonary fibrosis: histopathologic study on lung explant specimens and correlations with pulmonary hemodynamics. Hum Pathol 2007;38:60–65.

60. Bignon J, Hem B, Molinier B. Morphometric and angiographic studies in diffuse interstitial pulmonary fibrosis. Prog Redspir Res 1975;8:141–160.
61. Renzoni EA, Walsh DA, Salmon M, Wells AU, Sestini P, Nicholson AG, Veeraraghavan S, Bishop AE, Romanska HM, Pantelidis P, et al. Interstitial vascularity in fibrosing alveolitis. Am J Respir Crit Care Med 2003;167:438–443.
62. Keane MP, Belperio JA, Burdick M, Lynch JP, III, Fishbein MF, Strieter RM. ENA-78 is an important angiogenic factor in idiopathic pulmonary fibrosis. Am J Respir Crit Care Med 2001;164:2239–2242.
63. Nakayama S, Mukae H, Ishii H, Kakugawa T, Sugiyama K, Sakamoto N, Fujii T, Kadota J, Kohno S. Comparison of BALF concentrations of ENA-78 and IP10 in patients with idiopathic pulmonary fibrosis and nonspecific interstitial pneumonia. Respir Med 2005;99:1145–1151.
64. Arcasoy SM, Christie JD, Ferrari VA, Sutton MS, Zisman DA, Blumenthal NP, Pochettino A, Kotloff RM. Echocardiographic assessment of pulmonary hypertension in patients with advanced lung disease. Am J Respir Crit Care Med 2003;167:735–740.
65. Leuchte HH, Neurohr C, Baumgartner R, Holzapfel M, Giehrl W, Vogeser M, Behr J. Brain natriuretic peptide and exercise capacity in lung fibrosis and pulmonary hypertension. Am J Respir Crit Care Med 2004;170:360–365.
66. Chang JA, Curtis JR, Patrick DL, Raghu G. Assessment of health-related quality of life in patients with interstitial lung disease. Chest 1999;116:1175–1182.
67. Raghu G, Brown KK, Bradford WZ, Starko K, Noble PW, Schwartz DA, King TE Jr; Idiopathic Pulmonary Fibrosis Study Group. A placebo-controlled trial of interferon gamma-1b in patients with idiopathic pulmonary fibrosis. N Engl J Med 2004;350:125–133.
68. Charbeneau RP, Peters-Golden M. Eicosanoids: mediators and therapeutic targets in fibrotic lung disease. Clin Sci (Lond) 2005;108:479–491.
69. Wright L, Tuder RM, Cool CD, Lepley RA, Voelkel NF. 5-Lipoxygenase and 5-lipooxygenase activating protein (FLAP) immunoreactivity in lungs from patients with primary pulmonary hypertension. Am J Respir Crit Care Med 1998;157:219–229.
70. Budhiraja R, Tuder RM, Hassoun PM. Endothelial dysfunction in pulmonary hypertension. Circulation 2004;109:159–165.
71. Tuder RM, Cool CD, Geraci MW, Wang J, Abman SH, Wright L, Badesch DB, Voelkel NF. Prostacyclin synthase expression is decreased in lungs from patients with severe pulmonary hypertension. Am J Respir Crit Care Med 1999;159:1925–1932.
72. Badesch DB, McLaughlin VV, Delcroix M, Vizza CD, Olschewski H, Sitbon O, Barst RJ. Prostanoid therapy for pulmonary arterial hypertension. J Am Coll Cardiol 2004;43(12 Suppl 5):56S–61S.
73. Rubin LJ, Badesch DB, Barst RJ, Galie N, Black CM, Keogh A, Pulido T, Frost A, Roux S, Leconte I, Landzberg M, Simonneau G. Bosentan therapy for pulmonary arterial hypertension. N Engl J Med 2002;346:896–903.
74. Barst RJ, Langleben D, Badesch D, Frost A, Lawrence EC, Shapiro S, Naeije R, Galie N; STRIDE-2 Study Group. Treatment of pulmonary arterial hypertension with the selective endothelin-A receptor antagonist sitaxsentan. J Am Coll Cardiol 2006;47:2049–2056.
75. Galiè N, Ghofrani HA, Torbicki A, Barst RJ, Rubin LJ, Badesch D, Fleming T, Parpia T, Burgess G, Branzi A, Grimminger F, Kurzyna M, Simonneau G; Sildenafil Use in Pulmonary Arterial Hypertension (SUPER) Study Group. Sildenafil citrate therapy for pulmonary arterial hypertension. N Engl J Med 2005;353:2148–2157.
76. Olschewski H, Ghofrani HA, Walmrath D, Schermuly R, Temmesfeld-Wollbruck B, Grimminger F, Seeger W. Inhaled prostacyclin and iloprost in severe pulmonary hypertension secondary to lung fibrosis. Am J Respir Crit Care Med 1999;160:600–607.
77. Giaid A, Michel RP, Stewart DJ, Sheppard M, Corrin B, Hamid Q. Expression of endothelin-1 in lungs of patients with cryptogenic fibrosing alveolitis. Lancet 1993;341:1550–1554.
78. Saleh D, Furukawa K, Tsao MS, Maghazachi A, Corrin B, Yanagisawa M, Barnes PJ, Giaid A. Elevated expression of endothelin-1 and endothelin-converting enzyme-1 in idiopathic pulmonary fibrosis: possible involvement of proinflammatory cytokines. Am J Respir Cell Mol Biol 1997;16:187–193.

79. Trakada G, Spiropoulos K. Arterial endothelin-1 in interstitial lung disease patients with pulmonary hypertension. Monaldi Arch Chest Dis 2001;56:379–383.
80. King Jr TE, Behr J, Brown KK, du Bois RM, Lancaster L, de Andrade JA, Stahler G, Leconte I, Roux S, Raghu G. BUILD-1: a randomized placebo-controlled trial of bosentan in patients with idiopathic pulmonary fibrosis. Am J Respir Crit Care Med 2007;177:75–78.
81. Sebkhi A, Strange JW, Phillips SC, Wharton J, Wilkins MR. Phosphodiesterase type 5 as a target for the treatment of hypoxia-induced pulmonary hypertension. Circulation 2003;107: 3230–3235.
82. Zhao L, Mason NA, Morrell NW, Kojonazarov B, Sadykov A, Maripov A, Mirrakhimov MM, Aldashev A, Wilkins MR. Sildenafil inhibits hypoxia-induced pulmonary hypertension. Circulation 2001;104:424–428.
83. Maloney JP. Advances in the treatment of secondary pulmonary hypertension. Curr Opin Pulm Med 2003;9:139–143.
84. Ghofrani HA, Wiedemann R, Rose F, Schermuly RT, Olschewski H, Weissmann N, Gunther A, Walmrath D, Seeger W, Grimminger F. Sildenafil for treatment of lung fibrosis and pulmonary hypertension: a randomized controlled trial. Lancet 2002;360:895–900.
85. Collard HR, Anstrom KJ, Schwarz MI, Zisman DA. Sildenafil improves walk distance in idiopathic pulmonary fibrosis. Chest 2007;131:897–899.
86. Kawut SM, Horn EM, Berekashvili KK, Garofano RP, Goldsmith RL, Widlitz AC, Rosenzweig EB, Kerstein D, Barst RJ. New predictors of outcome in idiopathic pulmonary arterial hypertension. Am J Cardiol 2005;95:199–203.
87. Bignon J, Hem B, Molinier B. Morphometric and angiographic studies in diffuse interstitial pulmonary fibrosis. Prog Respir Res 1975;8:141–160.
88. Kubo H, Nakayama K, Yanai M, Suzuki T, Yamaya M, Watanabe M, Sasaki H. Anticoagulant therapy for idiopathic pulmonary fibrosis. Chest 2005;128:1475–1482.
89. Orens JB, Estenne M, Arcasoy S, Conte JV, Corris P, Egan JJ, Egan T, Keshavjee S, Knoop C, Kotloff R, Martinez FJ, Nathan S, Palmer S, Patterson A, Singer L, Snell G, Studer S, Vachiery JL, Glanville AR; Pulmonary Scientific Council of the International Society for Heart and Lung Transplantation. International guidelines for the selection of lung transplant candidates: 2006 update—a consensus report from the Pulmonary Scientific Council of the International Society for Heart and Lung Transplantation. J Heart Lung Transplant 2006;25:745–755.

Chapter 4
Lung Pathology

Andre L. Moreira and William D. Travis

Introduction

Interstitial lung disease (ILD) is a term that can be applied to many different pathological entities, both idiopathic or of a known cause. In a simplistic way, the term represents diffuse parenchymal lung disease in which there is expansion of the pulmonary interstitium by inflammation with or without fibrosis.

The role of the pathologist in the workup of interstitial lung disease is to try to categorize the histopathological changes present in the biopsy specimen into groups of entities that have implications for the clinical management of the patient, prognosis, and response to therapy.

The histologic patterns found in interstitial pneumonias are distinctive but, unfortunately, they are not specific and can be observed in a variety of other conditions. For example, the histologic pattern noted in usual interstitial pneumonia (UIP) can be detected in collagen vascular diseases as well as in asbestosis or drug reactions. Therefore, the recognition of UIP-like histologic pattern on a lung biopsy raises a differential diagnosis that includes idiopathic UIP, respectively, as well as several other conditions.

Surgical biopsies for the diagnosis and classification of ILD are uncommon, which prevents most general pathologists from developing critical knowledge of the histopathological criteria to be able to discriminate the subtle changes among the considerable overlap of histological appearance in ILD. To achieve an accurate pathological diagnosis, it is essential to correlate the findings in the lung biopsy specimen with clinical, high-resolution computed tomography scans, laboratory, and pulmonary function abnormalities. This correlation requires communication between the pathologist and clinical and radiologist colleagues. In this chapter, we discuss the histopathological findings of the most common interstitial pneumonias and the evolving concepts leading to their histopathological classification.

R.P. Baughman et al. (eds.), *Pulmonary Arterial Hypertension and Interstitial Lung Diseases,*
© Humana Press, a part of Springer Science + Business Media, LLC 2009

Histological Classification of Idiopathic Interstitial Pneumonias (IIPs)

The IIPs represent the most common and important group of ILDs. In approximately 30% of the cases, the cause of the interstitial pneumonia is found. In this small group, however, the etiological factors are also heterogeneous and vary from collagenous vascular disease, infection, or injury by toxic agents and drugs. The concept of the histological classification of interstitial pneumonia is still evolving. Many of the histological patterns described are very helpful for the clinical management of the patients independent of whether this is an idiopathic process or not.

The American Thoracic Society and European Respiratory Society have sponsored a panel of experts in the field of thoracic pathology, radiology, and pulmonologists who proposed a multidisciplinary approach in an attempt to correlate specific histological subsets with prognosis and response to therapy [1]. In this classification of ILD, there are paired lists of pathologic terms matched to clinical terms (Table 4.1). The major entities include UIP/idiopathic pulmonary fibrosis (IPF)/cryptogenic fibrosing alveolitis (CFA), nonspecific interstitial pneumonia (NSIP), organizing pneumonia/cryptogenic organizing pneumonia (COP), diffuse alveolar damage/acute interstitial pneumonia (DAD/AIP), respiratory bronchiolitis/respiratory bronchiolitis-interstitial lung disease (RB-ILD), desquamative interstitial pneumonia (DIP), and lymphocytic interstitial pneumonia (LIP).

There is a subset of patients with interstitial pneumonia that remain unclassifiable even after extensive clinical, radiologic, and/or pathological examination. This problem often exists in cases where some critical piece of data is unavailable; examples include inadequate clinical information or inadequate chest radiologic images; an inadequate or nondiagnostic lung biopsy as the result of its small size (a bronchoscopic or needle biopsy), poor sampling; or the presence of only a nondiagnostic pattern of end-stage fibrosis with honeycombing on the specimen. In some cases, the data are completely conflicting.

Table 4.1 American Thoracic Society and European Respiratory Society Histologic and Clinical Classification of Idiopathic Interstitial Pneumonias*

Histologic patterns	Clinicoradiological–pathologic diagnoses
Usual interstitial pneumonia	Idiopathic pulmonary fibrosis/Cryptogenic fibrosing alveolitis
Nonspecific interstitial pneumonia	Nonspecific interstitial pneumonia
Organizing pneumonia	Cryptogenic organizing pneumonia
Diffuse alveolar damage	Acute interstitial pneumonia
Respiratory bronchiolitis	Respiratory bronchiolitis interstitial lung disease
Desquamative interstitial pneumonia	Desquamative interstitial pneumonia
Lymphocytic interstitial pneumonia	Lymphocytic interstitial pneumonia
Unclassifiable interstitial pneumonia	

*From Travis et al. [1].

UIP

UIP is the most important of all the ILDs because it carries a poor prognosis and no effective therapy is recognized. Therefore, when evaluating a pulmonary biopsy for ILD, the pathologist must determine whether it shows histological features of a UIP or a non-UIP pattern. However, the UIP histologic pattern occurs in a variety of clinical settings, particularly in patients with collagen vascular diseases.

The diagnosis of UIP can be rendered on the clinical and radiographic basis without the need for open lung biopsy. Biopsies are recommended, when there are atypical clinical and/or radiographic features that are suspicious for another interstitial pneumonia other than UIP or when the clinical diagnosis of UIP is uncertain [2,3].

Histologic Features

The histologic hallmark of the UIP is patchy interstitial fibrosis often in a subpleural and/or paraseptal distribution alternating with areas of normal lung (Fig. 4.1) [4–9]. The fibrosis is heterogeneous, with old, established fibrosis and areas of recent fibrosis. The old fibrosis is characterized by dense fibrous bands of scar tissue that causes remodeling of the lung architecture resulting in collapse of alveolar walls and formation of cystic spaces. This pattern is called honeycombing.

The recent fibrosis consists of fibroblastic foci, a loose type of connective tissue that contains myofibroblasts within a myxoid stroma and few collagen fibers (Fig. 4.2). Smooth muscle proliferation may be found in areas of dense fibrotic scarring.

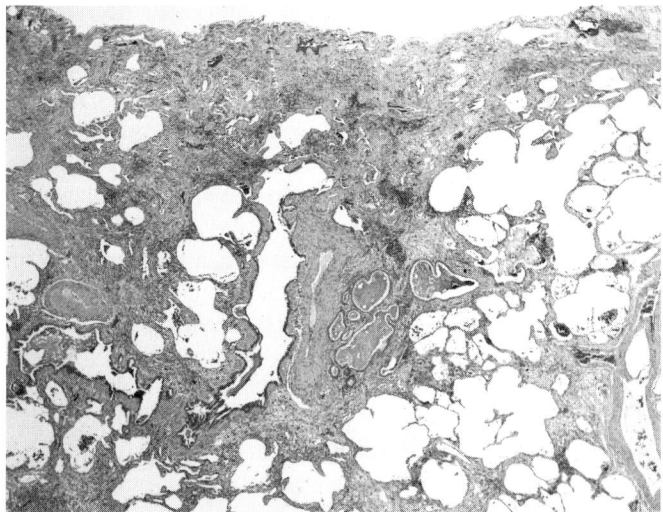

Fig. 4.1 Photomicrograph of UIP shows patchy involvement of the pulmonary parenchyma by a fibrotic process. Note that the fibrosis is mostly subpleural and there are areas of spared normal appearing lung (*See Color Plates*)

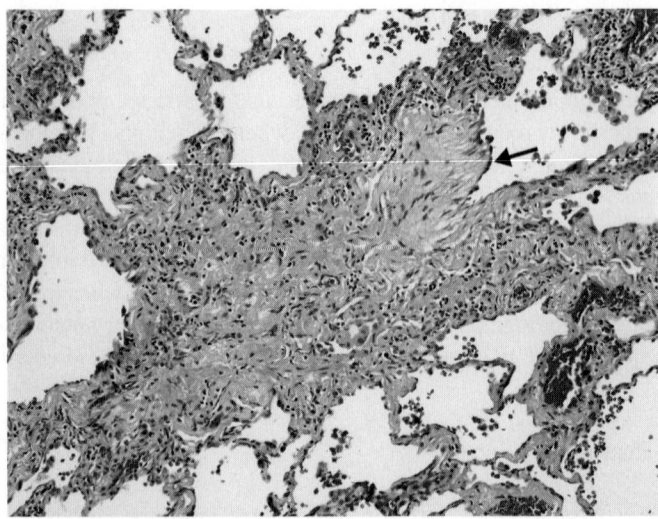

Fig. 4.2 Photomicrograph of UIP shows a fibroblastic foci (arrow) arising in an area of expanded alveolar septa and relatively normal lung (*See Color Plates*)

The temporal heterogeneity that characterizes UIP is favored to be the histological correlate of lesions in different healing stages as a result of multiple or continuous injury [10].

The fibrotically thickened alveolar septa tend to be lined by hyperplastic cuboidal epithelial cells, bronchiolar epithelium, or squamous metaplastic epithelium. Sometimes the epithelial cells overlying the fibroblastic foci show reactive cellular atypia with abundant cytoplasm, large hyperchromatic nuclei, and prominent nucleoli. Acute exacerbation of UIP can occur [11,12]. In these cases, the lung biopsy often shows a pattern of diffuse alveolar damage with formation of hyaline membranes, superimposed in a UIP pattern [12]. Patients with acute exacerbation of UIP usually are associated with rapidly progressive respiratory failure and worse prognosis.

Because one of the most important criteria for the histologic diagnosis of UIP is patchy process with temporal variegation, one of the most limiting factors for the diagnosis of this entity is sampling. It is important that the surgeon is made aware to include in the biopsy areas of relatively normal lung; otherwise, if only areas of honeycomb fibrosis are biopsied, one may only be able to identify a pattern of end-stage fibrosis without a more specific diagnosis.

The histological heterogeneity of UIP also accounts for overlapping patterns with other interstitial lung diseases. A NSIP pattern could be observed in 25% of cases [13] when multiple biopsies from different lobes are obtained and up to 80% of explanted specimens from UIP patients undergoing transplantation where there is more extensive sampling [14]. Therefore, the pathologist may report the diagnosis of UIP using different levels of certainty. The following approach can be useful: (1) definite UIP, (2) probable UIP, (3) possible UIP, and (4) definitely not UIP [13].

Differential Diagnosis

A marked interstitial inflammatory infiltrate or the presence of granulomatous inflammation in a lung biopsy showing a possible UIP pattern should raise the consideration of hypersensitivity pneumonitis, pneumoconiosis, drug-induced pneumonitis, infection, or collagen vascular disease. If there is a suspicion for asbestos exposure, iron stains should be performed unless asbestos bodies are seen on hematoxylin and eosin-stained sections. Polarization microscopy may also help to identify birefringent particles that could suggest significant dust deposits.

NSIP

The concept of NSIP resulted from the recognition that a group of interstitial pneumonia did not share histological characteristics recognized for the major interstitial lung diseases. In 1994, Katzenstein and Fiorelli [15] reported a series of 64 patients with similar lung biopsy findings and proposed these cases be called "nonspecific interstitial pneumonia." There was a wide range of histologic pattern of NSIP, which occurred in different clinical settings, such as collagen-vascular diseases, slowly resolving DAD, and a variety of environmental exposures [15]. The importance of the histological diagnosis of NSIP is that it has a more favorable prognosis than UIP [6,7,15–18].

Pathologic Features

The NSIP pattern is characterized by uniform interstitial inflammation and fibrosis. NSIP is separated into two groups: cellular NSIP and fibrosing NSIP. Cellular NSIP has a predominance of interstitial inflammatory infiltration over fibrosis, and fibrosing NSIP is predominantly fibrotic. Separation of cellular from fibrosing patterns of NSIP is important due to the significantly better prognosis associated with the former pattern [19]. The NSIP pattern also overlaps with a broad spectrum of different histologic patterns.

   NSIP is distinguished from UIP by its uniform involvement of the pulmonary parenchyma, in contrast to the patchy infiltrate and temporal heterogeneity of UIP. It generally lacks honeycomb fibrosis. NSIP is thought to represent a reaction to a one-time injury to the lungs.

NSIP, Cellular Pattern

The NSIP, cellular pattern consists primarily of mild-to-moderate interstitial chronic inflammation, usually with lymphocytes and a few plasma cells. The lung, contrary to UIP, is usually uniformly involved, but the distribution of the lesions may be patchy. The infiltrate typically involves the alveolar interstitium but is less severe than the extensive diffuse alveolar septal infiltration observed in lymphocytic interstitial pneumonia. Intraalveolar organizing fibrosis may be present giving a pattern of cellular NSIP and organizing pneumonia.

NSIP, Fibrosing Pattern

The hallmark of the NSIP, fibrosing pattern is the presence of dense or loose interstitial fibrosis and the lack of temporal heterogeneity characteristic of UIP. Honeycombing is not typical of fibrosing NSIP. Fibroblastic foci, the key lesion that gives the UIP pattern the appearance of temporal heterogeneity, should be inconspicuous or absent. In some cases, the pattern of fibrosis is patchy in distribution, causing remodeling of the lung architecture, sometimes with a subpleural distribution. In such cases, the lack of fibroblastic foci is especially important in distinguishing from the UIP pattern. Foci of proliferation of interstitial smooth muscle may be seen. Lymphoid aggregates are common.

Differential Diagnosis

The histologic and etiologic differential diagnosis for the NSIP pattern is listed in Table 4.2. Unfortunately in many cases, NSIP is a diagnosis of exclusion when the histological findings in the biopsy material cannot be classified into any known interstitial lung disease pattern.

COP

COP is also known as bronchiolitis obliterans organizing pneumonia (BOOP). Historically, BOOP has commonly been used and in the absence of any specific cause it has sometimes been referred to as idiopathic BOOP. The term COP is preferred because it conveys the essential features of the syndrome described below and avoids confusion with other airway diseases. There are many causes of the organizing pneumonia pattern on biopsy, so these must be excluded before making the diagnosis of COP. Some of the more common ones are summarized in Table 4.3.

Table 4.2 Differential Diagnosis of Nonspecific Interstitial Pneumonia, Cellular and Fibrosing Patterns

Usual interstitial pneumonia
Organizing pneumonia
Fibrotic phase of other interstitial disorders
  Hypersensitivity pneumonitis
  Histiocytosis X
  Desquamative interstitial pneumonia/respiratory bronchiolitis
  Diffuse alveolar damage
Eosinophilic pneumonia
Lymphocytic interstitial pneumonia
Possible etiologies
  Collagen vascular disease
  Drug-induced pneumonitis
  Infection

In the appropriate clinical setting and with characteristic chest imaging studies, the diagnosis may be established by obtaining a transbronchial lung biopsy that shows consistent histopathologic features. However, if the follow-up and response to therapy are not appropriate, alternative diagnoses should be considered.

Histologic Features

The organizing pneumonia pattern is patchy and consists of polypoid plugs of loose organizing connective tissue involving alveolar ducts and alveoli with or without bronchiolar intraluminal polyps (Fig. 4.3) [8,20,21]. The lung architecture is preserved. The majority of changes are centered on small airways. A small amount of airspace fibrin may be focally present.

Table 4.3 Causes of the Organizing Pneumonia Pattern Other Than COP

Organizing diffuse alveolar damage
Organizing infections
Organization distal to obstruction, aspiration pneumonia
Organizing drug reactions, fume, and toxic exposures
Collagen vascular disease
Extrinsic allergic alveolitis/hypersensitivity pneumonitis
Eosinophilic lung disease
As a reparative reaction around other processes (including abscesses, Wegener's granulomatosis, neoplasm, etc)

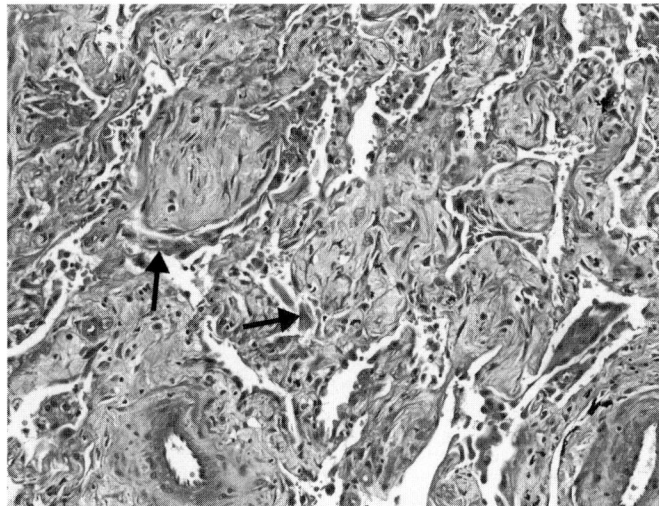

Fig. 4.3 The organizing pneumonia pattern is characterized by polypoid plugs of loose connective tissue that protudes into the alveolar space (arrows) (*See Color Plates*)

Histological Differential Diagnosis

The following histologic features are against a diagnosis of COP: airspace neutrophils, acute bronchiolitis, granulomas, necrosis, hyaline membranes, vasculitis, and prominent infiltration of eosinophils. The major histologic differential diagnostic considerations for the organizing pneumonia pattern include DAD, NSIP, DIP, and UIP patterns. DAD is characterized by more uniform and diffuse lung injury with marked edematous thickening and organization in alveolar walls and, often, hyaline membranes.

Respiratory Bronchiolitis-Associated Interstitial Lung Disease (RB-ILD)

RB is a common histologic lesion characterized by the presence of pigmented intraluminal macrophages within respiratory bronchioles. It is very often an incidental histologic pattern in the lungs of smokers. However, RB-ILD is a form of ILD associated with the histologic finding of respiratory bronchiolitis in patients with significant pulmonary symptoms, abnormal pulmonary function, and imaging abnormalities [8,22–25]. RB-ILD and DIP are thought to represent ends of a spectrum of smoking-associated interstitial lung disease [23,24].

Pathologic Features

In RB-ILD, the changes are patchy and have a bronchiolocentric distribution. Respiratory bronchioles, alveolar ducts, and peribronchiolar alveolar spaces contain clusters of dusty brown macrophages (Fig. 4.4). Mild peribronchiolar fibrosis is also observed, with expansion into contiguous alveolar septa, which are lined by hyperplastic type 2 cells and cuboidal bronchiolar-type epithelium.

Histologic Differential Diagnosis

The histologic differential diagnosis of the RB-ILD pattern includes DIP, bronchiolitis, and NSIP [26]. DIP and RB represent the ends of a spectrum, and overlap is common as one views multiple fields in a single specimen.

DIP

DIP is thought to represent part of a spectrum of cigarette smoking-related lung disease. However, it is thought to have sufficient distinctive clinical, radiographic, and histologic features to retain it as a separate category of IIP [1,8].

Color Plates

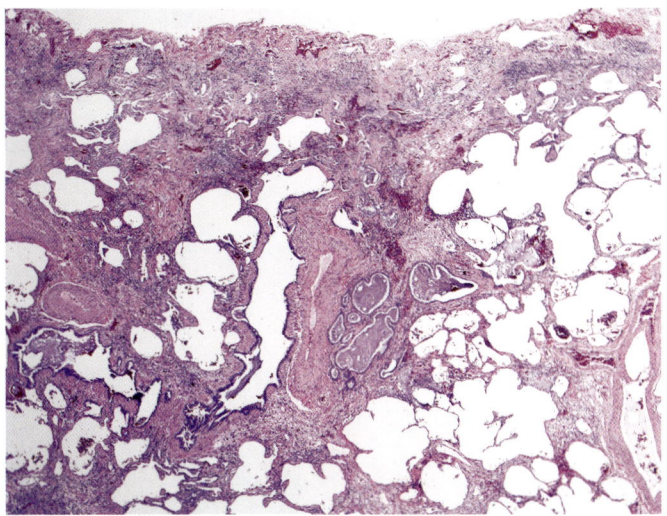

Fig. 4.1 Photomicrograph of UIP shows patchy involvement of the pulmonary parenchyma by a fibrotic process. Note that the fibrosis is mostly subpleural and there are areas of spared normal appearing lung

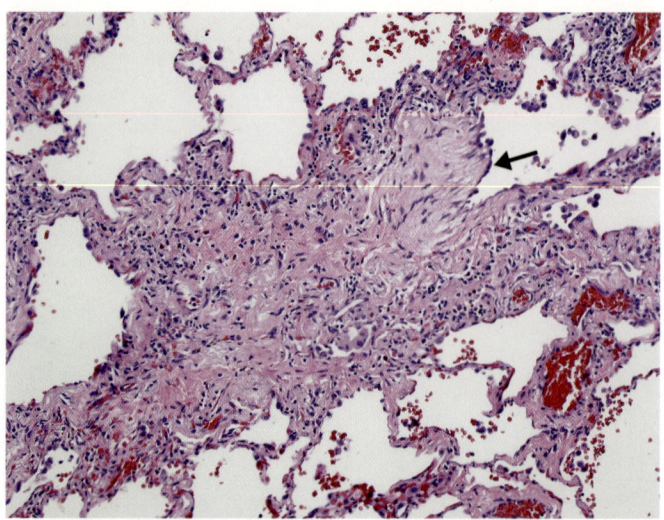

Fig. 4.2 Photomicrograph of UIP shows a fibroblastic foci (arrow) arising in an area of expanded alveolar septa and relatively normal lung

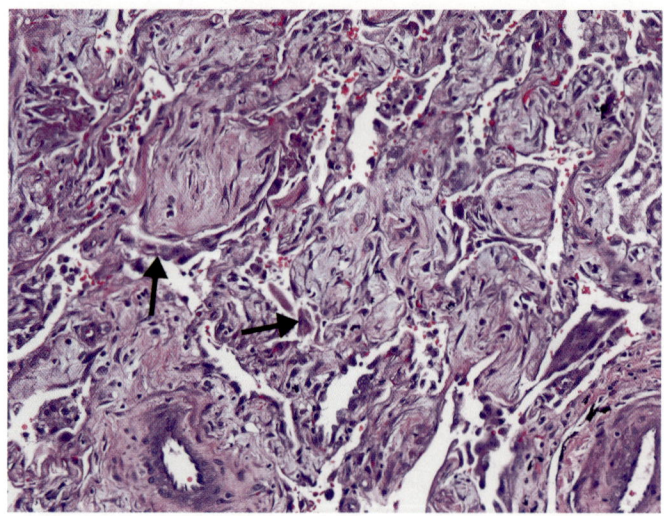

Fig. 4.3 The organizing pneumonia pattern is characterized by polypoid plugs of loose connective tissue that protudes into the alveolar space (arrows)

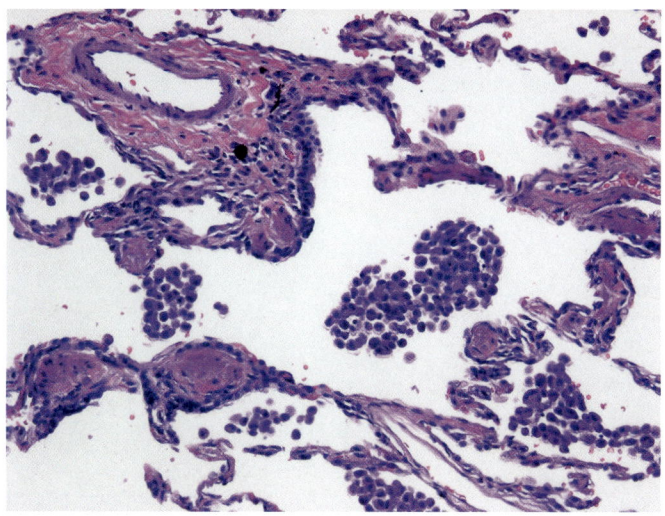

Fig. 4.4 RB-ILD: There is focal accumulation of pigmented alveolar macrophages in the peribronchiolar region and mild fibrosis of the bronchiolar wall

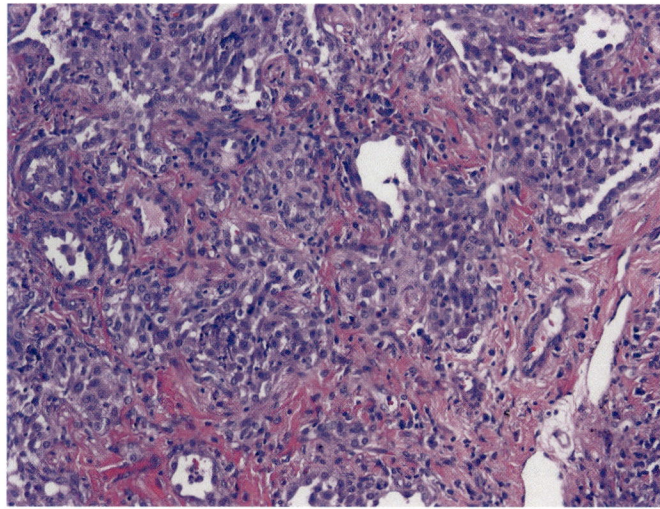

Fig. 4.5 In DIP, there is diffuse involvement of the lung by the accumulation of numerous alveolar macrophages within the alveolar sacs and mild fibrosis of the alveolar wall

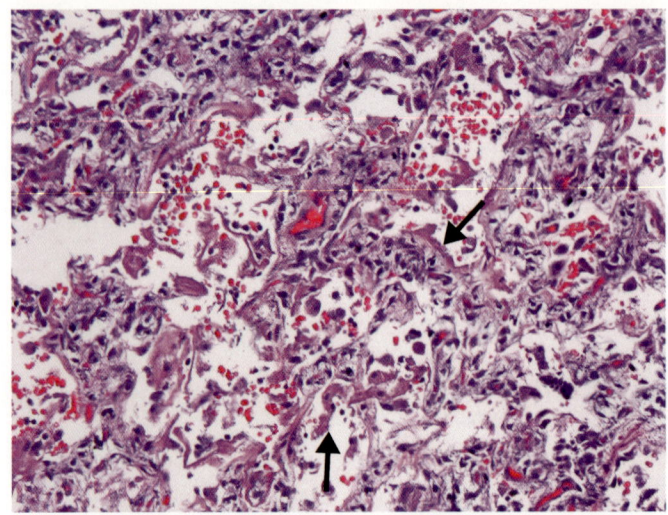

Fig. 4.6 In DAD, the alveolar walls are distended by edema, there is hyperplasia of type II pneumocytes and hyaline membranes. Hyaline membranes are pink fibrinous material that lines the alveolar wall (arrow)

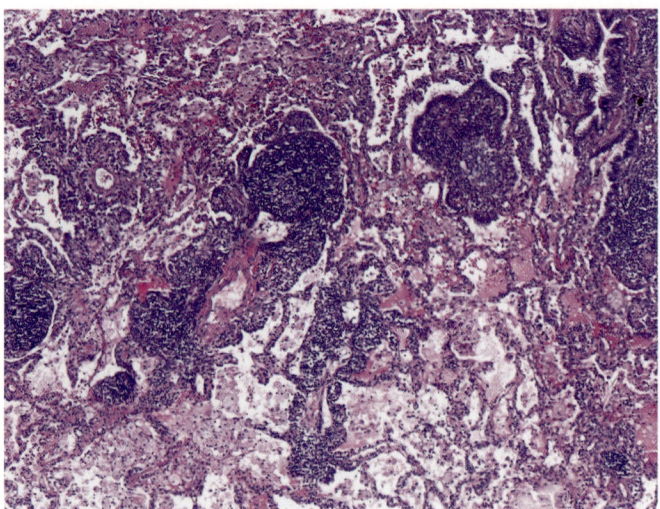

Fig. 4.7 Collagenous vascular disease. The presence of peribronchiolar and interstitial lymphoid follicles, although not specific, is commonly seen in cases of collagenous vascular disease

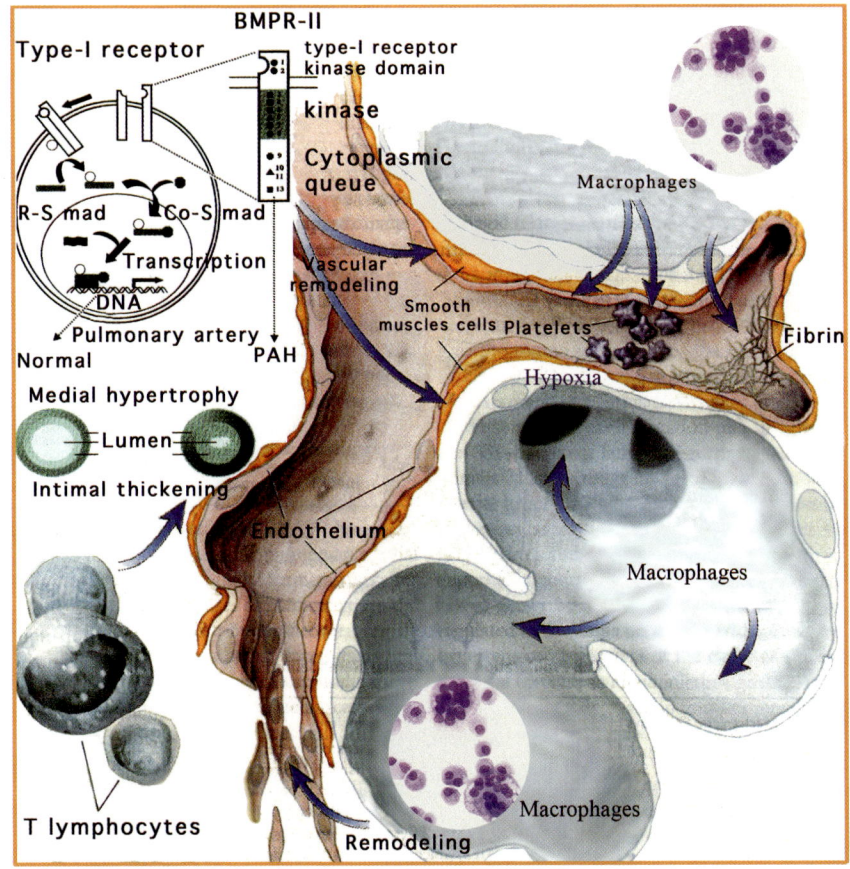

Fig. 5.1 Consequences of bone morphogenetic protein type-2 receptor (BMPR2) mutations implicated in PPH pathogenesis. A model pulmonary arteriolar system and alveolus with vasoconstriction, remodeling of the pulmonary vessel wall, and thrombosis increasing pulmonary vascular resistance in PAH are illustrated. The process of pulmonary vascular remodeling is complicated by all cellular heterogeneity types, such as endothelial, smooth muscle, fibroblast, T-lymphocytes, macrophages, and platelets. Hypoxia and pulmonary hypertension are the conclusion of the proliferation of the cellular processes involved

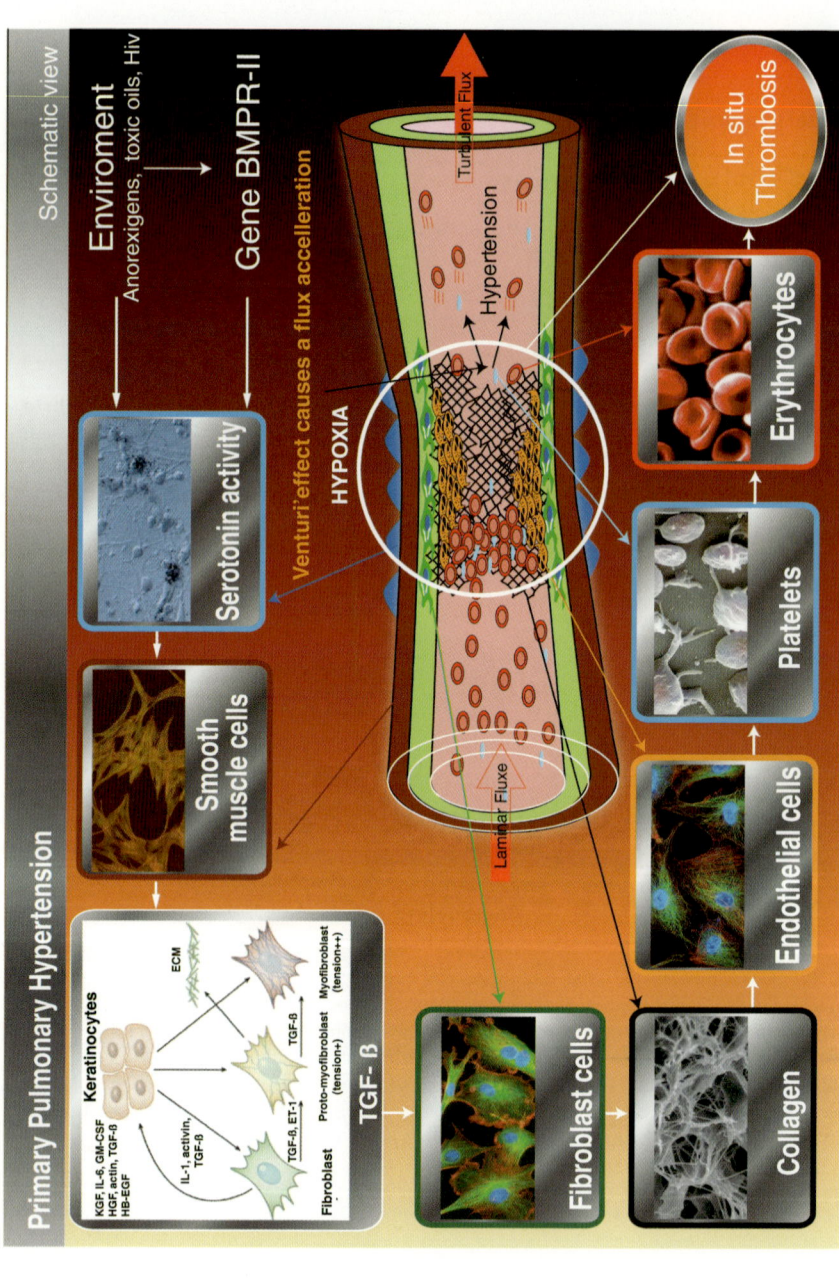

Fig. 5.2 A schematic view of PPH pathophysiology process. Vasoconstriction and in situ thrombosis and BMPR2 are shown

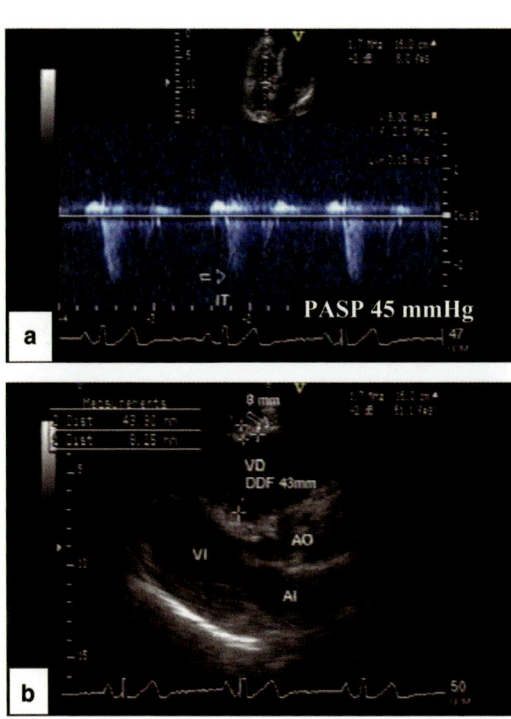

Fig. 7.3 Echocardiography in HP patients showing tricuspid insufficiency and increased pulmonary artery systolic pressure (**A**) and dilation and hypertrophy of right ventricle (**B**)

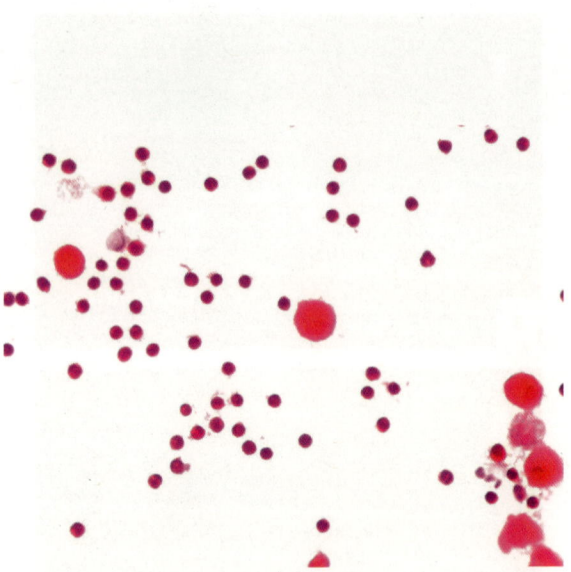

Fig. 7.4 BAL from a patient with subacute HP. Most of the lavaged cells are lymphocytes (hematoxylin & eosin [H&E], original magnification ×20)

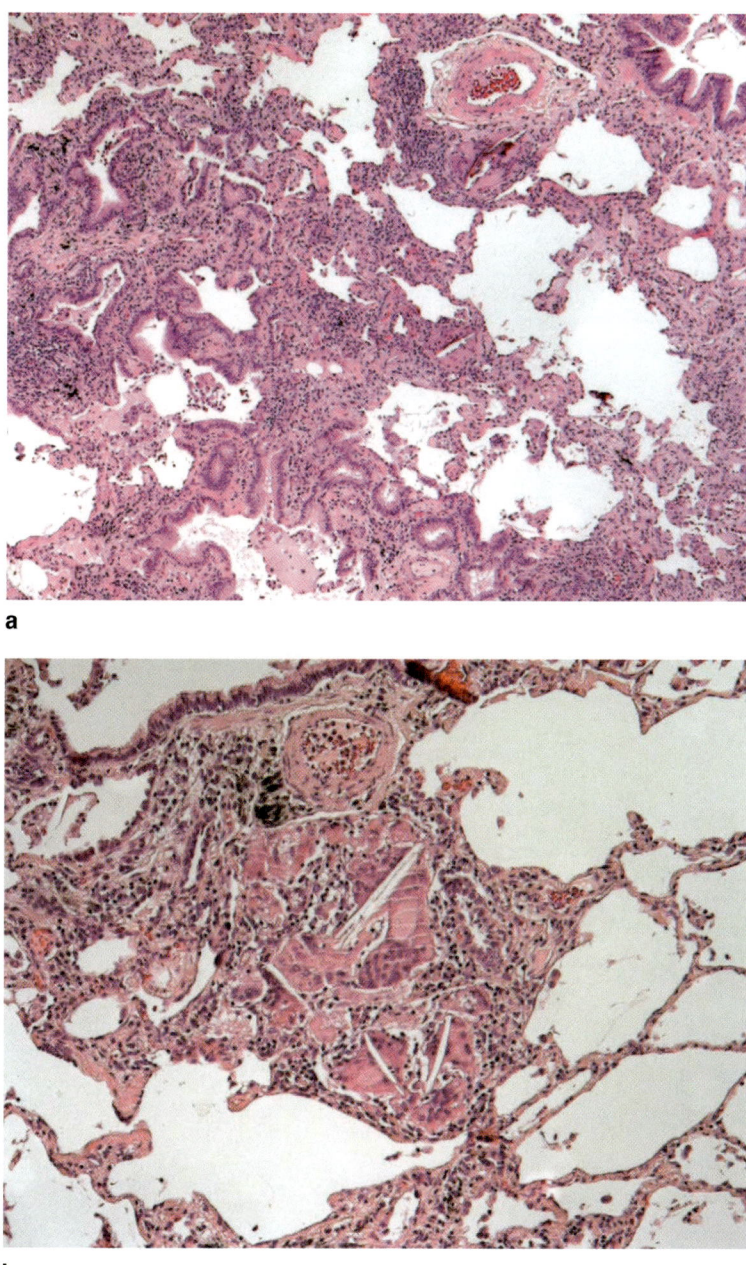

a

b

Fig. 7.5 **A** Photomicrograph of histopathologic specimen of a patient with subacute hypersensitivity pneumonitis showing, diffuse, chronic lymphocytic inflammatory infiltrate (H&E ×10X). **B** Another patient with subacute disease showing a granulomatous lesion with several multinucleated giant cells (H&E, ×40)

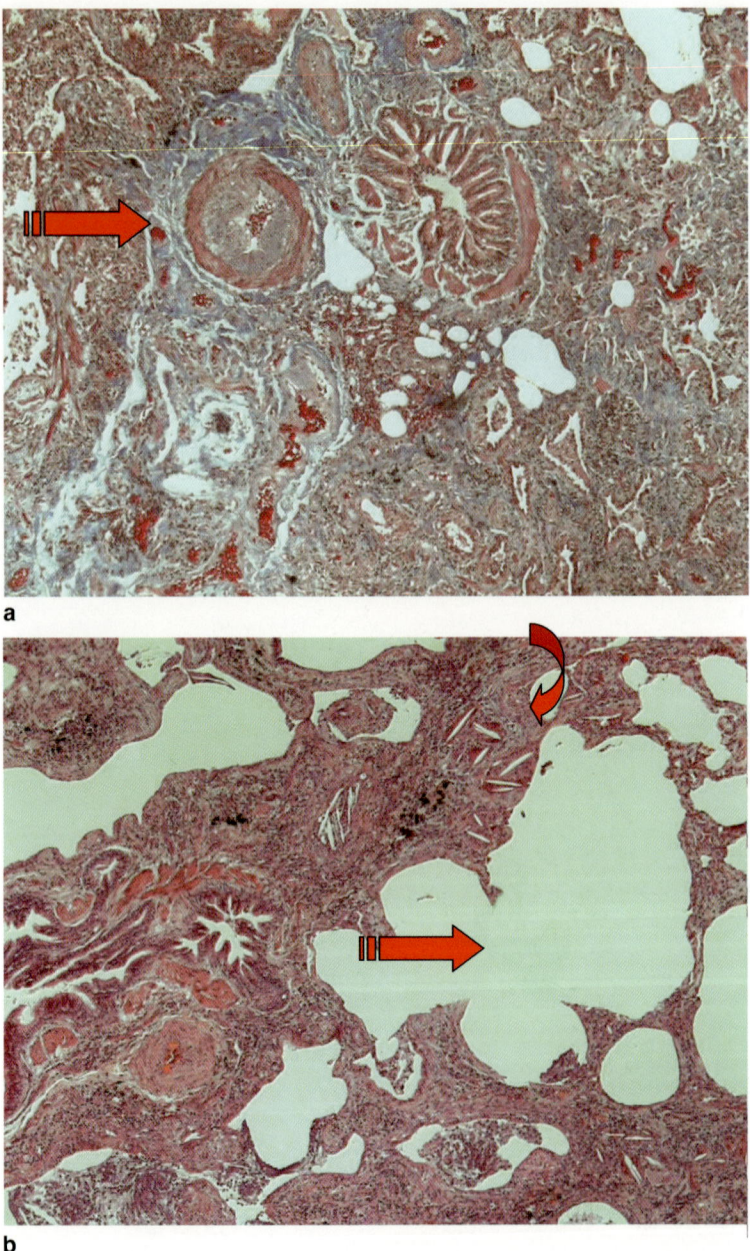

Fig. 7.6 Photomicrographs of histopathologic samples from two patients with (**A**) chronic HP showing collagen deposit (Masson's thrichrome, ×10) and (**B**) honeycomb changes (H&E, ×10). It can be noticed the vascular remodeling (arrows). In **B**, There is moderate inflammatory infiltrate and a small granuloma (curved arrow)

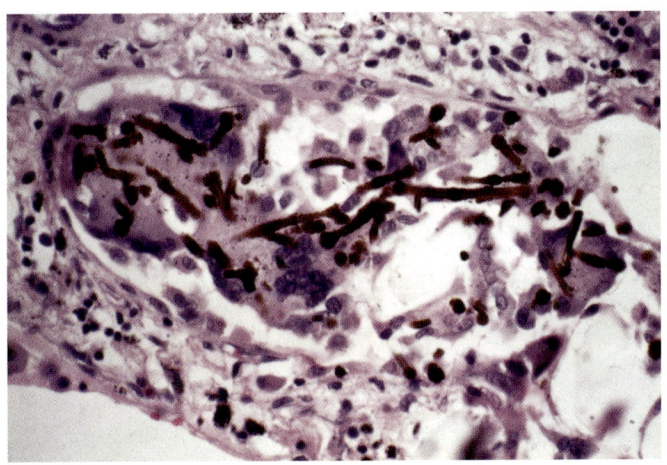

Fig. 10.1 Asbestosis. Photomicrograph demonstrates asbestos bodies ("ferruginous bodies") and adjacent macrophages in lung biopsy from a patient with asbestosis

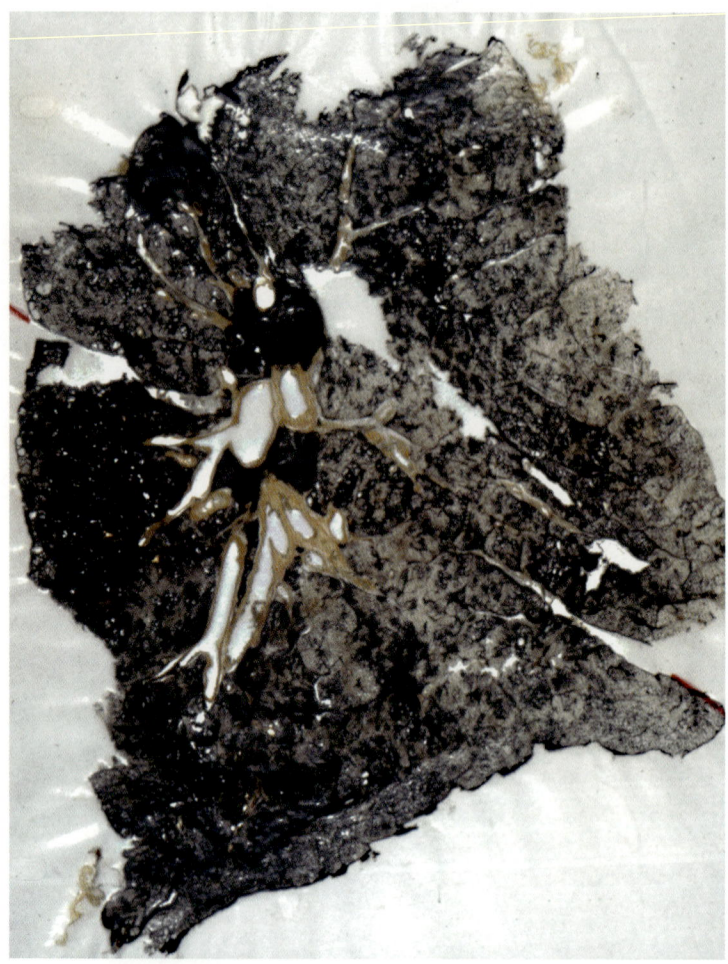

Fig. 10.4 Coal workers' pneumoconiosis. This Goff section through the entire lung of a deceased coalminer demonstrates the advanced stages of coal workers' pneumoconiosis. Note the extensive pigmentation, presence of coal macules, coalescence of these macules into conglomerate masses, and PMF in the upper lobe. Adjacent to the macules are areas of emphysema and bronchiectasis

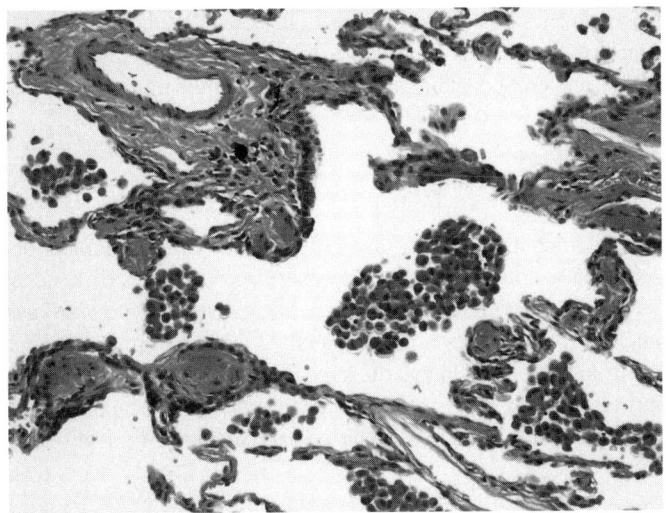

Fig. 4.4 RB-ILD: There is focal accumulation of pigmented alveolar macrophages in the peribronchiolar region and mild fibrosis of the bronchiolar wall (*See Color Plates*)

Histologic Features

The DIP pattern is characterized by diffuse involvement of the lung by numerous macrophage accumulations within most of the distal air spaces (Fig. 4.5). The alveolar septa are thickened by a sparse inflammatory infiltrate that often includes plasma cells and occasional eosinophils, and they are lined by plump cuboidal pneumocytes. The main

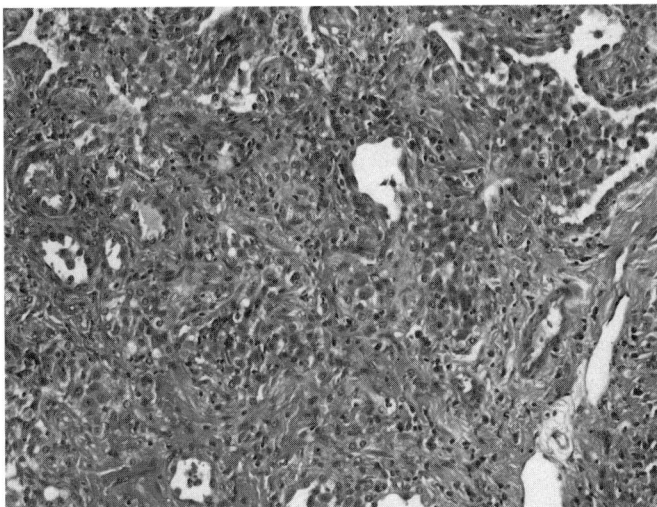

Fig. 4.5 In DIP, there is diffuse involvement of the lung by the accumulation of numerous alveolar macrophages within the alveolar sacs and mild fibrosis of the alveolar wall (*See Color Plates*)

feature that distinguishes DIP from RB is that DIP affects the lung in a uniform diffuse manner and lacks the bronchiolocentric distribution seen in RB. The intraluminal macrophages in DIP frequently contain dusty brown pigment identical to that seen in RB.

Histologic Differential Diagnosis

The histologic differential diagnosis of the DIP pattern includes a number of interstitial lung diseases because intra-alveolar macrophage accumulation or focal nonspecific "DIP-like" reaction is an expected consequence of cigarette smoking, and many patients with other interstitial lung diseases are frequently current or former smokers. The DIP pattern differs from that of UIP in that the interstitial changes are more diffusely distributed; the fibrotic reaction has a more uniform temporal appearance without dense widespread fibrosis, fibroblastic foci, architectural remodeling or honeycomb change.

DAD/AIP

AIP is an interstitial pneumonia characterized by widespread acute lung injury and a rapidly progressive clinical course [1,8]. DAD is the histologic manifestation. DAD usually is associated with known causes, such as infection, sepsis, collagen vascular disease, uremia, or drug toxicity. When the etiology is undetermined, AIP is the appropriate clinicopathologic term [1,27].

Pathologic Features

The lung pathology of AIP is identical to that of the acute and/or organizing phases of DAD [27–29]. There is typically diffuse histologic involvement of the lung, but the severity may vary in different areas. Edema, hyaline membranes and interstitial acute inflammation characterize the acute phase (Fig. 4.6). Loose organizing fibrosis mostly within alveolar septa and type II pneumocyte hyperplasia characterize the organizing phase [30]. Small to medium-sized pulmonary arterioles commonly show organized thrombi [27–29]. The lung may return to normal in DAD if the patient survives, but progression to endstage fibrosis may also occur.

Histologic Differential Diagnosis

The major histologic differential diagnostic considerations include other patterns of diffuse parenchymal lung disorders such as organizing pneumonia, acute eosinophilic pneumonia and UIP as well as potential etiologic considerations such as infection. When hyaline membranes are prominent, the DAD pattern is usually readily recognizable. However, because patients with AIP often undergo surgical lung biopsy during

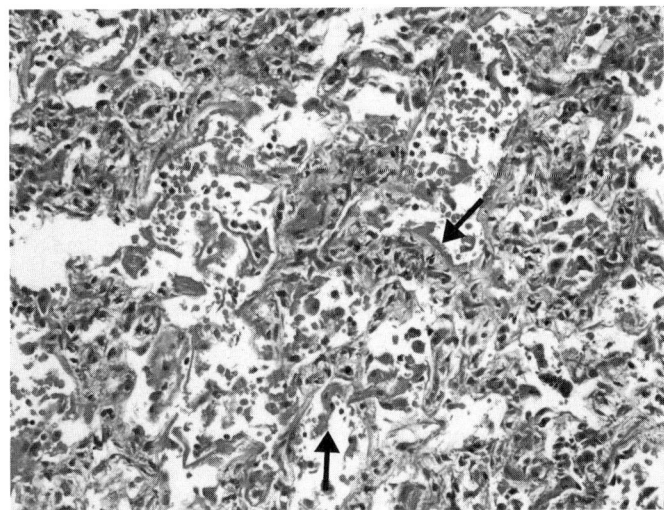

Fig. 4.6 In DAD, the alveolar walls are distended by edema, there is hyperplasia of type II pneumocytes and hyaline membranes. Hyaline membranes are pink fibrinous material that lines the alveolar wall (arrow) (*See Color Plates*)

the organizing phase, hyaline membranes may be difficult to identify. The findings of granulomas, viral inclusions, foci of necrosis or neutrophilic abscesses suggest infection. Special stains for microorganisms should routinely be performed to investigate infection. The diagnosis of AIP requires considerable clinical information. Much of the clinical evaluation to exclude specific causes of the DAD is likely to be completed after the lung biopsy has been finalized. In fact, studies on AIP have been based on cases that have been excluded on the basis of information that was probably not available at the time the biopsy diagnosis [31]. Therefore, the best diagnosis many pathologists may be able to make in cases of AIP is "DAD, etiology undetermined." The final diagnosis of AIP cannot be made unless a detailed history is provided. Even after making a careful diagnosis of AIP, an underlying condition such as a collagen vascular disease may declare itself after the initial pulmonary presentation and the original diagnosis of AIP revised.

LIP

LIP is a rare and controversial form of IIP. The entity is controversial because many patients included in Liebow's original description as having LIP were subsequently reclassified into distinct lymphoproliferative disorders like low-grade extranodal marginal zone lymphomas. In many cases, pulmonary infiltrate with pattern of LIP are in fact pulmonary manifestation of chronic systemic disease such as autoimmune diseases or human immunodeficiency virus infection [32]. However, LIP has been maintained in the American Thoracic Society/European Respiratory Society classification partly because of idiopathic cases (1). The histological diagnosis of LIP should prompt a clinical search for possible causes of the disease.

Pathologic Features

LIP is characterized histologically by the presence of dense and diffuse lympho-plasmacytic infiltrate within the alveolar septa. Germinal centers and a few nonca-seating granulomas may be present. Cases of LIP with a predominant nodular distribution have been described [32]; however, these should be evaluated for the presence of a low-grade lymphoma.

Histologic Differential Diagnosis

The histological pattern of LIP is observed most often as a pulmonary manifesta-tion of systemic collagen vascular disease, HIV infection, or after bone marrow transplantation. It is very difficult to distinguish histologically LIP from cellular NSIP; in general, the presence of an intense lymphoplasmacytic infiltrate in the former is the only differential criterion. The presence of small granulomata raises the suspicion for hypersensitivity pneumonitis or pulmonary manifestation of drug toxicity. Molecular analysis of immunoglobulin gene rearrangement is a useful tool in the differentiation of idiopathic LIP from pulmonary involvement by a low-grade lymphoma.

Pulmonary Manifestations of Collagen Vascular Diseases

Pulmonary manifestation of collagen vascular diseases are common and may be the major cause of morbidity and mortality in these diseases. There are no specific histologic patterns in the lung for collagen vascular diseases, which makes it almost impossible for the pathologist to make a specific diagnosis. The presence of lym-phoid follicles within the pulmonary parenchyma, although not a specific finding, is commonly seen in cases of collagen vascular disease (Fig. 4.7). In most cases, the histologic patterns are similar to those found in idiopathic interstitial lung dis-ease, such as UIP, NSIP, COP, LIP, and DAD [8]. In addition, pulmonary hemor-rhagic syndromes, and vasculitis can also be present in collagen vascular diseases. Therefore, clinical, radiographic, and pathological correlations are essential for the accurate diagnosis of the pulmonary alterations.

Among the idiopathic ILD patterns that can be seen in collagen vascular disease, NSIP and organizing pneumonia are the most common, especially in patients with scleroderma, rheumatoid arthritis, and polymyositis/dermatomyositis. Fortunately, these two manifestations, like their idiopathic counterpart, have a tendency to respond well to steroids and are associated with better survival than patients that present with

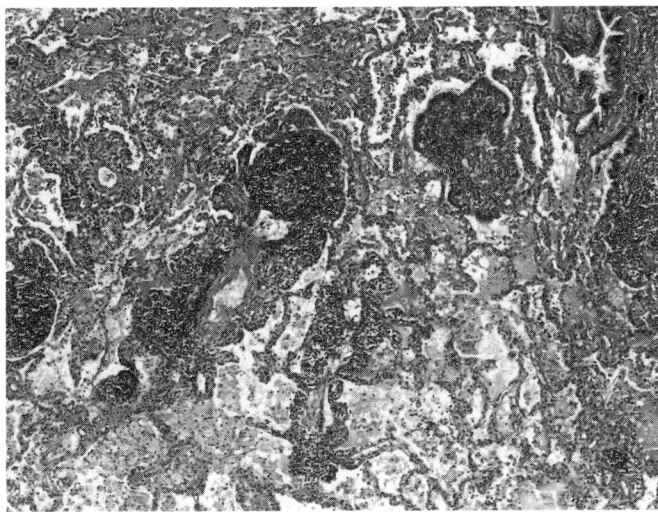

Fig. 4.7 Collagenous vascular disease. The presence of peribronchiolar and interstitial lymphoid follicles, although not specific, is commonly seen in cases of collagenous vascular disease (*See Color Plates*)

a pattern of UIP, which can also be seen in the same disease group. In contrast, LIP is a pattern most commonly found in patients with Sjorgren's syndrome.

Pulmonary manifestation of drug toxicity is also an important factor in the histological evaluation of lung biopsies from patients with collagen vascular disease. Many of these patients receive immunosuppressive drugs which will prone them to bacterial, fungal and mycobacterial infections. Although most of these infections can be diagnosed without a lung biopsy, granulomatous diseases with an atypical clinicoradiographical presentation may require a biopsy for diagnosis. Viral infections and fungal infections such as *Pneumocystis carinii* can present as acute respiratory distress syndrome, and a biopsy will show a pattern of DAD. Methotrexate, penicillamine, and gold are the most common drugs used in the treatment of collagen vascular disease that can cause toxicity in the lung. The pulmonary manifestation of these drug reactions are multiple and range from eosinophilic pneumonia to interstitial fibrosis mimicking UIP. Therefore, a strong suspicion for drug toxicity in the setting of collagen vascular disease must be given to the pathologist for correct evaluation of the biopsy material. ILD is relatively uncommon in patients with systemic lupus erythematous compared with other collagen vascular diseases, but all the histological patterns of interstitial lung disease have been described to occur in systemic lupus erythematous.

Rheumatoid nodules frequently are found in patients with rheumatoid arthritis. They consist of granulomas with a central area of necrosis surrounded by palisading histiocytes. Vasculitis can be seen in adjacent tissue. The combination of granulomatous inflammation and vasculitis brings infectious granulomas as well as Wegener's granulomatosis (WG) and bronchocentric granulomas into the histological differential diagnosis.

WG

WG is an idiopathic vasculitis syndrome that affects the upper and lower respiratory tract and the kidney, although it can involve any part of the body. Like any idiopathic disease, the histologic diagnosis of WG requires clinicoradiographical correlation. The use of the serum antineutrophil cytoplasmic antibody (ANCA) test [33,34] has revolutionized the diagnoses of vasculitis. Two patterns of staining can occur: the cytoplasmic (C-ANCA) and perinuclear (P-ANCA) [35]. The C-ANCA pattern is most common in WG. The P-ANCA pattern can be seen in WG, but it is more characteristic of other idiopathic vasculitis syndromes such as Churg-Strauss syndrome and microscopic polyangiitis. Therefore, a positive C-ANCA test associated with the characteristic clinical picture and histologic findings in a lung biopsy is diagnostic of WG. The ANCA test is also helpful in the differential diagnosis of WG when the histological features are not typical such as in cases of lung biopsies taken early in the course of the disease or after some course of therapy.

Histologic Features

The major histologic features of WG consist of a triad of necrosis, vasculitis, and inflammation [36]. Most often, the inflammatory infiltrate forms nodules of consolidation consisting of a mixture of neutrophils, lymphocytes, plasma cells, macrophages, giant cells, and eosinophils often with the formation of ill-defined granulomas. In WG, the inflammatory infiltrate extends beyond the area of granuloma with almost no normal intervening lung parenchyma. Parenchymal necrosis is manifested as neutrophilic microabscesses or large zones of geographic necrosis. Multinucleated giant cells scattered randomly or in loose clusters are typical. The vasculitis of WG may affect arteries, veins, or capillaries (neutrophilic capillaritis). The inflammation in the blood vessels is often focal and eccentrically involves the vessel wall. Destruction of the vascular elastic laminae frequently is found.

Differential Diagnosis

The differential diagnosis of WG in lung biopsies includes granulomatous infection [37], rheumatoid nodules [38], bronchocentric granulomatosis [38–40], and diffuse pulmonary hemorrhagic syndromes [41,42], such as seen in collagen vascular diseases.

One of the most important considerations in the diagnosis of WG is the exclusion of infection. Both tuberculosis and fungal infection can cause necrotizing granulomatous inflammation with secondary vasculitis resembling that seen in WG. Therefore, special stains for acid fast bacilli and fungi must be performed in biopsies with granulomatous inflammation where the diagnosis of WG is being considered.

Because WG can have a bronchocentric pattern of lung involvement, it must be considered in the differential diagnosis of bronchocentric granulomatosis (BCG). BCG is more of a histological pattern than a separate entity, because the histological changes found in BCG can be present in allergic bronchopulmonary fungal disease, other bacterial and parasitic infections, rheumatoid arthritis, and WG [37,38]. BCG is characterized by granulomatous inflammation involving the walls of bronchi or bronchioles. Contrary to WG, BCG is not associated with a positive ANCA test and it does not have involvement of the upper respiratory tract and the kidney. For the diagnosis of idiopathic BCG, the clinical features of allergic bronchopulmonary aspergillosis, rheumatoid arthritis and WG should be excluded and a careful search for microorganisms must be performed.

References

1. Travis WD, King TE, Bateman ED, Lynch DA, Capron LF, Colby TV. ATS/ERS International Multidisciplinary Consensus Classification of Idiopathic Interstitial Pneumonia. Am J Respir Crit Care Med 2002;165:277–304.
2. Lynch JP 3rd, Wurfel M, Flaherty K, White E, Martinez F, Travis W, Raghu G. Usual interstitial pneumonia. Semin Respir Crit Care Med 2001;4:357–386.
3. Hunninghake GW, Lynch DA, Galvin JR, Gross BH, Muller N, Schwartz DA, King TE Jr, Lynch JP 3rd, Hegele R, Waldron J, Colby TV, Hogg JC. Radiologic findings are strongly associated with a pathologic diagnosis of usual interstitial pneumonia. Chest 2003;124:1215–1223.
4. Katzenstein AL, Askin FB. Surgical Pathology of non-neoplastic lung disease. Philadelphia: WB Saunders, 1997.
5. Crystal RG, Fulmer JD, Roberts WC, Moss ML, Line BR, Reynolds HY. Idiopathic pulmonary fibrosis. Clinical histologic, radiographic, physiologic, scintigraphic, cytologic, and biochemical aspects. Ann Intern Med 1976;85:769–788.
6. Bjoraker JA, Ryu JH, Edwin MK, Myers JL, Tazelaar HD, Schroeder DR, Offord KP. Prognostic significance of histopathologic subsets in idiopathic pulmonary fibrosis. Am J Respir Crit Care Med 1998;157:199–203.
7. Müller NL, Colby TV. Idiopathic interstitial pneumonias: high-resolution CT and histologic findings. Radiographics 1997;17:1016–1022.
8. Travis WD, Colby TV, Koss MN, Müller NL, Rosado-de-Christenson ML, King TE, Jr. Nonneoplastic disorders of the lower respiratory tract. Washington, DC: American Registry of Pathology, 2002.
9. King TE Jr, Costabel U, Cordier JF, Dopico GA, du Bois RM, Lynch D, Lynch III JP, Myers J, Panos R, Raghu G, Schwartz D, Smith CM. Idiopathic pulmonary fibrosis: diagnosis and treatment. Am J Respir Crit Care Med. 2000;161:646–664.
10. Katzenstein AL, Meyers JL. Idiopathic pulmonary fibrosis: clinical relevance of pathologic classification. Am J Respir Crit Care Med 1998;18:1301–1315.
11. Leslie KO. Historical perspective: a pathologic approach to the classification of idiopathic interstitial pneumonias. Chest 2006;128:513–519.
12. Kim DS, Park JH, Park BK, Lee JS, Nicholson AG, Colby T. Acute exacerbation of idiopathic pulmonary fibrosis: frequency and clinical features. Eur Respir J 2006; 27:143–150.
13. Flaherty KR, Travis WD, Colby TV, Toews GB, Kazerooni EA, Gross BH, Jain A, Strawderman RL, Flint A, Lynch JP, Martinez FJ. Histopathologic Variability in Usual and Nonspecific Interstitial Pneumonias. Am J Respir Crit Care Med 2001;164:1722–1727.

14. Katzenstein AL, Zisman DA, Litzky LA, Nguyen BT, Kotloff RM. Usual interstitial pneumonia: histologic study of biopsy and explant specimens. Am J Surg Pathol 2002; 26: 1567–1577.
15. Katzenstein AL, Fiorelli RF. Nonspecific interstitial pneumonia/fibrosis. Histologic features and clinical significance. Am J Surg Pathol 1994; 18:136–147.
16. Daniil ZD, Gilchrist FC, Nicholson AG, Hansell DM, Harris J, Colby TV, du Bois RM. A histologic pattern of nonspecific interstitial pneumonia is associated with a better prognosis than usual interstitial pneumonia in patients with cryptogenic fibrosing alveolitis. Am J Respir Crit Care Med 1999;160:899–905.
17. Fujita J, Yamadori I, Suemitsu I, Suemitsu I, Yoshinouchi T, Ohtsuki Y, Yamaji Y, Kamei T, Kobayashi M, Nakamura Y, Takahara J. Clinical features of non-specific interstitial pneumonia. Respir Med 1999; 93:113–118.
18. Martinez FJ. Idiopathic Interstitial pneumonias. Usual interstitial pneumonia versus nonspecific interstitial pneumonia. Proc Am Thorac Soc 2006;3:81–95.
19. Travis WD, Matsui K, Moss JE, Ferrans VJ. Idiopathic nonspecific interstitial pneumonia: prognostic significance of cellular and fibrosing patterns. Survival comparison with usual interstitial pneumonia and desquamative interstitial pneumonia. Am J Surg Pathol 2000;24: 19–33.
20. Epler GR, Colby TV, McLoud TC, Carrington CB, Gaensler EA. Bronchiolitis obliterans organizing pneumonia. N Engl J Med 1985; 312:152–158.
21. Oikonomou A, Hansell DM. Organizing pneumonia: the many morphological faces. Eur Radiol 2002;12:1486–1496.
22. Myers JL, Veal CF, Jr., Shin MS, Katzenstein AL. Respiratory bronchiolitis causing interstitial lung disease. A clinicopathologic study of six cases. Am Rev Respir Dis 1987;135: 880–884.
23. Heyneman LE, Ward S, Lynch DA, Remy-Jardin M, Johkoh T, Muller NL. Respiratory bronchiolitis, respiratory bronchiolitis-associated interstitial lung disease, and desquamative interstitial pneumonia: different entities or part of the spectrum of the same disease process? AJR Am J Roentgenol 1999;173:1617–1622.
24. Yousem SA, Colby TV, Gaensler EA. Respiratory bronchiolitis-associated interstitial lung disease and its relationship to desquamative interstitial pneumonia. Mayo Clin Proc 1989;64: 1373–1380.
25. Fraig M, Shreesha U, Savici D, Katzenstein AL. Respiratory bronchiolitis: a clinicopathologic study in current smokers, ex-smokers, and never-smokers. Am J Surg Pathol 2002; 26:647–653.
26. Craig PJ, Wells AU, Doffman S, Rassl D, Colby TV, Hansell DM, du Bois RM, Nicholson AG. Desquamative interstitial pneumonia, respiratory bronchiolitis and their relationship to smoking. Histopathology 2004;45:275–282.
27. Katzenstein AL, Myers JL, Mazur MT. Acute interstitial pneumonia. A clinicopathologic, ultrastructural, and cell kinetic study. Am J Surg Pathol 1986;10:256–267.
28. Tomashefski JFJ. Pulmonary pathology of the adult respiratory distress syndrome. Clin Chest Med 1990;11:593–619.
29. Rice AJ, Wells AU, Bouros D, du Bois RM, Hansell DM, Polychronopoulos V, Vassilakis D, Kerr JR, Evans TW, Nicholson AG. Terminal diffuse alveolar damage in relation to interstitial pneumonias. An autopsy study. Am J Clin Pathol 2003;119:709–714.
30. Olson J, Colby TV, Elliott CG. Hamman-Rich syndrome revisited. Mayo Clin.Proc 1990; 65:1538–1548.
31. Nicholls JM, Poon LL, Lee KC, Ng WF, Lai ST, Leung CY, Chu CM, Hui PK, Mak KL, Lim W, Yan KW, Chan KH, Tsang NC, Guan Y, Yuen KY, Peiris JS. Lung pathology of fatal severe acute respiratory syndrome. Lancet 2003;361:1773–1778.
32. Cha SI, Fessler MB, Cool CD, Schwarz MI, Brown KK. Lymphoid interstitial pneumonia: clinical features, associations, and prognosis. Eur Respir J 2006;28:364–369.
33. Harper L, Savage CO. Pathogenesis of ANCA-associated systemic vasculitis. J Pathol 2000; 190:349–359.

34. Schultz DR, Diego JM. Antineutrophil cytoplasmic antibodies (ANCA) and systemic vasculitis: update of assays, immunopathogenesis, controversies, and report of a novel de novo ANCA-associated vasculitis after kidney transplantation. Semin Arthritis Rheum 2000;29: 267–285.
35. Davenport A, Lock RJ, Wallington TB. Clinical relevance of testing for antineutrophil cytoplasm antibodies (ANCA) with a standard indirect immunofluorescence ANCA test in patients with upper or lower respiratory tract symptoms. Thorax 1994;49:213–217.
36. Travis WD, Colby TV, Koss MN, Rosado-de-Christenson M, Müller NL, King TE, Jr. Pulmonary Vasculitis. In: King DW, editor. Nonneoplastic disorders of the lower respiratory tract. Washington, DC: American Registry of Pathology, 2002. p. 233–264.
37. Ulbright TM, Katzenstein AL. Solitary necrotizing granulomas of the lung: differentiating features and etiology. Am J Surg Pathol 1980;4:13–28.
38. Churg A. Pulmonary angiitis and granulomatosis revisited. Hum Pathol 1983;14:868–883.
39. Koss MN, Robinson RG, Hochholzer L. Bronchocentric granulomatosis. Hum Pathol 1981; 12:632–638.
40. Yousem SA. Bronchocentric injury in Wegener's granulomatosis: a report of five cases. Hum Pathol 1991;22:535–540.
41. Mark EJ, Ramirez JF. Pulmonary capillaritis and hemorrhage in patients with systemic vasculitis. Arch Patho Lab Med 1985;109:413–418.
42. Travis WD, Colby TV, Lombard CM, Carpenter HA. A clinicopathologic study of 34 cases of diffuse pulmonary hemorrhage with lung biopsy confirmation. Am J Surg Pathol 1990;14:1112–2115.

Chapter 5
Primary Pulmonary Hypertension

Roberto G. Carbone and Giovanni Bottino

Introduction

The most common causes of pulmonary hypertension (PH) are related to the impairment of cardiac and pulmonary function. Impaired pulmonary venous drainage caused by left heart failure, left ventricular diastolic dysfunction, and mitral valve disease are among the most frequently encountered causes; however, remarkably, severe pulmonary hypertension resulting from heart failure is not a common finding. Chronic hypoxemia associated with structural and functional disorders of the lung is also a major cause of pulmonary hypertension. Crucially, it is reversible with long-term oxygen therapy. An update of this subject at the World Symposium on Pulmonary Arterial Hypertension (Venice 2003) classified PH in five classes, as shown in Table 5.1. [1] Genetic factors, pulmonary vascular physiology, pathophysiology, PH, as well as interstitial lung diseases (ILD), diagnosis, and management of the secondary forms of pulmonary hypertension are reviewed in Chapter 2. In this chapter, a clinical view of epidemiology, pathophysiology, diagnosis, natural history, and the management of idiopathic pulmonary artery hypertension (IPAH), formerly known as primary pulmonary hypertension (PPH), will be reviewed. Although IPAH is a rare condition, because of its pathogenetic link with the use of anorexigen medications such as fenfluramine, phentermine, and dexfenfluramine, all physicians should be aware of this potentially fatal disease.

PPH

Background

PPH is a rare and usually rapidly progressive disorder characterized by an increase in pulmonary resistance which, if untreated leads to right ventricular failure and death within a few years. The diagnostic criteria developed by the National Institutes of Health Registry include a mean pulmonary artery (PAPm) pressure greater than 25 mmHg at rest, or 30 mmHg with exercise, determined by right

R.P. Baughman et al. (eds.), *Pulmonary Arterial Hypertension and Interstitial Lung Diseases,*
© Humana Press, a part of Springer Science + Business Media, LLC 2009

Table 5.1 Clinical Classification of Pulmonary Hypertension (Venice 2003)

Pulmonary arterial hypertension (PAH)
- Idiopathic (IPAH) or primary pulmonary hypertension (PPH)
- Familial (APAH)
- Associated with APAH
- Collagen vascular disease
- Congenital systemic-to-pulmonary shunts
- Portal hypertension
- HIV infection
- Drug and toxins
- Other (thyroid disorders, glycogen storage disease, Gaucher disease, hereditary hemorrhagic telangiectasia, hemoglobinopathies, myeloproliferative disorders, splenectomy)
- Associated with significant venous or capillary involvement
- Pulmonary veno-occlusive disease (PVOD)
- Pulmonary capillary hemangiomatosis (PCH)
- Persistent pulmonary hypertension of the newborn

Pulmonary hypertension with left heart disease
- Left-sided atrial or ventricular heart disease
- Left-sided valvular heart disease

Pulmonary hypertension associated with lung disease and/or hypoxemia
- Interstitial lung disease
- Chronic obstructive pulmonary disease (COPD)
- Sleep-disordered breathing
- Alveolar hypoventilation disorders
- Chronic exposure to high altitude
- Development abnormalities

Pulmonary hypertension caused by chronic thrombotic and/or embolic disease
- Thromboembolic obstruction of proximal arteries
- Thromboembolic obstruction of distal pulmonary arteries
- Non-trhombotic pulmonary embolism (tumor, parasites, foreign material)

Miscellaneous
- Sarcoidosis
- Lymphangiomatosis
- Hstiocytosis X
- Compression of pulmonary vessel (fibrosing mediastinitis, tumor, adenopathy)

heart catheterization [2], and no evidence of left-sided myocardial, valvular, or congenital heart disease (with the exception of high flow and low pressure shunts, as will be discussed), no clinically significant lung disease, pulmonary emboli, or active vasculitis. PPH is often not suspected and the diagnosis can be delayed for more than 2 years after the onset of symptoms [3]. The three classic pathologic signs are pulmonary arteriolar hypertrophy with obliterating arteriolar plexiform lesions and, much less commonly, pulmonary veno occlusive disease and pulmonary hemangiomatosis.

Shortly after the initial reports describing young women with "idiopathic" (primary) severe pulmonary hypertension and unusual arteriolar plexiform lesions, PH with plexiform lesions was attributed to the drug aminorex fumarate, an anorectic agent used in Europe in the 1960s. The same pathologic and clinical syndrome has been associated with the newer weight-reducing agents [4]. Since the early 1970s, autosomal-dominant familial forms of PPH have been described along with several other exogenous triggers active in susceptible individuals.

Epidemiology

PPH is a rare disease, with an estimated incidence of one to two cases per million in the general population. Approximately 400 new cases are diagnosed annually in the USA. PPH is most prevalent in patients who are in their twenties through their forties, and no racial differences in the rate of occurrence have been observed [3]. When diagnosed during childhood, it affects both sexes equally; however, after puberty, the condition is more common in women (ratio 1.7:1). In a number of cases, PPH may be associated with other disorders such as HIV (0.5% of infected patients) [5], liver cirrhosis (2–4%), and portal hypertension. In addition, 10–20% of patients with systemic scleroderma may develop PPH [6].

In 17 PAH referral centers of the French national prospective registry (ItinerAIR-HTAP) from October 2002 to October 2003, an investigation of 674 patients (mean ± SD age, 50 ±15 years; female 65.3%) indicated that 52.6% of those enrolled presented either primary (39.2%), familial (3.9%), or anorexigen-associated PH (9.5%). Systemic scleroderma or other autoimmune diseases, appetite suppressants, congenital heart disease, portal hypertension, and human deficiency virus infection accounted for 15.3%, 11.3%, 10.4%, and 6.2% of population, respectively. Most patients had severe disease at the time of diagnosis (New York Heart Association [NYHA] class IV, 12%; NYHA class III, 63%; NYHA class I–II, 25% respectively) [7].

A number of studies suggest that the postmortem diagnosis is greater than the clinical diagnosis and is in the region of 1/1,000. The sporadic form of PPH is two to five times more common in women than men. This female predominance is not observed in the childhood form of PPH. These observations, together with the frequent peripartum presentation and association with oral contraceptives, indicate that estrogens may play a role in the initiation or progression of the disease. The average adult age of onset is the early to mid-thirties. The classic paradigm is a young, obese woman with a past history of migraine headaches and/or Reynaud's phenomenon who presents with fatigue, dyspnoea, chest pain, and/or syncope.

We have idiopathic, familial, and then, we have pulmonary arterial hypertension related to a number of conditions. The most frequent are the connective tissue diseases and, of those, scleroderma spectrum of disease. PPH is also triggered by several common conditions, including HIV infection, portal hypertension and cirrhosis, exposure to cocaine, L-tryptophan, and anorectic agents was showed in Table 5.2. The widespread use of the anorectic dexfenfluramine was predicted to increase the incidence of PPH by 20- to 50-fold or 1 per 16,000 users [4].

Fortunately, with the withdrawal of the drug from the US market, the epidemic of PPH that was previously anticipated may not come true.

Table 5.2 Classification of PPH

Plexiform pulmonary arteriopathy
Familial or sporadic
Exogenous triggered: fenfluramine and related drugs, cocaine, oral contraceptives, L-tryptophan, toxic rapeseed oil
Other triggers: atrial septal defect (ASD), cirrhosis, HIV infection, scleroderma spectrum of disease
Pulmonary veno-occlusive disease
Pulmonary hemangiomatosis

Along with the pulmonary vascular effects of the fenfluramine derivatives, there has also been report of an association with tricuspid and mitral valve insufficiency, as seen in carcinoid heart disease and with ergot alkaloid [8]. It is now recommended that all individuals with a history of exposure to these drugs (especially those exposed for more than three months) undergo a thorough evaluation focusing on signs and symptoms of PH and valvular insufficiency. Those patients with abnormal findings should have an echocardiogram and be referred for further evaluation if abnormal.

Pathophysiology

Histopathologic and clinical studies suggest that PPH is a disease of the genetically predisposed individual in whom various triggers initiate the characteristic vascular lesions. Twenty percent of patients previously classified as having PPH are now thought to have a familiar form of the disease. There are indications that the PPH1 gene, a bone morphogenic protein receptor 2 gene (BMPR2), may be implicated in the pathogenesis of the disease (Fig. 5.1). The genetic background of this disease will be better elucidated in Chapter 2. Vasoconstriction followed by remodeling of the pulmonary vessels is a primary event in the pathogenesis of pulmonary artery hypertension (PAH) (Fig. 5.2). Additional pathogenetic mechanisms such as inflammation suggest that increased of LIGHT levels, i.e., mediated prothrombotic effects in endothelial cells, could contribute to disease progression in PAH [9].

Triggers include hypobaric hypoxia (high altitude), autoimmune disorders, drugs/toxins, increased pulmonary blood flow with or without increased pulmonary pressure and shear stress, lung injury, and increased sympathetic tone resulting in catecholamine-induced injury. Regardless of the trigger, endothelial damage, coagulation abnormalities, platelet aggregation, smooth muscle cell migration, and in situ thrombosis result and contribute to the pathophysiology of the disease.

Diagnosis

Consensus diagnostic criteria for PPH were developed based on the National Institutes of Health and Mayo Clinic series [2,10]. The diagnosis requires a resting or exercise mean pulmonary artery pressures of 25 and 30 mmHg, respectively, with no evidence of secondary causes.

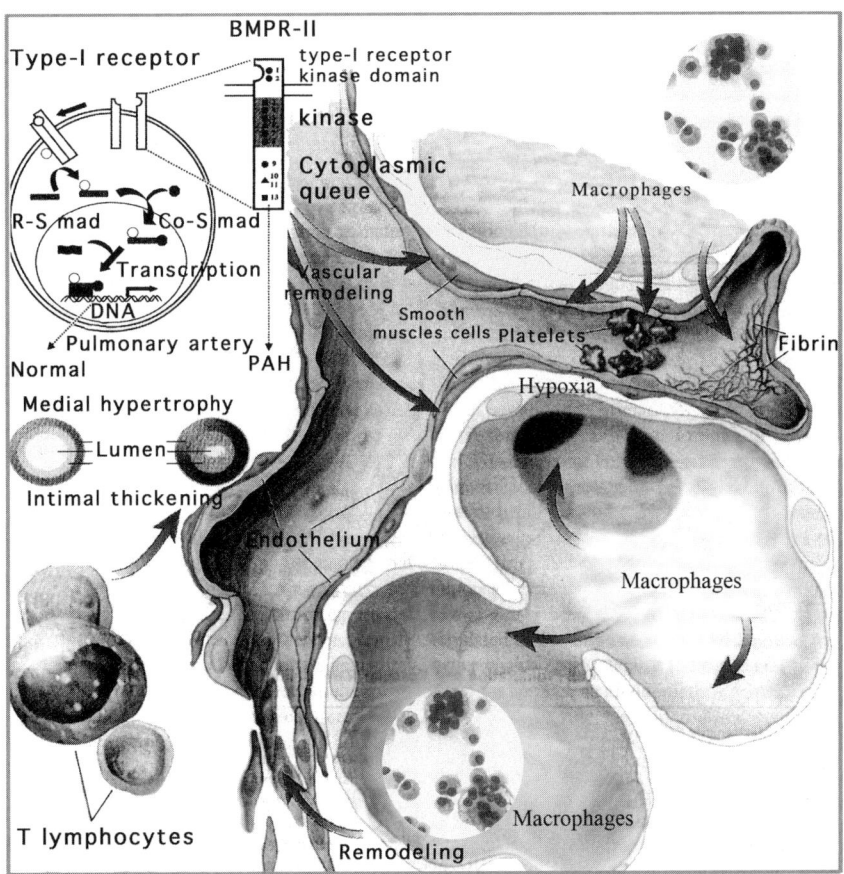

Fig. 5.1 Consequences of bone morphogenetic protein type-2 receptor (BMPR2) mutations implicated in PPH pathogenesis. A model pulmonary arteriolar system and alveolus with vasoconstriction, remodeling of the pulmonary vessel wall, and thrombosis increasing pulmonary vascular resistance in PAH are illustrated. The process of pulmonary vascular remodeling is complicated by all cellular heterogeneity types, such as endothelial, smooth muscle, fibroblast, T-lymphocytes, macrophages, and platelets. Hypoxia and pulmonary hypertension are the conclusion of the proliferation of the cellular processes involved (*See Color Plates*)

The symptoms associated with PPH do not differ from those of secondary PH (Table 5.3). The common striking finding is the symptoms of dyspnoea and fatigue disproportionate to the clinical appearance of the patient. HIV-positive patients with dyspnoea should be investigated for PAH, which is diagnosed in 85% of these patients. Recently, a screening algorithm based on a dyspnoea questionnaire, transthoracic Doppler echocardiography, and right heart catheterization was applied in routine clinical practice and showed good results identifying different degrees of PAH severity [11].

In PPH, most symptoms are attributable to reduced cardiac output. Lightheadedness, syncope, and presyncope with effort and Valsalva's manoeuvres are the result of systemic vasodilatation without accompanying increase in right heart

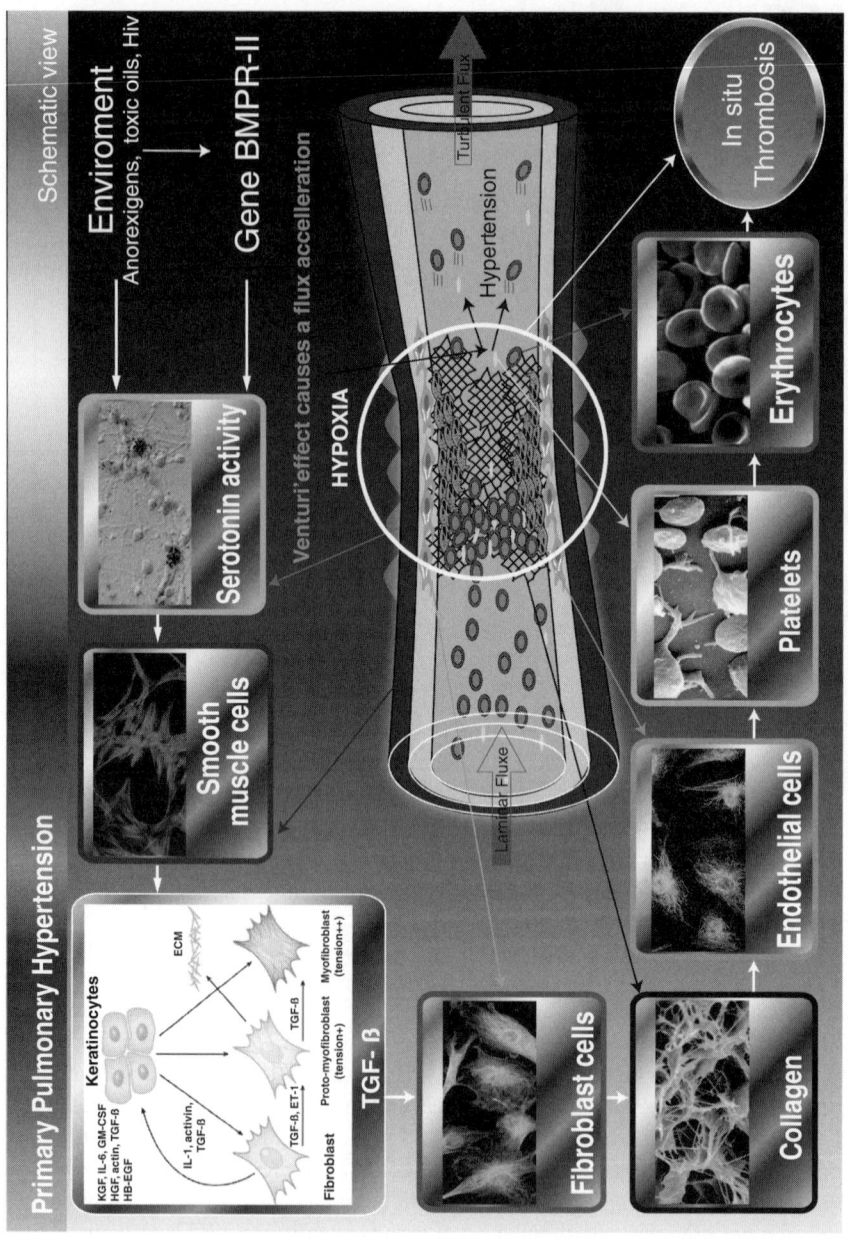

Fig. 5.2 A schematic view of PPH pathophysiology process. Vasoconstriction and in situ thrombosis and BMPR2 are shown (*See Color Plates*)

Table 5.3 Symptoms and Signs of PH

Common Symptoms
  Dyspnea, fatigue, angina, presyncope, syncope, weakness, palpitations, abdominal fullness, leg swelling, Raynaud's phenomenon

Common signs
  Normal to low blood pressure (occasionally hypertension)
  Lung findings dependent upon parenchymal involvement
  Jugular venous distention with prominent a and v waves
  Increased split of s2 with increased p2
  Systolic murmur at left 4th ICS increasing with inspiration (tricuspid insufficiency)
  Soft diastolic decrescendo murmur of pulmonic regurgitation in left 3rd ICS
  Pulmonic ejection click, systolic ejection murmur at left 2nd or 3rd ICS
  RV lift, RV s4, and or RV s3
  Hepatomegaly, pulsatile liver, ascites, peripheral edema, cyanosis, clubbing

output and inadequate LV filling pressures. Anginal chest pains may result from RV ischemia or pulmonary artery distension. Patients with PPH are noticeably sensitive to both the increase in rate and loss of atrial filling pressure in atrial fibrillation or flutter. In the later stages of PPH, palpitations may be caused by ventricular tachy arrhythmias. Death can be attributable to primary ventricular fibrillation (VF), VF secondary to hypotension, or terminal right heart failure and cardiogenic shock.

The typical patient has been told by at least one physician the symptoms are the result of anxiety. Patients typically delay seeking medical attention for 6 months, but the interval between symptom onset and diagnosis is generally delayed by 2 years. A history of Reynaud's phenomenon is frequent, but may not exceed that observed in the general population.

Although the diagnosis is difficult, once symptoms are present, the physical examination is invariably consistent with pulmonary hypertension (Table 5.3). Peripheral oedema is rare (10%) until late in the disease. Cyanosis, a late finding, results from low cardiac output and peripheral vasoconstriction, or arterial desaturation via a right to left shunt through an atrial septal defect or probe patent foramen oval, or with classic Eisenmenger syndrome, reversal of shunt, right-to-left shunt. Digital clubbing and hypoxemia suggest cyanotic congenital heart or pulmonary diseases.

Natural History of PPH

Overall 5-year survival of untreated PPH is approximately 20% [8], with a median survival of 2.8 years (NYHA class I–II, 6 years; Class III, 2.5 years; Class IV, 6 months) [2]. It is nearly universally fatal with only a few reports of disease regression. The median survival of patients with PPH associated with systemic scleroderma was reported to be only one year [12,13]. Various parameters have been used to define the severity of disease for prognosis and mortality, including NYHA functional class, exercise capacity, and haemodynamics. Cardiac output, the right atrial (RA) PAPm, and NYHA class correlate inversely with survival, whereas the cardiac index is directly correlated [14]. The strongest negative prognostic indicator is the presence and severity of pericardial effusion on echocardiogram, [15] which may be a function of the severity of the right heart failure.

Algorithm for Cardiopulmonary Testing

The diagnostic algorithm for patients with the clinical presentation consistent with PPH is outlined in Fig. 5.3. Early in the clinical course, patients with NYHA class II (symptoms with every day activity) will have evidence on electrocardiogram of right ventricular hypertrophy (RVH). The R wave in V1 is often prominent (R/S ≥ 1) and QRS axis rightward to 70–100 degrees. The lateral chest x-ray demonstrates filling of

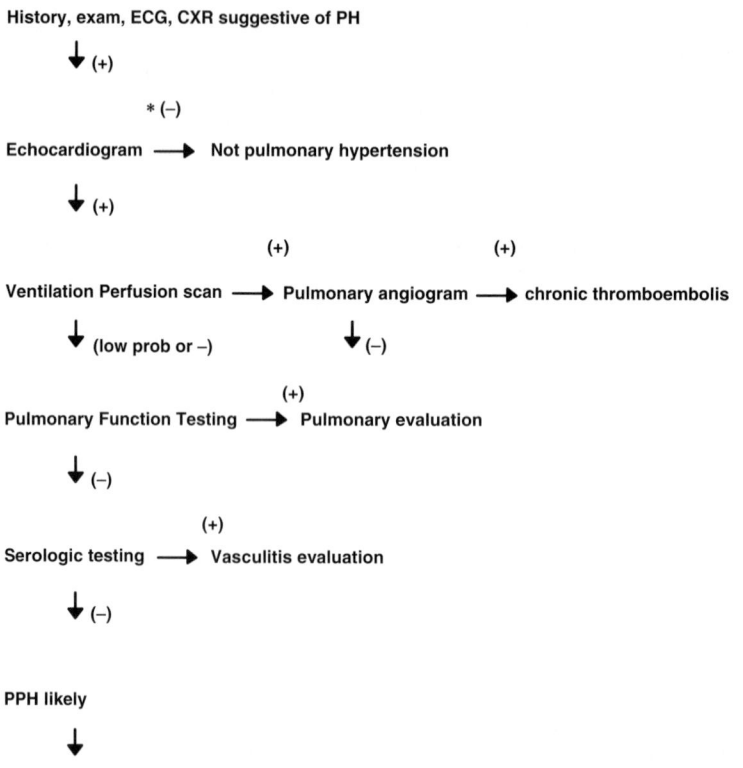

History, exam, ECG, CXR suggestive of PH

↓ (+)

* (−)

Echocardiogram ⟶ Not pulmonary hypertension

↓ (+)

(+)   (+)

Ventilation Perfusion scan ⟶ Pulmonary angiogram ⟶ chronic thromboembolis

↓ (low prob or −)   ↓ (−)

(+)

Pulmonary Function Testing ⟶ Pulmonary evaluation

↓ (−)

(+)

Serologic testing ⟶ Vasculitis evaluation

↓ (−)

PPH likely

↓

Right heart catheterization (to rule out right to left shunting and PVOD, to assess hemodynamics for prognosis, and perform vasodilator testing) and exercise testing for functional assessment.

* If intracardiac shunt or valvular disease suspected consider TEE and heart catheterization.

Fig. 5.3 Diagnostic algorithm for patients with PPH pulmonary hypertension suspected

the anterior mediastinal clear space, in the PA view the main and secondary pulmonary artery branches are enlarged, and the pulmonary vascularity is normal or reduced.

Pulmonary function testing (PFT) is usually normal, but in later stages (NYHA class ≥ III, symptoms with less than every day activity) can demonstrate a mild restrictive pattern and decrease in carbon monoxide diffusing capacity (DL_{CO}) as the result of low cardiac output. Particularly PFT with DL_{CO} may be useful in the presence of an isolated decrease of $DL_{CO} < 55\%$ of normal or an increase in the forced vital capacity (FVC)/DL_{CO} ratio (FVC/$DL_{CO} > 1.4$) [16]. However, moderate or severe abnormalities on PFT are unusual and should prompt consideration of other aetiologies for PH, particularly ILD.

Serologic studies are obtained to exclude rheumatologic diseases. The antinuclear antibody can be elevated in PPH, but rarely exceeds 1/320. An elevated sedimentation rate or ANA > 1/320 suggest systemic lupus, scleroderma, CREST, or mixed connective tissue disease. The only manifestation of lupus may be pulmonary hypertension. Patients with an established diagnosis of PPH should continually be suspect for occult scleroderma or lupus.

Anticardiolipin antibodies can be present in PPH. Increased plasma levels of a number of biochemical markers have been reported in patients with PAH, including uric acid, endothelin, and B-type natriuretic peptide. These markers showed correlations with prognostic factors for PAH, and some biochemicals have independent prognostic value [17–19]. Mutation in the BMPR2 gene has been identified in families with family PAH [20].

When pulmonary hypertension is suspected, an echo Doppler should be conducted to confirm an increase in the right ventricular systolic pressure (RVSP). Although the upper limit for RVSP on echo Doppler is 30–40 mmHg, even mildly symptomatic patients with PPH have an RVSP of 50–60 mmHg, the right ventricle is often dilated, and there is a degree of tricuspid insufficiency. The classic findings on echocardiography [21] include enlarged RA and RV, a normal-to-small LV, abnormal septal motion, and some increase in septal thickness. Mitral valve prolapse is common and explained by a change in the left ventricular size and geometry with RV dilation. If the RVSP is increased, contrast enhancement (injection of agitated saline) should be used to exclude an atrial septal defect and probe patent foramen oval. The latter should be suspected when cyanosis and or hypoxia are present. Transesophageal echocardiography may offer additional information regarding intracardiac shunts but is not essential.

Ventilation/perfusion (V/Q) scintigraphy is essential in the evaluation of PH. In PPH, the V/Q scan is normal or low probability with patchy defects. In contrast, chronic thromboembolic PH has at least one major ventilation perfusion mismatch [22]. Rare complications have occurred from macro aggregated albumin during V/Q scanning in persons with severe pulmonary hypertension and critically obstructed pulmonary vascular bed [23].

Pulmonary angiography is not necessary to confirm the diagnosis of PPH; however, it should be performed by experienced radiologists when thromboembolism is suspected. The pulmonary angiogram in PPH demonstrates symmetrically enlarged primary and secondary branches and pruning or loss of branching from tertiary vessels. Intraluminal filling defects and vascular webs are characteristic of chronic thromboembolic pulmonary hypertension. Magnetic resonance angiography and helical computer tomography are effective screening tools for excluding central thromboembolic PH, but do not exclude thromboembolic disease. Because in-situ thrombi occur in PPH, and chronic thromboemboli can result in severe PH, the differential diagnosis is not always possible. In this setting pulmonary angiography may be necessary but should be performed only by teams (radiology, thoracic surgery, and cardiology) with experience in pulmonary thromboendarterectomy.

A right heart catheterization is necessary in PPH to confirm the diagnosis, estimate prognosis, and perform a vasodilator trial to determine the therapeutic options. These studies should be performed by physicians experienced in the diagnosis and management of all forms of pulmonary hypertension. In moderate-to-severe PH, an increased pulmonary capillary wedge pressure suggests left heart failure (diastolic dysfunction) and mitral valve disease. If heart disease can be excluded, the PPH variant pulmonary veno-occlusive disease (PVOD) must be considered. When RV diastolic and RA pressures are >12–15 mmHg in PPH the pulmonary capillary wedge pressure is increased to 12–18 mmHg from compression of the LV. Intracardiac shunts are excluded by multiple site venous oxygen sampling and arterial blood gas analysis. Four deaths reported with right catheterization in the Mayo Clinic PPH series [10] emphasized the risk in these patients.

A lung biopsy is not essential for diagnosis of PPH and is rarely used in clinical practice. Exceptions include patients with a differential diagnosis of collagen vascular disease and PPH (lupus pulmonary vasculitis) and to distinguish PVOD for which therapy is considerably different.

Treatment

The American College of Chest Physicians (ACCP) Consensus statement [24] recommends that patients with PPH should be managed by teams of experienced specialists: "Because PPH is a rare disease whose complexity poses tremendous challenges to the treating physician, it is recommended that patients be referred to a center with experience in the management of this disease. The referring physician must, nevertheless, play a major role in the day to day care of these patients."

Once the diagnosis is established, counseling should focus on psychosocial adjustment to a changing life style and the stress of a life-threatening illness to the patient and significant others. The patient should refrain from activities that cause fatigue and exertion, with their activity guided by symptoms. Physical and mental stress increase sympathoadrenal discharge that increases pulmonary artery pressure and stresses the failing right ventricle. Airplane travel in pressurized cabins is safe if the patient's resting oxygen saturation is normal. The hemodynamic and hormonal changes of pregnancy are deleterious and necessitate measures to avoid conception. Unfortunately, oral contraceptives and estrogen supplements should be avoided because estrogens may promote or trigger the disease and increase the risk of in situ pulmonary artery thrombosis.

Recently the Health and Science Policy Committee of the ACCP authorized an update of the medical treatment guidelines published in 2004 [25] to describe and clarify new treatments which promise to open new therapeutic avenues [26]. When choosing a therapeutic option physicians should consider cardiopulmonary haemo dynamics, the results of a 6-minute walk test (6MWT), sign and symptoms of right-heart failure, side effect, drug–drug interaction, and the costs for every selected patient [26].

Basic Therapy

Medical therapy is both nonspecific (treating right heart failure) and specific (aimed at reducing pulmonary artery pressure). The nonspecific arm of treatment includes improving RV function, which reduces the dyspnoea, fatigue, and peripheral oedema. Digitalis is recommended to increase RV contractility. Because more than 75% of PPH patients are overweight or obese and cannot exercise, caloric restriction for weight reduction is critical. The diet should be low in saturated fat and salt ($\leq 2\,g$ of sodium), and caloric adjusted to reduce to ideal body weight. Obesity worsens the clinical course of PPH placing an incremental burden on the failing RV. Although excess physical activity is harmful, regular low-level exercise to maintain upper and lower body tone and strength is necessary.

Diuretics are effective for treating oedema, but caution with their use is necessary. Minimally decreased intravascular volume can result in profound hypotension and sudden death from underfilling of the left ventricle. Spironolactone is particularly effective for hepatic congestion and ascites, and can be used effectively in conjunction with loop diuretics.

Anticoagulation with warfarin is recommended (INR of 2–3) as pathologic studies indicate a major contribution of in situ thrombosis to the progression of PPH [27,28]. Markers of in vivo clotting and thrombolysis provide further evidence for reoccurring thrombosis in PPH [29]. Nonrandomized observational data suggest a salutary effect of anti-coagulants on prognosis [10,30]. The level of evidence for these medications to be used in PPH is level C, there are no randomized trials proving the efficacy of treatment. However, there is a strong recommendation for the use of diuretics, especially for patients with fluid overload. In this group, anticoagulants and digitalis are recommended and so is oxygen therapy in combination. The benefit of digitalis is uncertain and is grade IIB-C.

Calcium-Channel Antagonists

In patients with evidence of pulmonary vasodilator reserve (>20% reduction in PAPm or pulmonary vascular resistance [PVR]), the oral calcium channel blockers (CCBs) nifedipine and diltiazem may reduce symptoms and prolong life in selected patients [30]. The ACCP consensus statement strongly recommends a monitored therapeutic trial and not empiric use of CCBs [24]. The trial is performed in the catheterization laboratory with a balloon flotation catheter and arterial line. Inhaled nitric oxide, intravenous adenosine, or intravenous prostacyclins are administered to measure acute pulmonary vasodilator reserve. A reduction in PAPm and or PVR by ≥20% suggests that CCBs may be effective. However, if the PVR is >10–12 Wood units or right ventricle has failed represented by a high RA pressure or low cardiac output, CCBs should be avoided. Recently Sitbon et al. [31] further clarified the role of CCBs in the PPH population. As a result, a favourable response is now defined as fall in PAPm ≥ 10 mmHg to PAPm ≤ 40 mm Hg, with unchanged or increased cardiac output. PPH patients who meet these criteria may be treated with CCBs. Patients responding to CCBs and not on any other PPH treatment, were included in their corresponding NYHA functional class I or II [26]. Although approximately 25% of patients responded to oral therapy, even the initial administration of a small dose (10–20 mg) of nifedipine was associated with severe systemic hypotension and death (approximately 10% combined).

The optimal dose of CCBs is not known. Neither a dose finding nor randomized control trial comparing calcium channel blockade to placebo in patients with pulmonary vasodilator reserve has been performed. Although we have patients who are stable or improved on nifedipine for 1–15 years, it is possible that the pulmonary vasodilator reserve predicts a more benign form of the disease independent of treatment. Patients who demonstrate adequate pulmonary vasodilator reserve with nitric oxide, adenosine, or prostacyclin undergo a standardized hemodynamic trial of hourly nifedipine or diltiazem. After the trial, responders receive high-dose nifedipine (120–240 mg) or diltiazem (360–500 mg per day) with close monitoring. Long-acting nifedipine or diltiazem, or amlodipine are advisable. By contrast, verapamil should be avoided for its potential negative inotropic effects.

Prostanoids

Intravenous epoprostenol has markedly improved the quality of life and changed the natural history of PPH. Epoprostenol is a short-acting analogue of the naturally occurring vasodilator prostacyclin (PGI2), with a 3- to 5-min half-life. It can acutely reduce PVR and increases cardiac output and oxygen transport. The absence of an initial positive effect and reduction in PVR does not predict the subsequent benefit. The latter may be due to vascular remodeling, gradual improvement in RV function, and antiplatelet/thrombotic effects. When compared with conventional therapy in a 3-month trial, epoprostenol improved symptoms and short-term survival in class III and IV patients [32].

Most experts recommended intravenous epoproprostenol as the first-line of treatment for unstable patients in functional class NYHA IV, evidence A. Its short half-life and instability in low pH environments necessitate continuous intravenous administration usually through an indwelling catheter (subclavian Hickman or equivalent) with an automatic ambulatory pump. The vast majority of side effects encountered (rash, flushing, jaw claudication, thrombocytopenia, hypotension) are either tolerable, abate over time, or reverse with decreasing doses.

Although cumbersome, this single drug has, in many ways, revolutionized the treatment of PPH and has given hope to a large number of PPH patients who would otherwise have died while awaiting lung transplantation. In our experience, the majority of PPH patients (>90%) with advanced disease not only tolerates the drug but also has a markedly improved quality of life and survival [33,34].

Other prostanoids, such as treprostenil, intravenous treprostenil, and iloprost, were studied. Treprostenil was suggested for PPH patients with NYHA functional class II, III, and IV and was shown to improve exercise endurance as measured by 6MWT distance; however, its effects were dose related, and the necessity of administering the medication subcutaneously by infusion may be a limitation. Recently, the use of intravenous treprostinil showed a longer half-life compared to intravenous epoprostenol. In addition, there were modest improvements in haemodynamics and exercise endurance as measured by 6MWT, and the final dose was more than twice the dose of epoprostenol used at the start of the study. This treatment was suggested for PPH patients in NYHA functional class II, III, and IV in whom subcutaneous infusion is not tolerated.

Finally, iloprost via inhalation six to nine times per day appeared to improve by 10% the exercise endurance in the 6MWT distance and NHYA functional class in the absence of clinical deterioration or death. By contrast, long-term data regarding inhaled iloprost are conflicting. Iloprost is advised for the PPH patients in NYHA functional class III, IV with evidence A and B, respectively.

Endothelin Antagonists

As described in Chapter 2, the effects of endothelin are mediated by the receptors endothelin $(ET)_A$ and ET_B and include vasoconstriction, inflammation, fibrosis, and/or abnormal cells proliferations, these processes are associated with remodeling and mediate pathological conditions, including PAH, pulmonary fibrosis, connective tissue diseases, and heart failure. On the basis of these encouraging discoveries, the authors of a large Randomized trial of Endothelin Antagonist THErapy (BREATHE-1) with Bosentan, an orally active dual $(ET_A$ and $ET_B)$ endothelin-receptor antagonist, enrolled 213 patients suffering from PPH or PAH related to connective tissue disease.

Significant benefits in exercise capacity, Borg dyspnoea index, NYHA functional class, and improvement in cardiac haemodynamics and heart chamber remodeling were revealed by bosentan therapy, which also reduced the time to clinical worsening compared with placebo ($p = 0.002$) [35]. The clinical efficacy of bosentan has been demonstrated in a number of clinical trials in different patient populations and also in paediatric patients. In children with PPH and PAH associated with congenital heart disease or connective tissue disease, the Kaplan–Meier survival estimates at 1 year and 2 years were 98% and 91%, respectively, and PAPm and other PVR parameters decreased. In this study, children were treated with bosentan with or without concomitant intravenous epoprostenol or subcutaneous trepostinil. The median treatment with bosentan was 14 months. The NYHA functional class improved in 46% of the patients treated with bosentan [36].

A confirmation of the improvements in haemdodynamics parameter was showed in a multicenter double blind randomized and placebo-controlled study in patients with NYHA functional class III Einsenmenger syndrome (Bosentan Randomized Trial of Endothelin Antagonist Therapy for Pulmonary Hypertension–5) [37]. Moreover, in a randomized trial of 30 patients treated with epoprostenol (BREATHE-2), the addition of bosentan was well tolerated and resulted in greater improvements in haemodynamics than epoprostenol alone [38]. However, the ACCP guidelines for patients with PAH suggest that until additional evidence becomes available, combination therapy might be considered in the context of clinical trials [26]. The limitations of therapy may be the risk of abnormal hepatic function test findings, syncope, and flushing. Bosentan therapy was suggested for NYHA functional class III and IV PAH (Evidence A and B, respectively).

Recently, sitaxsentan, another oral endothelin A receptor selective antagonist, has been introduced. It has been used in patients with PAH at a dose of 100 mg once daily significantly, improving patients' 6MWT distance compared with placebo and was at least as effective as the use of twice-daily bosentan. Patients treated with sitaxsentan 100 mg experienced a 3% incidence of hepatic enzyme elevation in comparison with the Bosentan group, which had an 11% incidence [39].

Phosphodiesterase Inhibitors

Sildenalafil is a potent and specific phosphodiesterase 5 inhibitor that has been previously used for erectile dysfunctions. Patients with PAH treated with long-term sildenalafil may show some benefits. Sildenalfil reduced PAPm, improving NYHA functional class and exercise endurance measured by 6 MWT distance from baseline at 1 year. Sildenalafil long-term data were available only at 80 mg tid, in contrast with the dose approved by the Food and Drug Administration for PAH treatment that it was 20 mg tid. The therapy was suggested for NYHA functional class IV (Evidence C) [40]. Figure 5.4 shows a treatment algorithm for PAH evaluating NYHA functional class in comparison of PAH treatments and recommendations, respectively.

Surgical Treatment

In a minority of patients who respond poorly to medical therapy, the only alternative is lung or heart–lung transplantation. It is a strong recommendation, but the level of evidence is C, because there is no randomized trial available. Balloon atrial septostomy is also another therapeutic option. This procedure improves survival as compared with the estimated survival of control patients treated with conventional therapy; however, this procedure presents a high-risk and should be performed

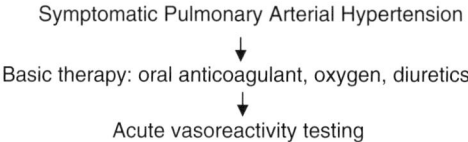

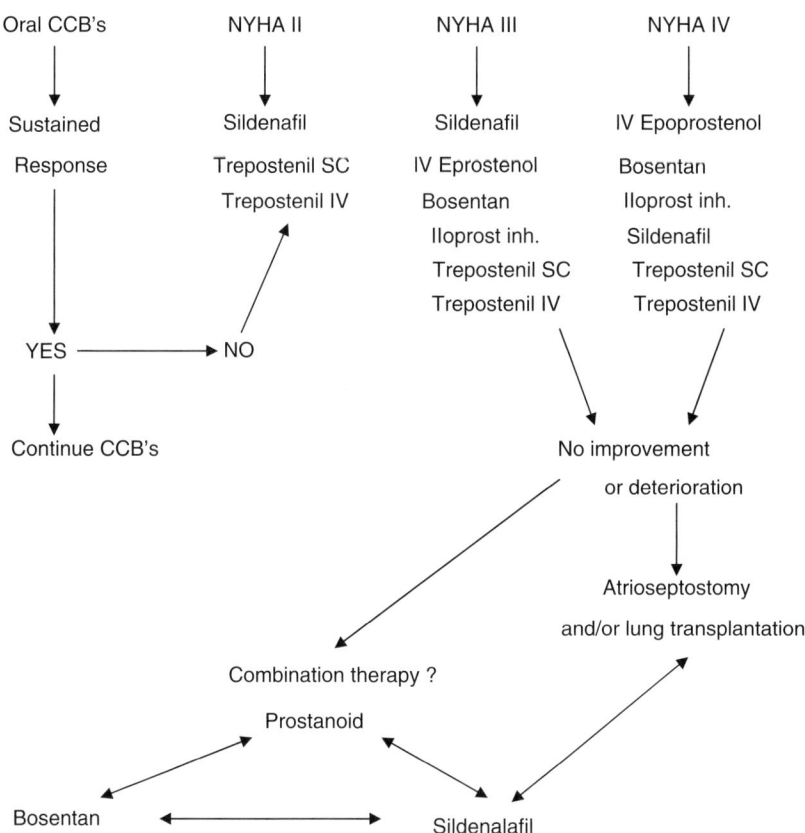

Fig. 5.4 Treatment algorithm for PAH. The therapies presented have been evaluated in PAH and PPH patients

only in expert centers. Current indications for atrial septostomy include failure of medical therapy with persistent RVF and/or recurrent syncope, bridging to transplantation, and the absence of other therapeutic options [41]. It is a grade of recommendation II-A and level of evidence C.

All Class III patients younger than 50 years of age are referred for transplant evaluation as part of the multidisciplinary approach for assessment and management. We rely on symptoms, physical examination with emphasis on estimated CVP, the presence of hepatomegaly and oedema, the echo Doppler RVSP and RV function, and distance walked in a 6-minute standard test at 6-month intervals to

Table 5.4 Survival After Lung And Heart Lung Transplantation (1990–2001) by Diagnosis of PPH and Type of Tansplant

| | PPH | |
Time	Lung transplantation (691 patients), %	Heart lung transplantation (302 patients), %
3 months	72	72
1 year	64	66
3 years	54	50
5 years	44	41
10 years	21	22

measure progress and need for further interventions. Because the waiting list for lung transplant is approximately 18 months and clinical deterioration may be rapid, it is imperative to monitor patients closely.

Combined heart–lung, double-lung, and single-lung transplantation have each been performed in PPH. Because of the limited availability of donors and reports of comparable (albeit relatively poor when compared to other diseases requiring lung transplantation) results, some feel single lung transplantation is acceptable [42]. The complications after single-lung transplantation for PPH are aggravated by the disparity between pulmonary flow, which is high in the transplanted lung, and minute ventilation, which is shared equally between the two lungs. Our institution and many others consider bilateral transplantation the preferred option. Operative survival for lung transplantation for PPH is more than 90%. However, the 1- and 5-year survival is relatively poor at 85% and 50%. Most transplant survivors are in NYHA class I or II. Actual survival is reported from US Scientific Registry and the International Society for Heart and Lung Transplantation (ISHLT) Registry [43,44]. Survival rates from ISHLT registry are presented in Table 5.4. No clearly significant difference in survival has been apparent among the procedures (single or bilateral lung transplantation, and heart–lung transplantation) in the ISHLT Registry.

Overlap PH Syndromes and PPH Variants

PH from all aetiologies can lead to in situ thrombosis and obliteration of the pulmonary vasculature, which makes the differentiation between PPH and chronic thromboembolic PH difficult. We and others treating a large number of patients with PH have encountered patients in whom the diagnosis remains unclear despite pulmonary angiography and open lung biopsy. One or more episodes of small pulmonary emboli may precipitate a rapidly progressive form of pulmonary vasculopathy, which is further aggravated by in situ thrombi appearing late in its course as PPH. Patients with biopsy-proven PPH have been shown to have large in situ thrombi.

Thrombotic PH is one of many variant forms of PPH triggered by disease states, which alone do not result in PH and are labelled PPH variants. Others include atrial septal defects (a high flow shunt should not cause severe PH), collagen diseases such as lupus, mild mitral stenosis, and milder forms of lung disease with mild to moderate hypoxemia such as sleep apnoea and restrictive lung disease accompanying obesity.

Summary

PPH presents a challenge to practicing physicians both in diagnosis and assessment. A high index of suspicion in patients exposed to anorectics and a careful examination in patients with dyspnoea and fatigue should prompt the use of the echo Doppler to screen for pulmonary hypertension. The burden on the practitioner is heavy considering how common the complaints of fatigue and dyspnoea are in the outpatient setting.

The discovery of prostanoids and endothelin antagonist especially as an effective treatment has revolutionized the approach to patients with PPH. The physician's role has changed from providing emotional support and 'hand-holding' for the dieing patient to that of chronic disease assessment.

Acknowledgment We thank Ivano Cantore for expert technical designer assistance and for help in the production of the figures.

References

1. Simonneau G, Galiè N, Rubin LJ, Langleben D, Seeger W, Domenighetti G, Gibbs S, Lebrec D, Speich R, Beghetti M, Rich S, Fishman A. Clinical classification of pulmonary hypertension. J Am Coll Cardiol 2004;43:5S–12S.
2. Rich S, Dantzker DR, Ayres SM, Bergofsky EH, Brundage BH, Detre KM, Fishman AP, Goldring RM, Groves BM, Koerner SK, et al. Primary pulmonary hypertension: a national prospective study. Ann Intern Med 1987;107:216–223.
3. Rubin LJ. Primary pulmonary hypertension (review). N Engl J Med 1997;336:111–117.
4. Abenhaim L, Moride Y, Brenot F, Rich S, Benichou J, Kurz X, Higenbottam T, Oakley C, Wouters E, Aubier M, Simonneau G, Bégaud B. Appetite-suppressant drugs and the risk of primary pulmonary hypertension. N Engl J Med 1996;335;609–616.
5. Speich R, Jenni R, Opravil M, Pfab M, Russi EW. Primary pulmonary hypertension in HIV infection Chest 1991;100:1268–1271.
6. Pan TL, Thumboo J, Boey ML. Primary and secondary pulmonary hypertension in systemic lupus erythematosus. Lupus 2000;9:338–342.
7. Humbert M, Sitbon O, Chaouat Ari, Bertocchi M, Habib G, Gressin V, Yaici A, Weitzenblum E, Cordier JF, Chabot F, Dromer C, Pison C, Reynaud-Gaubert M, Haloun A, Laurent M, Hachulla E, Simonneau G. Pulmonary arterial hypertension in France. Registry from a national Registry. J Respir Crit Care Med 2006;173:1023–1030.
8. Connolly HM, Crary JL, McGoon MD, Hensrud DD, Edwards BS, Edwards WD, Schaff HV. Valvular heart disease associated with fenfluramine-phentermine. N Engl J Med 1997:337;581–588.
9. Otterdal K, Andreassen AK, Yndestad A, Oie E, Sandberg WJ, Dahl CP, Pedersen TM, Ueland T, Gullestad L, Brosstad FR, Aukrust P, Damås JK. Raised LIGHT levels in pulmonary artery hypertension. Am J Respir Crit Care Med 2008;177:202–207.

10. Fuster V, Steele PM, Edwards WD, Gersh BJ, McGoon MD, Frye RL. Primary pulmonary hypertension: natural history and the importance of thrombosis. Circulation 1884;70:580–587.
11. Sitbon O. Prevalence of HIV-related pulmonary artery hypertension in the current antiretroviral therapy era. Am J Respir Crit Care Med 2008;177:108–113.
12. Koh ET, Lee P, Gladman DD, Abu-Shakra M. Pulmonary hypertension in systemic sclerosis: an analysis of 17 patients. Br J Rheumatol 1996;35:989–993.
13. Kawut SM, Taichman DB, Archer-Chicko CL, Palevsky HI, Kimmel SE. Hemodynamics and survival in patients with pulmonary arterial hypertension related to systemic sclerosis. Chest 2003;123:344–350.
14. Kanemoto N, Sasamoto H. Pulmonary hemodynamics in primary pulmonary hypertension. Jpn Heart J 1979;20:395–405.
15. Eysmann SB, Palevsky HI, Reichek N, Hackney K, Douglas PS. Two dimensional and Doppler-echocardiographic correlates of survival in primary pulmonary hypertension. Circulation 1989;80:353–360.
16. Steen VD, Graham G, Conte C, Owens G, Medsger TA Jr. Isolated diffusing capacity reduction in systemic sclerosis. Arthritis Rheum 1992;35:765–770.
17. Nagaya N, Ando M, Oya H, Ohkita Y, Kyotani S, Sakamaki F, Nakanishi N. Plasma brain natriuretic peptide as a noninvasive marker for efficacy of pulmonary thromboendarterectomy. Ann Thorac Surg 2002;74:180–184.
18. Rubens C, Ewert R, Halank M, Wensel R, Orzechowski HD, Schultheiss HP, Hoeffken G. Big endothelin-1 and endothelin-1 plasma levels are correlated with the severity of primary pulmonary hypertension. Chest 2001;120:1562–1569.
19. Nagaya N, Uematsu M, Satoh T, Kyotani S, Sakamaki F, Nakanishi N, Yamagishi M, Kunieda T, Miyatake K. Serum uric acid levels correlate with the severity and the mortality of primary pulmonary hypertension. Am J Respir Crit Care Med 1999;160:487–492.
20. Thomson JR, Machado RD, Pauciulo MW, Morgan NV, Humbert M, Elliott GC, Ward K, Yacoub M, Mikhail G, Rogers P, Newman J, Wheeler L, Higenbottam T, Gibbs JS, Egan J, Crozier A, Peacock A, Allcock R, Corris P, Loyd JE, Trembath RC, Nichols WC. Sporadic primary pulmonary hypertension is associated with germline mutations of the gene encoding BMPR-II, a receptor member of the TGF-beta family. J Med Genet 2000;37:741–745.
21. Goodman DJ, Harrison DC, Popp RL. Echocardiographic features of primary pulmonary hypertension. Am J Cardiol 1974;33:438–443.
22. Moser KM, Page GT, Ashburn WL, Fedullo PF. Perfusion lung scans provide a guide to which patients with apparent primary pulmonary hypertension merit angiography. West J Med 1988;148:167–170.
23. Child JS, Wolfe JD, Tashkin D, Nakano R. Fatal lung scan in a case of pulmonary hypertension due to obliterative pulmonary vascular disease. Chest 1975;67:308–310.
24. Rubin LJ. Primary pulmonary hypertension: ACCP consensus statement. Chest 1993;104:236–250.
25. Badesch DB, Abman SH, Ahearn GS, et al. American College of Chest Physicians. Medical therapy for pulmonary arterial hypertension: ACCP evidence-based clinical practice guidelines. Chest. 2004;126(1 Suppl):35S–62S.
26. Badesch DB, Abman SH, Simonneau G, Rubin LJ, McLaughlin VV. Medical therapy for pulmonary arterial hypertension: updated ACCP evidence-based clinical practice guidelines. Chest 2007;131:1917–1928.
27. Wagenvoort CA, Mulder PG. Thrombotic lesions in primary plexigenic arteriopathy. Chest 1993:103;844–849.
28. Pietra GG, Edwards WD, Kay JM, Rich S, Kernis J, Schloo B, Ayres SM, Bergofsky EH, Brundage BH, Detre KM, et al. Histopathology of primary pulmonary hypertension. Circulation 1989;80:1198–206.
29. Eisenberg PR, Lucore C, Kaufman L, Sobel BE, Jaffe AS, Rich S. Fibrinopeptide A levels indicative of pulmonary vascular thrombosis in patients with primary pulmonary hypertension. Circulation 1990;82:841–847.

30. Rich S, Kaufmann E, Levy PS. The effect of high doses of calcium channel blockers on survival in primary pulmonary hypertension. N Engl J Med 1992;327:76–81.
31. Sitbon O, Humbert M, Jaïs X, Ioos V, Hamid AM, Provencher S, Garcia G, Parent F, Hervé P, Simonneau G. Long-term response to calcium channel blockers in idiopathic pulmonary arterial hypertension. Circulation 2005;111:3105–3111.
32. Barst RJ, Rubin LJ, Long WA, McGoon MD, Rich S, Badesch DB, Groves BM, Tapson VF, Bourge RC, Brundage BH, et al. A comparison of continuous intravenous epoprostenol (prostacyclin) with conventional therapy for primary pulmonary hypertension. N Engl J Med 1996;334;296–302.
33. Sitbon O, Humbert M, Nunes H, Parent F, Garcia G, Hervé P, Rainisio M, Simonneau G.Long-term intravenous epoprostenol infusion in primary pulmonary hypertension: prognostic factors and survival. J Am Coll Cardiol 2002;40:780–788.
34. McLaughlin VV, Shillington A, Rich S. Survival in primary pulmonary hypertension: the impact of epoprostenol therapy. Circulation 2002;106:1477–1482.
35. Rubin LJ, Badesch DB, Barst RJ, Galie N, Black CM, Keogh A, Pulido T, Frost A, Roux S, Leconte I, Landzberg M, Simonneau G.Bosentan therapy for pulmonary arterial hypertension (erratum in: N Engl J Med 2002;346:1258). N Engl J Med. 2002;21;346:896–903.
36. Rosentzweig EB, Ivy DD, Widlitz A, Doran A, Claussen LR, Yung D, Abman SH, Morganti A, Nguyen N, Barst RJ. Effects of long-term bosentan in children with pulmonary arterial hypertension. J Am Coll Cardiol 2005;60:1025–1030.
37. Galie N, Beghetti M, Gatzoulis MA, Granton J, Berger RM, Lauer A, Chiossi E, Landzberg M; Bosentan Randomized Trial of Endothelin Antagonist Therapy-5 (BREATHE-5) Investigators. Bosentan therapy in patients with Eisenmenger syndrome: a multicenter, double-blind, randomized, placebo-controlled study. Circulation 2006;114:48–54.
38. Humbert M, Barst RJ, Robbins IM, Channick RN, Galiè N, Boonstra A, Rubin LJ, Horn EM, Manes A, Simonneau G. Combination of bosentan with epoprostenol in pulmonary arterial hypertension: BREATHE-2.Eur Respir J 2004;24:353–359.
39. Barst RJ, Langleben D, Badesch D, Frost A, Lawrence EC, Shapiro S, Naeije R, Galie N; STRIDE-2 Study Group. Treatment of pulmonary arterial hypertension with the selective endothelin-A receptor antagonist sitaxsentan. J Am Coll Cardiol 2006;47:2049–2056.
40. Galie N, Ghofrani HA, Torbicki A, Barst RJ, Rubin LJ, Badesch D, Fleming T, Parpia T, Burgess G, Branzi A, Grimminger F, Kurzyna M, Simonneau G; Sildenafil Use in Pulmonary Arterial Hypertension (SUPER) Study Group. Sildenalafil citrate therapy for pulmonary arterial hypertension. N Engl J Med 2005;353:2148–2157.
41. Sandoval J, Barst RJ, Rich S, Rothman A. Atrial septostomy for pulmonary hypertension. In: Rich S, editor. Primary pulmonary hypertension:e summary from the World Symposium on PPH 1998. Available at: http://www.Who.int/ncd/cvd/pph.html
42. Pasque MK, Trulock EP, Cooper JD, Triantafillou AN, Huddleston CB, Rosenbloom M, Sundaresan S, Cox JL, Patterson GA. Single lung transplantation for pulmonary hypertension. Circulation 1995;92:2252–2258.
43. 2001 Annual report of U.S. organ procurement and transplantation network and the scientific registry of transplant recipients: transplant data 1991–2000. Department of Health and Human Services, Health Resource and Service Administration Office of Special Programs, Division of transplantation, Rockville, MD; United Network for organ sharing; Richmond VA; University Renal Research and Education Association, Ann Arbor, MI.
44. Hertz MI, Taylor DO, Trulock EP, Boucek MM, Mohacsi PJ, Edwards LB, Keck BM. The registry of the International Society for Heart and Lung Transplantation: Nineteenth Official Report. J Heart Lung Transplant 2002;21:950–970.

Part II
Specific Lung Disorders

Chapter 6
Bronchiolar Disorders

Joseph P. Lynch, III, Rajeev Saggar, Robert D. Suh,
and Michael C. Fishbein

Bronchiolar Disorders: Anatomy and Definition

Bronchioles are small airways (diameter of ≤2 mm) lacking cartilage [1–3]. Bronchioles have a lining epithelium that includes ciliated cells, non-ciliated surfactant-secreting (clara) cells, mucin-secreting goblet cells, basal cells, and occasional neuroendocrine (Kulchitsky) cells [2]. The proximal bronchioles (membranous and terminal) are purely air-conducting, whereas the distal respiratory bronchioles contain alveolar tissue within their walls [4]. Respiratory bronchioles communicate directly with alveolar ducts and are in the range of 0.5 mm in diameter [5]. The gas-exchanging unit of the lung, termed the acinus or primary pulmonary lobule, comprises one terminal bronchiole, two to five generations of respiratory bronchioles, alveolar ducts, alveolar sacs, and alveoli [5]. Connective tissue anchors the bronchiole to the surrounding alveolar and perivascular interstitium [2]. Each bronchiole travels with an arteriole, forming a bronchovascular bundle; small lymphatics also course along the bronchovascular bundles [2].

Bronchiolar Disorders: Classification Schema

Bronchiolar inflammation and/or fibrosis can occur as a result of myriad disorders or injuries to the small airways [1,3,5]. Some causes of bronchiolar disorders include infections, connective tissue disease (CTD) [6]; inhalational injuries [7]; drug reactions [6]; lung transplant recipients (LTRs) with chronic allograft rejection [8]; hematopoietic stem cell transplantation (HSCT) [9]; diverse immunologic disorders [10]; large airway disorders [11]; and unknown causes [4,5]. Clinical classification is based on proven or presumptive etiology [4,12]. A clinical classification schema has been proposed (Table 6.1) [1], but it has not been universally adopted. In 2003, Rhu et al. [5] proposed classifying bronchiolar disorders into three major categories (see Table 6.2) [5]. In this schema, seven primary bronchiolar disorders are recognised (i.e., the process was limited to bronchioles anatomically): four bronchiolar disorders associated with interstitial lung disease and three disorders associated with large airways disease.

R.P. Baughman et al. (eds.), *Pulmonary Arterial Hypertension
and Interstitial Lung Diseases,*
© Humana Press, a part of Springer Science + Business Media, LLC 2009

Table 6.1 Clinical Classification of Bronchiolitis

Bronchiolitis involving the small conducting airways
- Inhalation bronchiolitis
    Toxic fume inhalation
    Irritant gases and mineral dusts
    Organic dusts
- Infectious and postinfectious bronchiolitis
- Drug-induced bronchiolitis
- Collagen vascular disease-associated bronchiolitis
- Posttransplant bronchiolitis
- Paraneoplastic pemphigus-associated bronchiolitis
- Neuroendocrine cell hyperplasia with bronchiolar fibrosis
- Diffuse panbronchiolitis
- Cryptogenic bronchiolitis
- Miscellaneous
    Lysinuric protein intolerance
    Ataxia-telangiectasia
    Familial form of immunodeficiency
    IgA nephropathy
- Organizing pneumonia (bronchiolitis obliterans organizing pneumonia)
- Idiopathic
- Focal
- Secondary

Reprinted with permission from Poletti and Costabel [1].

Table 6.2 Classification of Bronchiolar Disorders

Primary bronchiolar disorders
- Constrictive bronchiolitis (obliterative bronchiolitis)
- Acute bronchiolitis
- Diffuse panbronchiolitis
- Respiratory bronchiolitis (smoker's bronchiolitis)
- Mineral dust airway disease
- Follicular bronchiolitis
- Other forms of primary bronchiolitis

Bronchiolar involvement in interstitial lung disease (ILD)
- Hypersensitivity pneumonia (HP)
- Respiratory bronchiolitis-associated ILD (RB-ILD) and desquamative interstitial pneumonia (DIP)
- Cryptogenic Organizing Pneumonia (idiopathic bronchiolitis obliterans organizing pneumonia)
- Other ILDs (e.g., pulmonary Langerhans' cell histiocytosis; sarcoidosis, bronchiolocentric interstitial pneumonia)

Bronchiolar involvement in large airway disease
- Chronic bronchitis
- Bronchiectasis
- Asthma

Adapted from Ryu et al. [5].

Given the exhaustive differential diagnosis and spectrum of bronchiolar disorders, in this chapter we focus our discussion on two major histopathologic patterns of bronchiolar disorders, each of which may be observed in diverse clinical settings: (1) organizing pneumonia (OP) and (2) obliterative bronchiolitis (OB). These entities, OP and OB, differ dramatically clinically, radiographically, and prognostically. OP (whether idiopathic or associated with a specific disease) is characterized by a restrictive defect on pulmonary function tests (PFTs), consolidation on chest radiographs (mimicking pneumonia), and excellent prognosis and responsiveness to corticosteroid therapy [13–15]. In contrast, OB (formerly termed bronchiolitis obliterans) is characterised by severe airflow obstruction, the absence of parenchymal infiltrates on chest radiographs, poor responsiveness to therapy, and high mortality rates [4,5,16].

Bronchiolar Disorders: Histopathology

The histological spectrum of bronchiolitis is diverse (Fig. 6.1A–E and 6.2A–D). An initial classification schema published by Myers and Colby [17] included eight subtypes (Table 6.3). A more recent classification schema recognizes four main histological patterns (discussed in the sections to follow; also see Table 6.4) [1].

Cellular Bronchiolitis

Cellular bronchiolitis is a complication of numerous disorders or insults affecting the airways [18]. The spectrum of cellular bronchiolitis is wide; its features include necrosis of epithelial and inflammatory cells, necrotic debris and fibrin, submucosal oedema, microabscesses, nodular and granulomatous inflammation, and germinal center hyperplasia (follicular bronchiolitis) [2].

Infectious Bronchiolitis

Diverse infections (particularly viral) elicit acute bronchiolitis (e.g., respiratory syncytial virus [RSV], influenza A, adenovirus, measles, Bordetella pertussis, Mycoplasma pneumoniae, tuberculosis, etc.) [18,19]. Infectious bronchiolitis is characterized by acute bronchiolar injury, epithelial necrosis, inflammation and oedema of the bronchial wall, and intramural exduates (Fig. 6.1A) [18]. Infectious bronchiolitis is most often observed in infants and children (particularly as the result of RSV infections), but may affect adults. Symptoms include cough, wheezing, and dypsnea [5]. Postinfectious OP is rare [4,5].

OP

This histological hallmark of OP is inflammatory polyps of granulation tissue (termed Masson bodies) within the lumens of terminal and respiratory bronchioles;

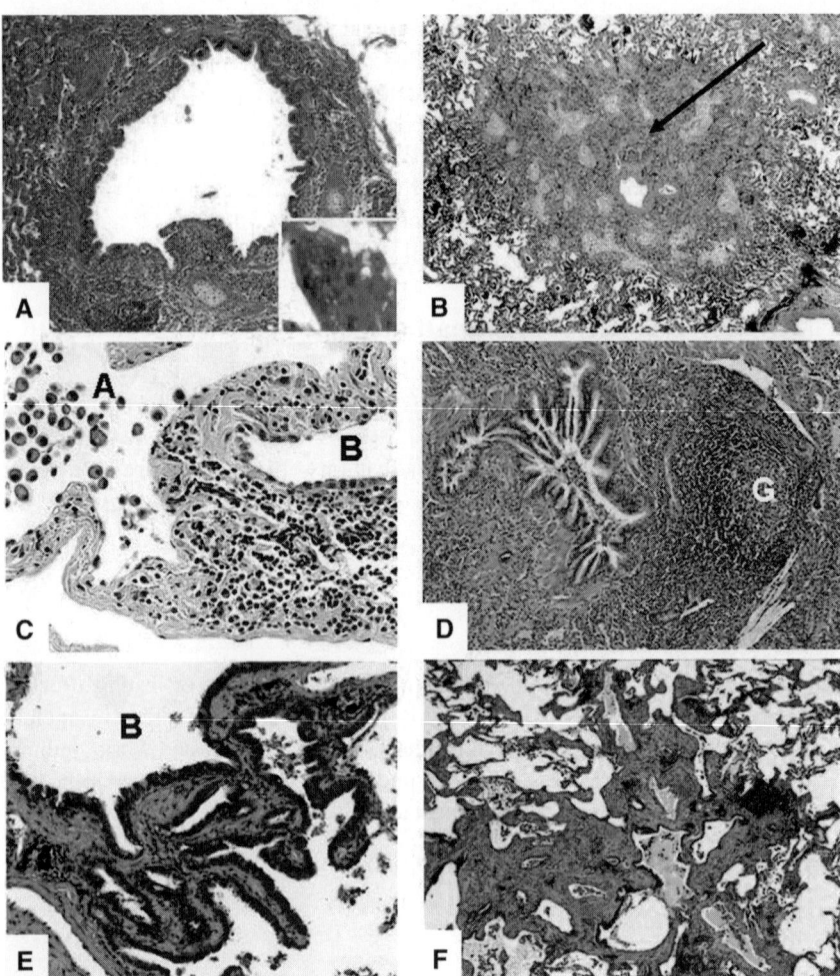

Fig. 6.1 Examples of bronchiolar disorders. **a** Inflammatory, infectious, bronchiolitis, in this case due to respiratory syncytial virus (×100), inset shows characteristic multinucleated giant cell. **b** COP with obliterated bronchiole (arrow) surrounded by alveoli filled with loose connective tissue (×40). **c** Respiratory bronchiolitis in a smoker. There is chronic inflammation around the terminal bronchiole and numerous macrophages in the adjacent alveolar tissue (A) (×200). **d** Follicular bronchiolitis from a patient with rheumatoid arthritis. Note peribronchiolar intense chronic inflammation with a germinal center (G) present (×100). **e** Peribronchiolar metaplasia (AKA Lambertosis) found in patients with small airway disease. Note the alveoli adjacent to the bronchiole (B) have similar bronchiolar type epithelium (×100). **f** Marked peribronchiolar and interstitial fibrosis characteristic of idiopathic bronchiolocentric interstitial pneumonia (×40) **a-f,** all hematoxylin and eosin stains.

extension into the alveolar ducts and alveoli represents the "organizing pneumonia" component (Fig. 6.1B) [2]. At low-power magnification, pale-shaped round or oval plugs of granulation tissue fill the bronchiolar lumens; these plugs contain proliferating fibroblasts, edema, fibrin, mucopolysaccharides, and immature connective

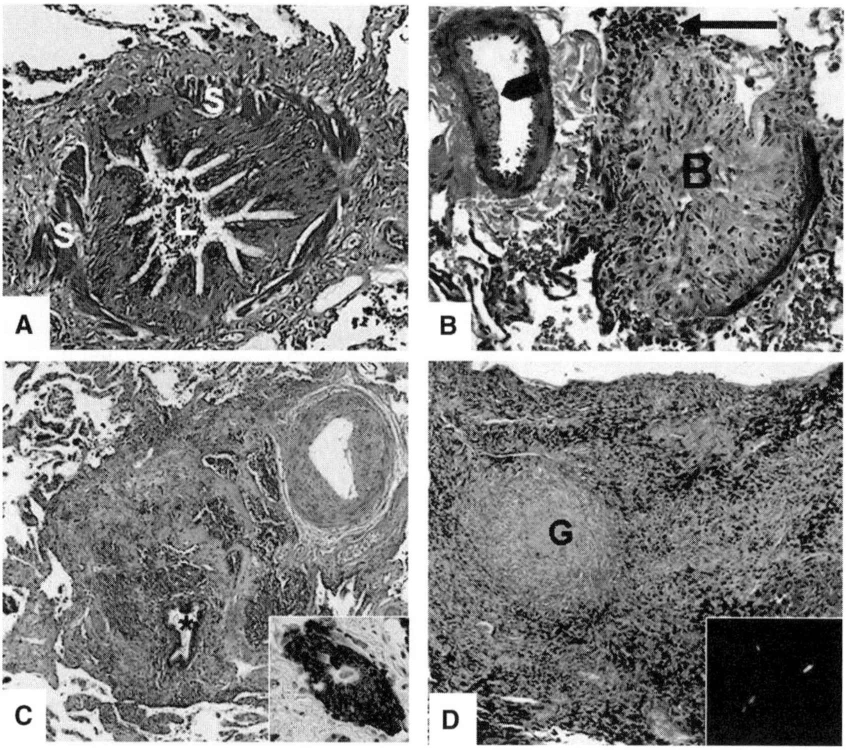

Fig. 6.2 Examples of OB. **A** trichrome stain of small airway with fibrosis (blue) between the bronchiolar epithelium and the bronchiolar smooth muscle (S), constricting the bronchiolar lumen (L) (×100). **B** Trichrome stain of completely occluded bronchiole (B) from lung transplant patient, note inflammation also present (arrow) and early graft vasculopathy (arrowhead) (×100). **C** Hematoxylin and eosin stain of markedly constricted bronchiole (asterisk) caused by diffuse idiopathic pulmonary neuroendocrine hyperplasia (DIPNECH) (×100). Inset shows chromogranin immunostain of neuroendocrine cells in the wall of the airway. **D** Peribronchiolar hyalinized granuloma (G) with surrounding anthracosis in a patient with silicosis (×100). Inset shows weak polarization of fibers.

Table 6.3 Histopathological Classification of Bronchiolitis

Acute (infectious) bronchiolitis
COP [formerly termed bronchiolitis obliterans organizing pneumonia (BOOP)]
Constrictive (obliterative) bronchiolitis
Adult bronchiolitis
RB-ILD
Mineral dust airways disease bronchiolitis
Follicular bronchiolitis
Diffuse panbronchiolitis

Adapted from Myers and Colby [17].

Table 6.4 Histopathological Classification of Bronchiolitis (adapted from Poletti and Costabel [1])

Cellular bronchiolitis
- Follicular bronchiolitis
- Respiratory bronchiolitis
- Diffuse panbronchiolitis

BOOP

Constrictive (cicatricial) bronchiolitis

Peribronchiolar fibrosis and bronchiolar metaplasia ("lambertosis")

tissue [2]. Ancillary features include chronic inflammation of alveolar walls and foamy alveolar macrophages [2]. The alveolar architecture is preserved, and fibrosis is not a prominent feature [17]. Organizing pneumonia exhibits bronchocentricity and patchy involvement; these features can be appreciated on low magnification of lung biopsy specimans [17].

Constrictive (Cicatricial) Bronchiolitis

Constrictive bronchiolitis (also termed OB) is a purely bronchiolar disorder, with few or no changes in the distal lung parenchyma [2]. Diverse conditions have been associated with OB (discussed later) [3–5]. The respiratory bronchioles in OB are concentrically narrowed and "obliterated" by collagen (Fig. 6.2). The fibrosing inflammatory process surrounds the bronchiolar lumens, resulting in extrinsic compression and obliteration of airways (Fig. 6.2B) [5]. Additional findings include distortion of the lumens; mucostasis; bronchiolar smooth muscle hypertrophy; and patchy, chronic inflammation [2]. These changes may be patchy and subtle, even in seriously affected patients [5]. Thus, transbronchial lung biopsies (TBBs) rarely substantiate the diagnosis. Surgical lung biopsy can be used to confirm the diagnosis when histological confirmation is necessary [5]. Elastic stains and serial sections may be necessary to appreciate the fibrotic component [5].

Respiratory Bronchiolitis (RB)

RB is a specific form of bronchiolitis in cigarette smokers characterized by pigmented macrophages within the lumens of respiratory bronchioles, alveolar ducts, and sacs (Fig. 6.1C) [20]. Macrophages in RB are characterized by eosinophilic cytoplasm with superimposed light brown and finely granular pigments that represent constituents of cigarette smoke [2]. Respiratory bronchiolitis is a relatively specific morphological marker of cigarette smoking [21]. Typically, RB is an incidental finding that is *not* associated with specific symptoms [20]. Progression of the lesion into distal airways spaces (termed RB-ILD) may be associated with cough, dyspnea, and restrictive defects on PFTs [22]. Chest computed tomographic (CT) scans reveal centrilobular micronodules [20]. The prognosis of RB or RB-ILD is generally good. Improvement occurs in most patients after cessation of smoking, but the disease progresses in a minority of patients [20]. Corticosteroids have been used, with anecdotal successes, in patients exhibiting worsening disease [20].

Mineral Dust Airways Disease

Inhalation of mineral dust, particulate matter, or pollutants may cause mineral dust-associated bronchiolitis, with associated fibrosis [2,23]. Asbestos, iron oxide, aluminum, talc, mica, silicate, silica, and coal may elicit this response [2,5]. Histological features include fibrotic thickening and distortion of bronchial walls; pigment in the small airways (particularly respiratory bronchioles); cellular infiltration, including macrophages; and smooth muscle hyperplasia [5]. The degree of fibrosis in the bronchiolar walls is linked to local dust burden [5. The use of high-resolution CT (HRCT) may reveal tiny ill-defined peribronchiolar opacities [5].

Follicular Bronchiolitis

Follicular bronchiolitis is defined as lymphoid hyperplasia of the bronchus-associated lymphoid tissue along bronchioles and bronchi (Fig. 6.1D) [24]. Grossly, lung show peribronchial nodules, 1 to 2 mm in diameter [5]. Most cases of follicular bronchiolitis are associated with CTD (particularly rheumatoid arthritis and Sjogren's syndrome) [18], acquired immunodeficiency syndromes [2], or hypersensitivity reactions [25]. Treatment is directed towards the underlying disease. For idiopathic cases, corticosteroids, bronchodilators, and macrolide antibiotic have been used, with anecdotal successes [5], but data are limited.

Diffuse Panbronchiolitis

Diffuse panbronchiolitis is a specific form of cellular bronchiolitis with a pronounced genetic component (principally observed in Japanese adults) [26]. Histological features include chronic inflammation of respiratory bronchioles and surrounding alveoli; mural infiltrate of mononuclear cells and neutrophils; foamy macrophages in the walls; and lumens of respiratory bronchioles and airspaces [2]. Clinical findings resemble cystic fibrosis, with chronic sinusitis and bronchiectasis, leading to infections caused by *Pseudomonas aeruginosa* and progressive respiratory insufficiency [26,27]. The course is ameliorated by macrolide antibiotics [26].

Peribronchiolar Fibrosis and Bronchiolar Metaplasia

In this disorder, metaplastic bronchiolar epithelium extends into the alveolar walls (called lambertosis); bronchiolar and peribronchiolar scarring are present concomitantly [2,28]. This process is bronchiolocentric. Some cases may represent the recently described entity, idiopathic bronchiolocentric interstitial pneumonia (Fig. 6.1F) [29]. These disorders are poorly understood but may reflect bronchiolar injury and scarring from an antecedent inflammatory process such as viral bronchitis or hypersensitivity pneumonia [2].

Radiographic Features of Bronchiolar Disorders

HRCT scans are critically important to discern patterns of bronchiolar disorders (Table 6.5) [1,25,30–32]. Normal bronchioles are not visible on HRCT, but diseased bronchioles with dilated lumens (>2 mm in diameter) or thickened walls can be visualised [25]. Muller and Miller [33] first classified bronchiolar disorders based on three CT patterns: (1) nodules and branching lines; (2) ground-glass attenuation and consolidation; and (3) low attenuation and mosaic perfusion [33]. V- or Y-shaped branching linear opacities (the so-called "tree-in-bud" pattern) [32] reflect inflammatory cells, mucus, or debris within bonchiolar lumens (Fig. 6.3A and 6.3B) [18]. Poorly defined centrilobular nodules or ground glass opacities (GGOs) reflect inflammatory cells within the peribronchiolar alveoli (Fig. 6.4A and 6.4B) [18]. Consolidation reflects extension of the inflammatory process into the lung parenchyma (Fig. 6.5). These CT findings (i.e., linear opacities, tree-in-bud pattern, centrilobular nodules, GGOs, consolidation) may be found in diverse infectious [12] or noninfectious [5,25] causes of bronchiolitis but may also be seen in lymphangitic spread of cancer, bronchoalveolar cell carcinoma, sarcoidosis, pulmonary edema, hypersensitivity pneumonia [34], vasculitis, etc. [25].

Characteristic CT features of constrictive bronchiolitis or OB include bronchial dilation or bronchial wall thickening; patchy areas of decreased lung attenuation (hyperlucency); mosaic pattern of perfusion (low and high areas of attenuation); and air-trapping (best appreciated on expiratory images) (Fig. 6.6A and 6.6B) [18]. The use of dynamic CT is more sensitive in detecting regional abnormalities and air-trapping [5]. The mosaic pattern is caused by hypoventilation of alveoli distal to the bronchiolar obstruction and resultant secondary vasoconstriction (i.e.,

---

Table 6.5 Cardinal HRCT Features of Bronchiolitis (Adapted from Poletti and Costabel [1])

- Centrilobular nodules and branching lines (tree in bud)
- Ground glass attenuation and/or alveolar consolidation
- Low attenuation (mosaic perfusion) and expiratory air-trapping

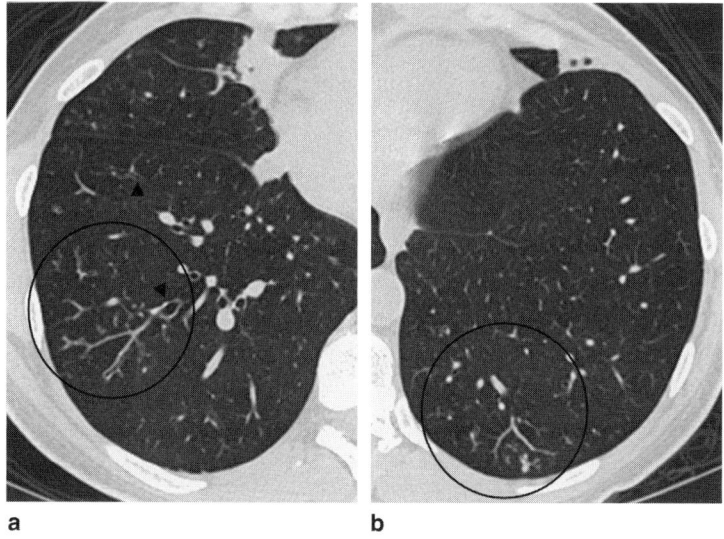

Fig. 6.3 "Tree-in-Bud" pattern (HRCT). **a** Clustered branching V- and Y-shaped linear and nodular opacities (circle), referred to as "tree-in-bud" pattern, within the right lower lobe of a patient with atypical mycobacteria. Associated peribronchial and peribronchiolar thickening (▲) is consistent with airway disease. **b** Another site of "tree-in-bud" pattern (circle) within the left lower lobe with accompanying end airways mucus impaction.

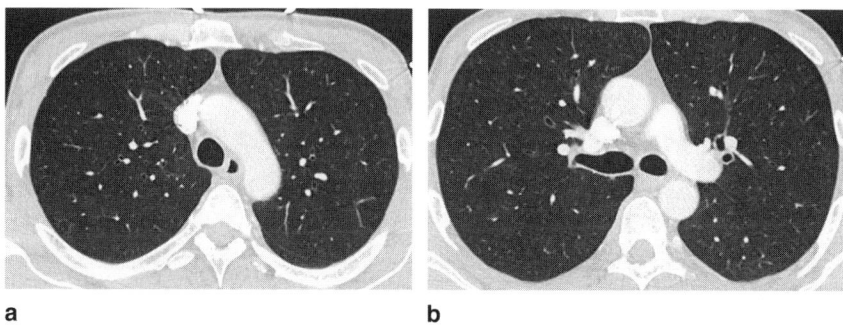

Fig. 6.4 C entrilobular nodules (HRCT). Axial HRCT images of the upper lobes in a symptomatic smoker demonstrate numerous poorly defined centrilobular ground glass nodular opacities, reflecting inflammatory cells within the peribronchiolar alveoli. Diffuse peribronchial thickening involves the larger airways.

reduced perfusion and low attenuation on CT) in the affected lung [5]. Uninvolved segments of lung show normal or increased perfusion with resultant normal or increased attenuation [5]. Mosaic perfusion is not specific for bronchiolar disorders but may be caused by pulmonary vascular obstruction [5,25,35].

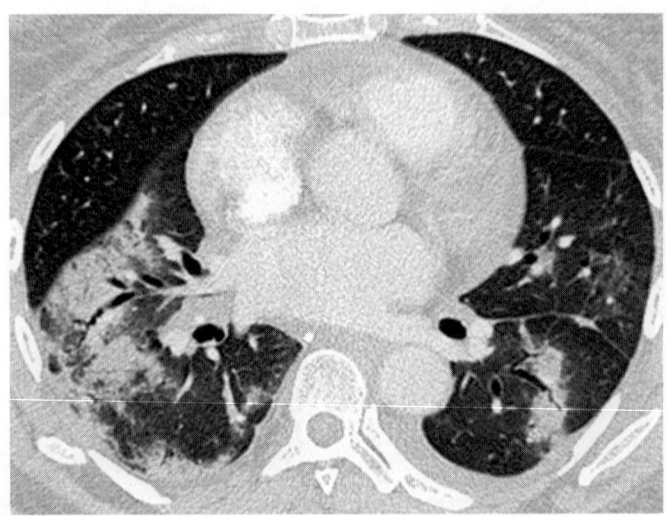

Fig. 6.5 Pulmonary consolidation (HRCT). In a patient with OP, air space parenchymal consolidations reside within both lower lobes with notable peribronchial thickening of the subtending bronchi.

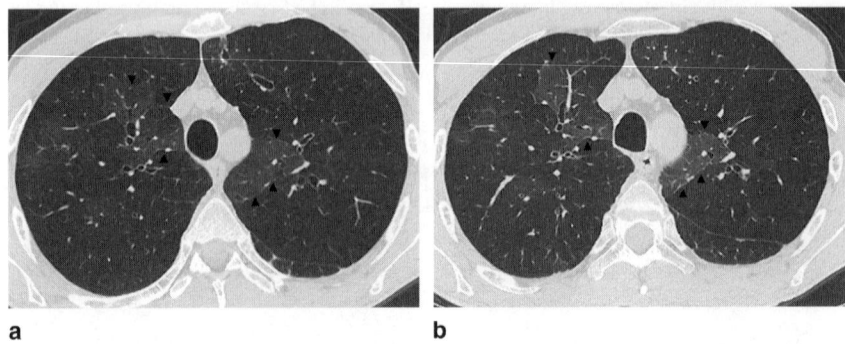

a   b

Fig. 6.6 Mosaic hypoperfusion (HRCT). **A** Full inspiratory axial HRCT image demonstrates patchy geographic alternations of hypo- (▲) and hyperlucent parenchyma and scattered bronchiectasis and bronchiolectasis. **B** Expiratory HRCT at a comparable level confirms the presence of diffuse air-trapping, the hypo- (▲) and hyperlucent lung becoming accentuated and more obvious.

OP

OP is a histological pattern that may be observed in the context of specific medical disorders (e.g., radiation or chemotherapy-induced injury; HSCT or lung transplant recipients; inhalation injury; CTD; idiopathic) [4,13–15]. The term cryptogenic organizing pneumonia (COP) was introduced by Davison et al. in 1983 [36]. The term bronchiolitis obliterans organizing pneumonia (BOOP), cited in a classic article in 1985 [37], is synonymous with OP. In 2002, a consensus statement published by the American Thoracic Society/European Respiratory Society advocated using the term COP to refer to the idiopathic variant [38]. Comprehensive reviews of diverse bronchiolar disorders have been published elsewhere [4,15].

COP

Clinical manifestations of COP include cough, malaise, dyspnea, low-grade fever, and focal lobar or segmental infiltrates on chest radiographs (often with air-bronchograms) [13,14,37,39]. Extrapulmonary involvement does not occur. The course is subacute or chronic, developing over the course of 2 to 12 weeks [13,14,37,39]. An antecedent respiratory tract infection precedes the onset of symptoms in one-third of patients [13,14,37,39]. Physical examination reveals rhonchi and "mid-inspiratory squeaks" or rales; however, wheezing is not a feature [14,37]. The constellation of these features mimics an infectious etiology. The diagnosis is usually not suspected until patients fail to respond to antibiotic therapy.

Radiographic Features

Chest radiographs reveal focal or segmental alveolar infiltrates, often in the periphery of the lung (Fig. 6.7A and 6.7B) [13,14]. Any lobe may be involved, but a basilar predominance is more common [13,14]. A more diffuse pattern, with a reticulonodular pattern, may be observed in 10–30% of patients with COP [13,14]. Pleural effusions, cavitation, or intrathoracic lymphadenopathy are not features of

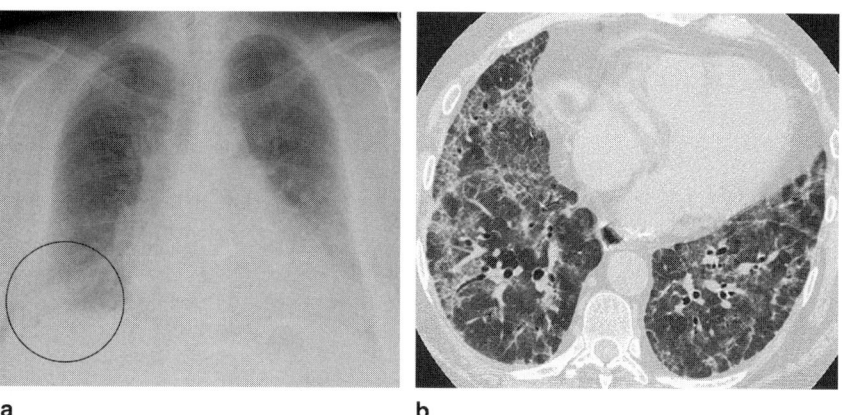

a   b

Fig. 6.7 COP. **A** Frontal chest radiograph shows poorly defined multifocal segmental and subsegmental air space opacities throughout both lungs, most confluent within the right lung base periphery (circle). **B** Axial HRCT through the lung bases confirms the presence of multifocal parenchymal consolidations with peribronchial and peribronchiolar thickening of the adjacent and subtending airways.

COP. Chest CT scans in COP demonstrate peripheral consolidations (80–95%) and GGOs (>80%), with subpleural and/or peribronchial predominance [40–42]. Bronchial dilation is noted in 50–60% of cases; nonseptal linear or reticular opacities, in 45% [43]. Honeycomb change is not a feature of COP (Fig. 6.8A and 6.8B) [40–42]. Chest radiographs or CT scans typically improve dramatically within days after the institution of corticosteroid therapy (Fig. 6.9A and 6.9B).

Pulmonary Function Tests

Pulmonary function tests in COP reveal reductions in lung volumes (forced vital capacity [FVC] and total lung capacity [TLC]) and diffusing capacity for carbon monoxide (DL$_{CO}$), and a widened alveolar-arterial oxygen gradient [6,13,14,37,39].

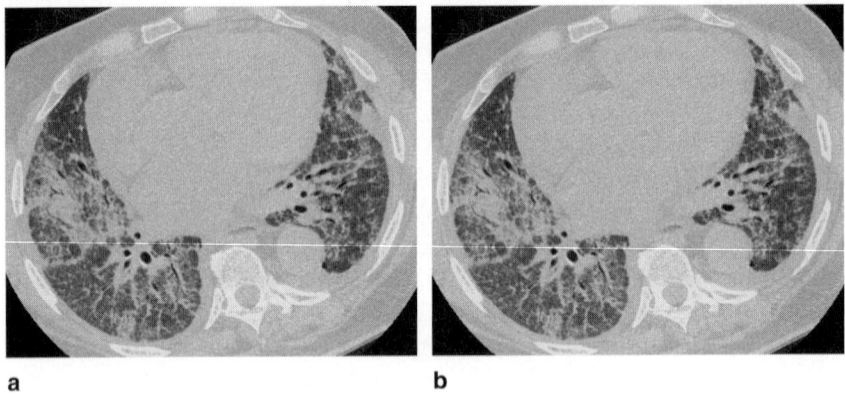

a   b

Fig. 6.8 COP with Fibrosis. On **A** and **B**, axial HRCT images, diffuse reticulation with architectural distortion and traction bronchiectasis and bronchiolectasis permeates both lower and right middle lobes, consistent with fibrosis but notable for lack of honeycombing.

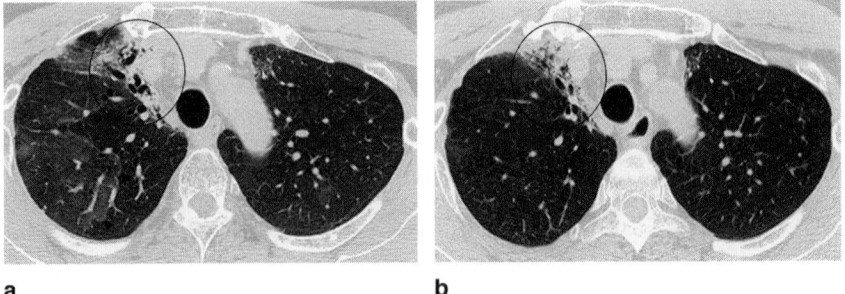

a   b

Fig. 6.9 OP with CS therapy response. After radiotherapy (circle) for thymic carcinoma, axial HRCT images at comparable levels (**A**) before and (**B**) after corticosteroid therapy demonstrate resolution of well-demarcated ground glass opacity (▲), representing organizing pneumonia, within the right upper lobe.

Despite the involvement of small airways, an obstructive component is lacking (except in smokers) [14,37]. Deficits usually reverse promptly with corticosteroid therapy [14,37].

Bronchoalveolar Lavage (BAL)

The use of BAL in patients with COP reveals increases in lymphocytes (mean 23–44% of cells), neutrophils (mean 4–14%), or eosinophils (mean 3–6%); foamy macrophages and plasma cells may also be present [6,13,14,37,39].

Pathogenesis

The cause of idiopathic COP is not known, but it likely represents an exaggerated response to a variety of inflammatory or injurious stimuli [6]. The uniformity of the histologic lesions and peribronchiolar distribution suggest that inhaled stimuli (e.g., possible inhaled antigens or noxious agents) initiate lung injury. The factors responsible for elicitating or down-regulating host immune responses in this context have not been elucidated.

Treatment

Corticosteroids (CS) are the cornerstone of therapy for COP and are highly efficacious. Complete resolution is achieved in more than three-quarters of patients [5,13,39]. The optimal dose and duration of therapy have not been studied in randomized trials. An initial dose of prednisone 40–60 mg/day or equivalent is adequate; lower doses may be used in patients at increased risk for side effects [13,14,39]. Responses are usually dramatic (within 24–72 h). Relapses occur in 50–80% of patients as CS are tapered or discontinued [13,14,39]. Some patients require long-term (sometimes indefinite) therapy with low-dose prednisone (e.g., 10–20 mg every other day) to maintain remissions. A minority of patients [10–15%] have progressive disease that is recalcitrant to CS therapy [14,39,44]. Immunosuppressive or cytotoxic agents (e.g., azathioprine, cyclophosphamide, mycophenolate mofetil, etc.) are reserved for patients who are unresponsive to or who are experiencing adverse effects from CS. Data evaluating these agents are limited to anecdotal cases. Fatalities attributed to COP were noted in 2–8% of patients [13,14,39].

Rapidly Progressive OP

Rapidly progressive COP with severe hypoxemic respiratory failure developing within a few days or weeks is exceptionally rare [45,46]. In this context, lung biopsies show typical histological features of OP; in addition; diffuse alveolar damage (DAD) is a prominent concomitant feature [45,46]. Mortality rates are high (>50%), even with CS therapy [45,46]. Pulse methylprednisolone (1,000 mg daily intravenously for 3 days), followed by high-dose prednisone, with taper) is recommended, but data are limited to a few cases.

OP Complicating Radiation Therapy

OP occurs in approximately 2.5% of women treated with radiation therapy for breast cancer [47–51]. The incidence of OP appears to be lower in patients treated with thoracic radiation for lung cancer or other malignancies [15,52]. Fever, cough, dyspnea, and peripheral alveolar opacities on chest radiographs develop 1–12 months after completion of radiation therapy [51,53]. Migratory infiltrates, initially observed in the irradiated area, spread to nonirradiated areas in the ipsilateral lung and to the contralateral lung [51,53]. This migratory pattern distinguishes OP from radiation pneumonitis. Chest CT scans reveal peripheral air-space opacities with air-bronchograms [53]. Lymphocytosis on BAL is typical; BAL neutrophilia or eosinophilia is present in a minority of patients [51,53]. Lymphocytic alveolitis on BAL (predominantly CD4+ T cells) may also be observed in radiation-induced pneumonitis [50,51,54].

CS are the cornerstone of therapy. CSs usually affect clinical and radiographic improvement within 1–2 weeks, but relapses may occur while tapering or stopping CS [51,53]. Immunosuppressive agents are not required. Macrolides were effective in three cases for OP complicating radiation therapy [49]. The salutorious effect of macrolides likely reflects immunomodulatory and antiinflammatory properties [55,56].

Complications of OP in LT

Constrictive (obliterative) bronchiolitis is the hallmark of chronic allograft rejection among LTRs (discussed in detail later) [8,57]. OP has also been described among LTRs, and is believed to represent a form of acute allograft rejection [58–60]. Early reports of OP in LTRs often were associated with infection [58–60]. Subsequent series found that OP was often associated with acute allograft rejection and may progress to bronchiolitis obliterans syndrome (BOS) or OB [61]. In one review, histological features of OP were found in 17 of 163 (10%) LTRs; acute rejection was present concurrently in 11 (65%) [61]. Ten of the 17 patients (59%) with OP eventually developed OB. Other investigators detected OP in 34% of biopsies from LTRs; OP was associated with an increased risk of BOS [hazards ratio of 1.75] [62]. Gastroesophageal reflux has been suggested as a cause of both OP and OB in LTRs [63–66], but this link is controversial [67].

OP Complicating Collagen Vascular Disorders

OP or OB may rarely complicate CTDs [6,68–73]. Clinical, radiographic, and histopathological features are similar to OP or OB complicating other disorders [6]. Although data are limited, CS are usually efficacious for OP whereas OB is unresponsive to therapy [6].

OP Complicating Inhalation Injury

Exposure to toxic gases, fumes, or irritants (e.g., nitrogen dioxide [18], chlorine gas [19], volatile flavoring agents [74,75], and nylon flock [75 76]) may cause airway injury and bronchiolitis [19,77]. Inhalation injuries to the bronchioles typically are associated with OB; OP is rare [19].

Constrictive (Obliterative) Bronchiolitis

Constrictive (obliterative) bronchiolitis is the prototype of an obstructive bronchiolar disorder resulting in airflow obstruction [78]. The term bronchiolitis obliterans (no longer used) is synonynous with OB. Clinical features include cough, dyspnea, irreversible airflow obstruction (reduced expiratory flow rates) and, in some cases, fatal respiratory insufficiency [78]. The most common causes of OB are chronic lung allograft rejection [8,57] or graft versus host disease among HSCT recipients [9,79,80]. Myriad other etiologies of OB include CTD [6]; drugs [6]; chronic hypersensitivity pneumonia [34]; inhalation injury [7,77]; inhalation of mineral dust, particulate matter or pollutants [2,23']; IgA nephropathy [81]; ataxia telangiectasia [82]; lysinuric protein intolerance [83]; consumption of uncooked leaves of *Sauropus androgynus* [84]; idiopathic inflammatory bowel disease [10,85]; HIV infection [78]; gastroesophageal reflux [86]; diffuse neuroendocrine cell hyperplasia [87,88]; exposure to a volatile agent (diacetyl) in workers in microwave-popcorn plants [74,75]; and exposure to massive amount of ambient dust by firefighters and workers in New York City on September 11, 2001 [77]. When no cause is identified, the term cryptogenic obliterative (constrictive) bronchiolitis is used [89]. Given the rarity of OB, we limit our discussion to OB complicating organ transplantation (lung or HSCT).

BOS Complicating Lung Transplantation

BOS, a manifestation of chronic allograft rejection, is the leading cause of death among LTRs after the first year [57,90]. The terms OB, bronchiolitis obliterans, and constrictive bronchiolitis are synonymous [8]. Elicitation of inflammatory mediators, immune cells, and cytokines may give rise to an exuberant fibroproliferative process, leading to granulation tissue within the lumen of the allograft airways and ultimately collagenous obliteration of the airways [8]. Recipient bone marrow-derived fibroblasts and myofibroblasts contribute to the fibrotic process [91]. Lymphocytic bronchitis or bronchiolitis is often a precursor to BOS [92]. Clinically, BOS is characterized by progressive decline in lung function and ultimately, fatal respiratory failure [8,57]. Although BOS is rare within the first year after lung transplantation (LT), the cumulative incidence of OB post-LT ranges from 43% to 80% [8,67]. In early studies among LTRs, 58% of adults developed BOS [93] and 63% of children [94] by 3 years. At 5 years, 75% of adults had developed BOS [93]. In more-recent studies, the incidence of BOS decreased modestly.

The International Society of Heart Lung Transplantation (ISHLT) Registry in 2005 analyzed 7,775 LTRs followed between 1994 and 2005 [95]. In that cohort, freedom from BOS was 91% at 1 year, 71% at 3 years, and 57% at 5 years after LT [95]. The lower incidence of BOS in recent surveys may reflect more aggressive prophylaxis against cytomegalovirus (CMV), and earlier detection and treatment of episodes of acute rejection (AR). Even a single episode of mild AR increases the risk of BOS [96–98]. Further, treating AR decreases the risk of OB. These data support the role of surveillance bronchoscopy among LTRs [96], aiming to identify and treat even asymptomatic episodes of minimal or mild rejection [98–100]. However, the value of surveillance bronchoscopy remains controversial [57].

Risk Factors for BOS

The dominant risk factor for BOS or BO is acute allograft rejection [90,97]. Multiple or severe episodes of AR or late-onset AR increase the risk of BOS [62,97,101,102]. However, additional co-factors play contributory roles, including CMV and non-CMV community-acquired respiratory infections) [90,103–105]; injury to the allograft or airways [106–108]; human leukocyte antigen (HLA) mis-matching [57]; organizing pneumonia [8,62,102]. Marked HLA mismatches was associated with greater rates of late graft failure and OB in some studies [62,109–111], but analysis of >3,500 LTRs from the ISHLT database found no significant association between HLA mismatching and development of BOS [112]. This lack of association likely reflects the fact >95% of LTRs have more than 2 HLA mis-matches [112]. This high degree of HLA mismatching reflects the need to harvest donor organs within a few hours, precluding HLA matching between donors and recipients prior to transplantation [57]. Plausible, but unproven, risk factors for BOS include nonimmune injury to the lung allograft or airway [106–108]. The pathogenesis of BOS among LTRs is complex and involves myriad cell types and release of diverse cytokines and chemokines [8,113].

Diagnosis of BOS

Confirming the diagnosis of OB histologically is difficult. Because of the patchy nature of OB, and small sample size, the yield of TBBs in detecting OB is low

(<15–48%) [114–116]. Surgical lung biopsy has a greater yield but is infrequently performed. A diagnosis of BOS is presumed when LTRs develop progressive airflow obstruction not explained by other etiologies.

Pulmonary function tests in patients with OB demonstrate a decrease in expiratory flow rates (e.g., forced expiratory volume in one second [FEV_1] or maximum midexpiratory flow rates [$MMEF_{25-75}$]) [117]. Typically, there is no improvement followed inhaled bronchodilators. Spirometry is useful to diagnose and follow the course of BOS. In 1993, a consensus committee sponsored by the ISHLT proposed a clinical definition of BOS among LTRs; identification of BOS and severity was based on spirometric values [118]. In a later publication, BOS was divided into five stages, based on severity of pulmonary dysfunction [119]. Further, subtypes were identified as follows: "a": no pathological material available; "b": pathological evidence for OB.

Spirometry remains the key surrogate parameter to identify patient with BOS, and follow-the course of the disease. In two recent studies, serial FEV_1 values were as sensitive and specific as $MMEF_{25-75}$ criteria [120,121]. Exhaled nitric oxide [122], exhaled breath condensate [122], single breath washout tests [123], and serum or urine biomarkers [57] have been applied to detect acute or chronic lung allograft rejection, but these sophisticated studies have not been shown to be superior to spirometry.

The use HRCT scans demonstrates dilation of proximal bronchi, bronchial wall thickening, patchy areas of low attenuation (hyperlucency), and a mosaic pattern of attenuation in 62–80% of LTRs with OB [8,124–126]. End-expiratory images are more senstitive than inspiratory CT scans [124–126]. The extent of air-trapping on expiratory CT correlated with BOS severity, but spirometry is superior to CT in this regard [124]. However, CT has an adjunctive role to exclude other causes of airflow obstruction from BOS (e.g., anastomotic complications or stenosis, infection, hyperinflation of the contralateral lung, to name a few). The use of BAL demonstrates the presence of increased neutrophils [127–130] and up-regulation of certain cytokines [8,129–133] in patients with BOS or at risk for BOS. However, the clinical value of BAL is controversial.

Clinical Course and Features of BOS

The onset of BOS is variable, ranging from 3 months to >9 years after LT [8,57,134]. Progressive airflow obstruction, recurrent lower respiratory tract infections and, ultimately, fatal respiratory insufficiency, is typical [57,62,92,135]. Physical examination is often unrevealing. Rales, wheezing, rhonchi, and inspiratory "squeaks" are late findings. Late in the course of BOS, superinfection and/or colonization with *Pseudomonas aeruginosa* or *Aspergillus spp* is common.

Five-year mortality post-onset of BOS ranges from 57% to 74% [57,62,92,134–136]. However, the course is variable [134,136]. BOS may present insidiously or suddenly [57,134,136]. In some LTRs, a gradual and inexorable downhill course ensues. In others, the disease is quiescent after an initial abrupt decrease in lung function, with prolonged periods of stability (months or even years). Respiratory viral infections may be associated with an abrupt onset of BOS and precipitous decline in lung function [62,103,104]. Early-onset" BOS (defined as within the first 3 years of LT) has a more rapid decline in FEV_1, greater need for oxygen dependency, and mortality compared with late-onset BOS (i.e., >3 years) [134,136]. It is possible that differences in clinical course and prognosis reflect differences in cellular profiles and pathogenic mechanisms in accelerated versus chronic OB.

Therapy for BOS

Unforunately, no therapy for BOS has been shown to improve survival [57]. Intensification (augmentation) of immunosuppression is the cornerstone of therapy for AR, but it has not been shown to alter the outcome of BOS or BO [57,137]. Pulse methylprednisolone, adding or altering immunosuppressive regimens, the addition of methotrexate [138], cyclophosphamide [139], rapamycin [140,141], cytolytic agents (e.g., OKT3 antibody, antilymphocyte globulin, antithymocyte globulin) [142], interleukin-2 receptor antagonists (e.g., daclizumab, basiliximab) [142,143], total lymphoid irradiation [144], extracorporeal phototherapy [145], and aerosolized cyclosporin A [146] have been used [57], but none of these regimens has been proven to influence pulmonary function or survival. Data regarding treatment for OB or BOS are limited to small nonrandomized studies and anecdotal reports.

Recently, azithromycin has been used, with anecdotal successes, in LTRs with BOS [147–150]. In the sentinel study, five of six LTRs with BOS improved their FEV_1 (by a mean of 17%) [147]. In a subsequent prospective study, 14 LTRs with BOS were treated with azithromycin (in addition to conventional immunosuppression) for 3 months [149]. Overall, mean FEV_1 increased by 13% and BAL neutrophils and interleukin-8 levels decreased. Importantly, FEV_1 increased more than 10% above baseline in six patients (43%). By contrast, Shirit et al [150] cited stable FEV_1 (mean duration follow-up 10 months) among 11 LTRs with BOS treated with azithromycin in an open-label trial (nine were colonized with *Pseudomonas aeruginosa*). Although no patient improved, azithromycin may have slowed the rate of disease progression. Given the limited number of patients in these various studies, and the lack of placebo-controlled trials, the value of azithromycin remains unproven.

A link between gastroesophageal reflux (GER) and BOS has been suggested [67,151]. The incidence of GER increases after LT [65,66,152]. The mechanisms by which LT increases the incidence of GER is likely multifactorial, reflecting dysfunction of the vagus nerve and effects of immunosuppressive medications on gastric emptying and lower esophageal sphincter function [67]. Aggressive treatment of GER among LTRs may improve lung function [67,153]. In one study of LTRs with GER, fundoplication was shown to improve lung function and survival [153]. For patients with BOS who are unresponsive to medical therapy, retransplantation is an option. However, given the limited number of donor organs, the ethics and role of retransplantation is this context is controversial.

Pulmonary Complications of HSCT

HSCT is associated with myriad pulmonary complications, including infections; diffuse alveolar hemorrhage; pre-engraftment respiratory distress; acute pulmonary edema; idiopathic pulmonary syndrome (i.e., diffuse alveolar damage); delayed pulmonary toxicity syndrome; pulmonary embolism; and bronchiolar disorders (both OP and OB) [9,80,154]. In this chapter, we limit our discussion to the bronchiolar disorders (OB and OP).

OB as a Complication of HSCT

OB is a late complication of allogeneic HSCT, occurring >3 months to years after HSCT [79,154–156]. The incidence of OB ranges from 4% to 26% among allogeneic HSCT recipients but is exceptionally rare after autologous HSCT [9,79,80,154,155]. Most cases are associated with chronic graft versus host disease [9,79,80]. The pathogenesis of OB may reflect bronchial epithelial injury induced by donor cytotoxic T cells [9]. However, recipient bone marrow-derived fibroblasts and myofibroblasts likely contribute to the fibrotic process [91]. Additional risk factors for OB include older donor and recipient age, myeloablative conditioning, methotrexate use, antecedent respiratory infection, and immunoglobulin deficiency [9,79]. Recurrent viral infections has also been implicated as a risk factor for OB among HSCT recipients [155].

Clinical features are consistent with OB in other disorders: irreversible airflow obstruction; dry cough; dyspnea; and wheezing [79,80]. Chest radiographs may be normal or show hyperinflation; HRCT may reveal bronchial dilation, centrilobular nodules, decreased lung attenuation, and expiratory air trapping [79]. BAL may show increases in neutrophils or lymphocytes or both [80,157]. Twenty percent of HSCT recipients with OB and abnormal PFTs are asymptomatic at the time of diagnosis [80]. Transbronchial lung biopsies are usually nondiagnostic. Surgical lung biopsies may show fibrous obliteration of bronchiolar lumens [79] but are rarely indicated because the diagnosis can be presumed without histological confirmation, provided the clinical features are characteristic and other causes have been excluded) [9,79,80,158,159].

The clinical course is variable. Disease progression may be rapid, whereas others exhibit a more protracted course [9,155]. CS or intensification of immunosuppression have been the mainstay of therapy, with favorable responses in 8–20% of treated patients [9,79,80,155,156,158,160]. One recent study cited improvement or stabilization with high-dose pulse methylprednisolone therapy in seven of nine children with OB complicating HSCT [161]. However, given the lack of randomized, controlled trials, the benefit of this approach is unproven. A favourable response to infliximab (a monoclonal antibody directed against tumour necrosis factor-α) was cited in a child with OB after HSCT [162]. Macrolide antibiotics have been used, but data are limited to small, uncontrolled trials. One study of eight HSCT recipients with OB cited benefit with azithromycin [156].

Irrespective of therapy, fatality rates among HSCT recipients with OB typically exceed 50% [79,80]. In one study of 47 HSCT recipients with OB, only 10% survived 5 years (compared with 40% without OB) [158]. LT may be an option for a patient with life-threatening OB recalcitrant to medical therapy [163].

OP as a Complication of HSCT

OP is a rare complication of HSCT. Only anecdotal case reports [79,80,164] and small series [13,159,165–167] have been published. Clinical, radiographic [166], and histopathological features are similar to COP [79,80]. PFTs demonstrate a restrictive defect, with no evidence for airflow obstruction [79,80]. Chest radiographs and CT show patchy, bilateral, consolidation, GGOs, and nodules [166]. Given the myriad other causes of "pneumonic-like" infiltrates in HSCT recipients, a definitive diagnosis of OP usually requires surgical lung biopsy [80].

CS are the mainstay of therapy, with favorable responses in 80% of patients [79,80]. However, in one study, case fatality rate was 19% among HRST recipients with OP [79]. A favourable response to macrolides plus CS were cited in one HSCT recipient with BOOP [164].

References

1. Poletti V, Costabel U. Bronchiolar disorders: classification and diagnostic approach. Semin Respir Crit Care Med 2003;24:457–464.
2. Couture C, Colby TV. Histopathology of bronchiolar disorders. Semin Respir Crit Care Med 2003;24:489–498.
3. Wright JL, Cagle P, Churg A, Colby TV, Myers J. Diseases of the small airways. Am Rev Respir Dis 1992;146:240–262.
4. Ryu JH. Classification and approach to bronchiolar diseases. Curr Opin Pulm Med 2006;12:145–151.
5. Ryu JH, Myers JL, Swensen SJ. Bronchiolar disorders. Am J Respir Crit Care Med 2003; 168:1277–1292.
6. White ES, Tazelaar HD, Lynch JP, 3rd. Bronchiolar complications of connective tissue diseases. Semin Respir Crit Care Med 2003;24:543–566.
7. Boswell RT, McCunney RJ. Bronchiolitis obliterans from exposure to incinerator fly ash. J Occup Environ Med 1995;37:850–855.
8. Belperio JA, Lake K, Tazelaar H, Keane MP, Strieter RM, Lynch JP, 3rd. Bronchiolitis obliterans syndrome complicating lung or heart-lung transplantation. Semin Respir Crit Care Med 2003;24:499–530.
9. Kotloff RM, Ahya VN, Crawford SW. Pulmonary complications of solid organ and hematopoietic stem cell transplantation. Am J Respir Crit Care Med 2004;170:22–48.
10. Mahadeva R, Walsh G, Flower CD, Shneerson JM. Clinical and radiological characteristics of lung disease in inflammatory bowel disease. Eur Respir J 2000;15:41–48.

11. Paganin F, Seneterre E, Chanez P, Daurés JP, Bruel JM, Michel FB, Bousquet J. Computed tomography of the lungs in asthma: influence of disease severity and etiology. Am J Respir Crit Care Med 1996;153:110–114.

12. Reittner P, Muller Nl, Heyneman L, Johkoh T, Park JS, Lee KS, Honda O, Tomiyama N. *Mycoplasma pneumoniae* pneumonia: radiographic and high-resolution ct features in 28 patients. AJR Am J Roentgenol 2000;174:37–41.

13. Alasaly K, Muller N, Ostrow DN, Champion P, FitzGerald JM. Cryptogenic organizing pneumonia. A report of 25 cases and a review of the literature. Medicine (Baltimore) 1995;74: 201–211.

14. Cordier JF. Organising pneumonia. Thorax 2000;55:318–328.

15. Schlesinger C, Koss MN. The organizing pneumonias: an update and review. Curr Opin Pulm Med 2005;11:422–430.

16. Schlesinger C, Veeraraghavan S, Koss MN. Constrictive (obliterative) bronchiolitis. Curr Opin Pulm Med 1998;4:288–293.

17. Myers JL, Colby TV. Pathologic manifestations of bronchiolitis, constrictive bronchiolitis, cryptogenic organizing pneumonia, and diffuse panbronchiolitis. Clin Chest Med 1993;14: 611–622.

18. Pipavath SJ, Lynch DA, Cool C, Brown KK, Newell JD. Radiologic and pathologic features of bronchiolitis. AJR Am J Roentgenol 2005;185:354–363.

19. King TE, Jr. Miscellaneous causes of bronchiolitis: inhalational, infectious, drug-induced, and idiopathic. Semin Respir Crit Care Med 2003;24:567–576.

20. Wells AU, Nicholson AG, Hansell DM, du Bois RM. Respiratory bronchiolitis-associated interstitial lung disease. Semin Respir Crit Care Med 2003;24:585–594.

21. Fraig M, Shreesha U, Savici D, Katzenstein AL. Respiratory bronchiolitis: a clinicopathologic study in current smokers, ex-smokers, and never-smokers. Am J Surg Pathol 2002;26:647–653.

22. Moon J, du Bois RM, Colby TV, Hansell DM, Nicholson AG. Clinical significance of respiratory bronchiolitis on open lung biopsy and its relationship to smoking related interstitial lung disease. Thorax 1999;54:1009–1014.

23. Churg A, Wright JL. Bronchiolitis caused by occupational and ambient atmospheric particles. Semin Respir Crit Care Med 2003;24:577–584.

24. Howling SJ, Hansell DM, Wells AU, Nicholson AG, Flint JD, Muller NL. Follicular bronchiolitis: thin-section CT and histologic findings. Radiology 1999;212:637–642.

25. Verschakelen JA. Imaging of the small airways. Semin Respir Crit Care Med 2003;24: 473–488.

26. Kudoh S, Keicho N. Diffuse panbronchiolitis. Semin Respir Crit Care Med 2003;24: 607–618.

27. Fitzgerald JE, King TE, Jr., Lynch DA, Tuder RM, Schwarz MI. Diffuse panbronchiolitis in the United States. Am J Respir Crit Care Med 1996;154:497–503.

28. Colby TV. Bronchiolitis. Pathologic considerations. Am J Clin Pathol 1998;109:101–109.

29. Yousem SA, Dacic S. Idiopathic bronchiolocentric interstitial pneumonia. Mod Pathol 2002;15:1148–1153.

30. Hansell DM, Rubens MB, Padley SP, Wells AU. Obliterative bronchiolitis: individual CT signs of small airways disease and functional correlation. Radiology 1997;203: 721–726.

31. Hansell DM. HRCT of obliterative bronchiolitis and other small airways diseases. Semin Roentgenol 2001;36:51–65.

32. Collins J, Blankenbaker D, Stern EJ. CT patterns of bronchiolar disease: what is "tree-in-bud"? AJR Am J Roentgenol 1998;171:365–370.

33. Muller NL, Miller RR. Diseases of the bronchioles: CT and histopathologic findings. Radiology 1995;196:3–12.

34. Adler BD, Padley SP, Muller NL, Remy-Jardin M, Remy J. Chronic hypersensitivity pneumonitis: high-resolution CT and radiographic features in 16 patients. Radiology 1992;185: 91–95.

35. Sherrick AD, Swensen SJ, Hartman TE. Mosaic pattern of lung attenuation on CT scans: frequency among patients with pulmonary artery hypertension of different causes. AJR Am J Roentgenol 1997;169:79–82.

36. Davison AG, Heard BE, McAllister WA, Turner-Warwick ME. Cryptogenic organizing pneumonitis. Q J Med 1983;52:382–394.

37. Epler GR, Colby TV, McLoud TC, Carrington CB, Gaensler EA. Bronchiolitis obliterans organizing pneumonia. N Engl J Med 1985;312:152–158.

38. American Thoracic Society/European Respiratory Society International Multidisciplinary Consensus Classification of the Idiopathic Interstitial Pneumonias. This joint statement of the American Thoracic Society (ATS), and the European Respiratory Society (ERS) was adopted by the ATS board of directors, June 2001 and by the ERS Executive Committee, June 2001. Am J Respir Crit Care Med 2002;165:277–304.

39. Lazor R, Vandevenne A, Pelletier A, Leclerc P, Court-Fortune I, Cordier JF. Cryptogenic organizing pneumonia. Characteristics of relapses in a series of 48 patients. The Groupe d'Etudes et de Recherche sur les Maladles "Orphelines" Pulmonaires (GERM"O"P). Am J Respir Crit Care Med 2000;162:571–577.

40. Ujita M, Renzoni EA, Veeraraghavan S, Wells AU, Hansell DM. Organizing pneumonia: perilobular pattern at thin-section CT. Radiology 2004;232:757–761.

41. Kim SJ, Lee KS, Ryu YH, et al. Reversed halo sign on high-resolution CT of cryptogenic organizing pneumonia: diagnostic implications. AJR Am J Roentgenol 2003;180: 1251–1254.

42. Lee JS, Lynch DA, Sharma S, Brown KK, Muller NL. Organizing pneumonia: prognostic implication of high-resolution computed tomography features. J Comput Assist Tomogr 2003;27:260–265.

43. Lee KS, Kullnig P, Hartman TE, Muller NL. Cryptogenic organizing pneumonia: CT findings in 43 patients. AJR Am J Roentgenol 1994;162:543–546.

44. Yousem SA, Lohr RH, Colby TV. Idiopathic bronchiolitis obliterans organizing pneumonia/ cryptogenic organizing pneumonia with unfavorable outcome: pathologic predictors. Mod Pathol 1997;10:864–871.

45. Cohen AJ, King TE, Jr., Downey GP. Rapidly progressive bronchiolitis obliterans with organizing pneumonia. Am J Respir Crit Care Med 1994;149:1670–1675.

46. Perez de Llano LA, Soilan JL, Garcia Pais MJ, Mata I, Moreda M, Laserna B. Idiopathic bronchiolitis obliterans with organizing pneumonia presenting with adult respiratory distress syndrome. Respir Med 1998;92:884–886.

47. Crestani B, Kambouchner M, Soler P, et al. Migratory bronchiolitis obliterans organizing pneumonia after unilateral radiation therapy for breast carcinoma. Eur Respir J 1995;8: 318–321.

48. Bayle JY, Nesme P, Bejui-Thivolet F, Loire R, Guerin JC, Cordier JF. Migratory organizing pneumonitis "primed" by radiation therapy. Eur Respir J 1995;8:322–326.

49. Stover DE, Mangino D. Macrolides: a treatment alternative for bronchiolitis obliterans organizing pneumonia? Chest 2005;128:3611–3617.

50. Takigawa N, Segawa Y, Saeki T, et al. Kataoka M, Ida M, Kishino D, Fujiwara K, Ohsumi S, Eguchi K, Takashima S. Bronchiolitis obliterans organizing pneumonia syndrome in breast-conserving therapy for early breast cancer: radiation-induced lung toxicity. Int J Radiat Oncol Biol Phys 2000;48:751–755.

51. Miwa S, Morita S, Suda T, Suzuki K, Hayakawa H, Chida K, Nakamura H. The incidence and clinical characteristics of bronchiolitis obliterans organizing pneumonia syndrome after radiation therapy for breast cancer. Sarcoidosis Vasc Diffuse Lung Dis 2004;21:212–218.

52. Kaufman J, Komorowski R. Bronchiolitis obliterans. A new clinical-pathologic complication of irradiation pneumonitis. Chest 1990;97:1243–1244.

53. Crestani B, Valeyre D, Roden S, Wallaert B, Dalphin JC, Cordier JF. Bronchiolitis obliterans organizing pneumonia syndrome primed by radiation therapy to the breast. The Groupe d'Etudes et de Recherche sur les Maladies Orphelines Pulmonaires (GERM"O"P). Am J Respir Crit Care Med 1998;158:1929–1935.

54. Roberts CM, Foulcher E, Zaunders JJ, et al. Radiation pneumonitis: a possible lymphocyte-mediated hypersensitivity reaction. Ann Intern Med 1993;118:696–700.
55. Rubin BK, Henke MO. Immunomodulatory activity and effectiveness of macrolides in chronic airway disease. Chest 2004;125(2 Suppl):70S–78S.
56. Labro MT, Abdelghaffar H. Immunomodulation by macrolide antibiotics. J Chemother 2001;13:3–8.
57. Knoop C, Estenne M. Acute and chronic rejection after lung transplantation. Semin Respir Crit Care Med 2006;27:521–533.
58. Abernathy EC, Hruban RH, Baumgartner WA, Reitz BA, Hutchins GM. The two forms of bronchiolitis obliterans in heart-lung transplant recipients. Hum Pathol 1991;22:1102–1110.
59. Yousem SA, Duncan SR, Griffith BP. Interstitial and airspace granulation tissue reactions in lung transplant recipients. Am J Surg Pathol 1992;16:877–884.
60. Milne DS, Gascoigne AD, Ashcroft T, Sviland L, Malcolm AJ, Corris PA. Organizing pneumonia following pulmonary transplantation and the development of obliterative bronchiolitis. Transplantation 1994;57:1757–1762.
61. Chaparro C, Chamberlain D, Maurer J, Winton T, Dehoyos A, Kesten S. Bronchiolitis obliterans organizing pneumonia (BOOP) in lung transplant recipients. Chest 1996;110:1150–1154.
62. Heng D, Sharples LD, McNeil K, Stewart S, Wreghitt T, Wallwork J. Bronchiolitis obliterans syndrome: incidence, natural history, prognosis, and risk factors. J Heart Lung Transplant 1998;17:1255–1263.
63. Reid KR, McKenzie FN, Menkis AH, Novick RJ, Pflugfelder PW, Kostuk WJ, Ahmad D. Importance of chronic aspiration in recipients of heart-lung transplants. Lancet 1990;336:206–208.
64. Miyagawa-Hayashino A, Wain JC, Mark EJ. Lung transplantation biopsy specimens with bronchiolitis obliterans or bronchiolitis obliterans organizing pneumonia due to aspiration. Arch Pathol Lab Med 2005;129:223–226.
65. Palmer SM, Miralles AP, Howell DN, Brazer SR, Tapson VF, Davis RD. Gastroesophageal reflux as a reversible cause of allograft dysfunction after lung transplantation. Chest 2000;118:1214–1217.
66. Hadjiliadis D, Duane Davis R, Steele MP, Steele MP, Messier RH, Lau CL, Eubanks SS, Palmer SM. Gastroesophageal reflux disease in lung transplant recipients. Clin Transplant 2003;17:363–368.
67. Verleden GM, Dupont LJ, Van Raemdonck DE. Is it bronchiolitis obliterans syndrome or is it chronic rejection: a reappraisal? Eur Respir J 2005;25:221–224.
68. Gammon RB, Bridges TA, al-Nezir H, Alexander CB, Kennedy JI, Jr. Bronchiolitis obliterans organizing pneumonia associated with systemic lupus erythematosus. Chest 1992;102:1171–1174.
69. Matteson EL, Ike RW. Bronchiolitis obliterans organizing pneumonia and Sjogren's syndrome. J Rheumatol 1990;17:676–679.
70. Mana F, Mets T, Vincken W, Sennesael J, Vanwaeyenbergh J, Goossens A. The association of bronchiolitis obliterans organizing pneumonia, systemic lupus erythematosus, and Hunner's cystitis. Chest 1993;104:642–644.
71. Kinney WW, Angelillo VA. Bronchiolitis in systemic lupus erythematosus. Chest 1982;82:646–649.
72. Yoshida K, Mouri T, Kuroda S, Suzuki J, Yamauch K, Inoue H, Saito R, Sawai T. A case of Sjogren syndrome associated with bronchiolitis obliterans organizing pneumonia [in Japanese]. Nippon Naika Gakkai Zasshi 2001;90:329–331.
73. Camus P, Piard F, Ashcroft T, Gal AA, Colby TV. The lung in inflammatory bowel disease. Medicine (Baltimore) 1993;72:151–183.
74. Akpinar-Elci M, Travis WD, Lynch DA, Kreiss K. Bronchiolitis obliterans syndrome in popcorn production plant workers. Eur Respir J 2004;24:298–302.
75. Kreiss K, Gomaa A, Kullman G, Fedan K, Simoes EJ, Enright PL. Clinical bronchiolitis obliterans in workers at a microwave-popcorn plant. N Engl J Med 2002;347:330–338.

76. Kern DG, Crausman RS, Durand KT, Nayer A, Kuhn C, 3rd. Flock worker's lung: chronic interstitial lung disease in the nylon flocking industry. Ann Intern Med 1998;129:261–272.
77. Mann JM, Sha KK, Kline G, Breuer FU, Miller A. World Trade Center dyspnea: bronchiolitis obliterans with functional improvement: a case report. Am J Ind Med 2005;48:225–229.
78. Schlesinger C, Meyer CA, Veeraraghavan S, Koss MN. Constrictive (obliterative) bronchiolitis: diagnosis, etiology, and a critical review of the literature. Ann Diagn Pathol 1998; 2:321–334.
79. Afessa B, Litzow MR, Tefferi A. Bronchiolitis obliterans and other late onset non-infectious pulmonary complications in hematopoietic stem cell transplantation. Bone Marrow Transplant 2001;28:425–434.
80. Afessa B, Peters SG. Major complications following hematopoietic stem cell transplantation. Semin Respir Crit Care Med 2006;27:297–309.
81. Hernandez JI, Gomez-Roman J, Rodrigo E, Olmos JM, González-Vela C, Ruiz JC, Val JF, Riancho JA. . Bronchiolitis obliterans and iga nephropathy. A new cause of pulmonary-renal syndrome. Am J Respir Crit Care Med 1997;156:665–668.
82. Ito M, Nakagawa A, Hirabayashi N, Asai J. Bronchiolitis obliterans in ataxia-telangiectasia. Virchows Arch 1997;430:131–137.
83. Parto K, Svedstrom E, Majurin ML, Harkonen R, Simell O. Pulmonary manifestations in lysinuric protein intolerance. Chest 1993;104:1176–1182.
84. Chang H, Wang JS, Tseng HH, Lai RS, Su JM. Histopathological study of Sauropus androgynus-associated constrictive bronchiolitis obliterans: a new cause of constrictive bronchiolitis obliterans. Am J Surg Pathol 1997;21:35–42.
85. Mahajan L, Kay M, Wyllie R, Steffen R, Goldfarb J. Ulcerative colitis presenting with bronchiolitis obliterans organizing pneumonia in a pediatric patient. Am J Gastroenterol 1997;92:2123–2124.
86. D'Ovidio F, Mura M, Tsang M, Waddell TK, Hutcheon MA, Singer LG, Hadjiliadis D, Chaparro C, Gutierrez C, Pierre A, Darling G, Liu M, Keshavjee S. Bile acid aspiration and the development of bronchiolitis obliterans after lung transplantation. J Thorac Cardiovasc Surg 2005;129:1144–1152.
87. Lee JS, Brown KK, Cool C, Lynch DA. Diffuse pulmonary neuroendocrine cell hyperplasia: radiologic and clinical features. J Comput Assist Tomogr 2002;26:180–184.
88. Aguayo SM, Miller YE, Waldron JA, Jr., Bogin RM, Sunday ME, Staton GW Jr, Beam WR, King TE Jr. Brief report: idiopathic diffuse hyperplasia of pulmonary neuroendocrine cells and airways disease. N Engl J Med 1992;327:1285–1288.
89. Kraft M, Mortenson RL, Colby TV, Newman L, Waldron JA, Jr., King TE, Jr. Cryptogenic constrictive bronchiolitis. A clinicopathologic study. Am Rev Respir Dis 1993;148:1093–1101.
90. Scott AI, Sharples LD, Stewart S. Bronchiolitis obliterans syndrome: risk factors and therapeutic strategies. Drugs 2005;65:761–71.
91. Brocker V, Langer F, Fellous TG, Mengel M, Brittan M, Bredt M, Milde S, Welte T, Eder M, Haverich A, Alison MR, Kreipe H, Lehmann U. Fibroblasts of recipient origin contribute to bronchiolitis obliterans in human lung transplants. Am J Respir Crit Care Med 2006; 173:1276–1282.
92. Estenne M, Hertz MI. Bronchiolitis obliterans after human lung transplantation. Am J Respir Crit Care Med 2002;166:440–444.
93. Meyers BF, Lynch J, Trulock EP, Guthrie TJ, Cooper JD, Patterson GA. Lung transplantation: a decade of experience. Ann Surg 1999;230:362–370; discussion 70–71.
94. Whitehead B, Rees P, Sorensen K, Bull C, Higenbottam TW, Wallwork J, Fabre J, Elliott M, de Leval M. Incidence of obliterative bronchiolitis after heart-lung transplantation in children. J Heart Lung Transplant 1993;12:903–908.
95. Trulock EP, Edwards LB, Taylor DO, Boucek MM, Keck BM, Hertz MI. Registry of the International Society for Heart and Lung Transplantation: twenty-second official adult lung and heart-lung transplant report—2005. J Heart Lung Transplant 2005;24:956–967.
96. Glanville AR. The role of bronchoscopic surveillance monitoring in the care of lung transplant recipients. Semin Respir Crit Care Med 2006;27:480–491.

97. Sharples LD, McNeil K, Stewart S, Wallwork J. Risk factors for bronchiolitis obliterans: a systematic review of recent publications. J Heart Lung Transplant 2002;21:271–281.

98. Khalifah AP, Hachem RR, Chakinala MM, Yusen RD, Aloush A, Patterson GA, Mohanakumar T, Trulock EP, Walter MJ. Minimal acute rejection after lung transplantation: a risk for bronchiolitis obliterans syndrome. Am J Transplant 2005;5:2022–2030.

99. Hachem RR, Khalifah AP, Chakinala MM, Yusen RD, Aloush AA, Mohanakumar T, Patterson GA, Trulock EP, Walter MJ. The significance of a single episode of minimal acute rejection after lung transplantation. Transplantation 2005;80:1406–1413.

100. Hopkins PM, Aboyoun CL, Chhajed PN, et al. Association of minimal rejection in lung transplant recipients with obliterative bronchiolitis. Am J Respir Crit Care Med 2004;170: 1022–1026.

101. Girgis RE, Tu I, Berry GJ, et al. Risk factors for the development of obliterative bronchiolitis after lung transplantation. J Heart Lung Transplant 1996;15:1200–1208.

102. Husain AN, Siddiqui MT, Holmes EW, Chandrasekhar AJ, McCabe M, Radvany R, Garrity ER. Analysis of risk factors for the development of bronchiolitis obliterans syndrome. Am J Respir Crit Care Med 1999;159:829–833.

103. Kumar D, Erdman D, Keshavjee S, Peret T, Tellier R, Hadjiliadis D, Johnson G, Ayers M, Siegal D, Humar A. Clinical impact of community-acquired respiratory viruses on bronchiolitis obliterans after lung transplant. Am J Transplant 2005;5:2031–2036.

104. Vilchez RA, Dauber J, McCurry K, Iacono A, Kusne S. Parainfluenza virus infection in adult lung transplant recipients: an emergent clinical syndrome with implications on allograft function. Am J Transplant 2003;3:116–120.

105. Gerna G, Vitulo P, Rovida F, Lilleri D, Pellegrini C, Oggionni T, Campanini G, Baldanti F, Revello MG. Impact of human metapneumovirus and human cytomegalovirus versus other respiratory viruses on the lower respiratory tract infections of lung transplant recipients. J Med Virol 2006;78:408–416.

106. Bando K, Paradis IL, Similo S, Konishi H, Komatsu K, Zullo TG, Yousem SA, Close JM, Zeevi A, Duquesnoy RJ, et al. Obliterative bronchiolitis after lung and heart-lung transplantation. An analysis of risk factors and management. J Thorac Cardiovasc Surg 1995;110:4–13; discussion-4.

107. King RC, Binns OA, Rodriguez F, et al. Reperfusion injury significantly impacts clinical outcome after pulmonary transplantation. Ann Thorac Surg 2000;69:1681–1685.

108. Fisher AJ, Wardle J, Dark JH, Corris PA. Non-immune acute graft injury after lung transplantation and the risk of subsequent bronchiolitis obliterans syndrome (BOS). J Heart Lung Transplant 2002;21:1206–1212.

109. Keogh A, Kaan A, Doran T, Macdonald P, Bryant D, Spratt P. HLA mismatching and outcome in heart, heart-lung, and single lung transplantation. J Heart Lung Transplant 1995;14:444–451.

110. Wisser W, Wekerle T, Zlabinger G, Senbaclavaci O, Zuckermann A, Klepetko W, Wolner E. Influence of human leukocyte antigen matching on long-term outcome after lung transplantation. J Heart Lung Transplant 1996;15:1209–1216.

111. Kroshus TJ, Kshettry VR, Savik K, John R, Hertz MI, Bolman RM, 3rd. Risk factors for the development of bronchiolitis obliterans syndrome after lung transplantation. J Thorac Cardiovasc Surg 1997;114:195–202.

112. Quantz MA, Bennett LE, Meyer DM, Novick RJ. Does human leukocyte antigen matching influence the outcome of lung transplantation? An analysis of 3,549 lung transplantations. J Heart Lung Transplant 2000;19:473–479.

113. Snyder LD, Palmer SM. Immune mechanisms of lung allograft rejection. Semin Respir Crit Care Med 2006;27:534–543.

114. Chamberlain D, Maurer J, Chaparro C, Idolor L. Evaluation of transbronchial lung biopsy specimens in the diagnosis of bronchiolitis obliterans after lung transplantation. J Heart Lung Transplant 1994;13:963–971.

115. Hopkins PM, Aboyoun CL, Chhajed PN, Malouf MA, Plit ML, Rainer SP, Glanville AR. Prospective analysis of 1,235 transbronchial lung biopsies in lung transplant recipients. J Heart Lung Transplant 2002;21:1062–1067.

116. Sundaresan S, Trulock EP, Mohanakumar T, Cooper JD, Patterson GA. Prevalence and outcome of bronchiolitis obliterans syndrome after lung transplantation. Washington University Lung Transplant Group. Ann Thorac Surg 1995;60:1341–1346; discussion 6–7.
117. Nathan SD, Barnett SD, Wohlrab J, Burton N. Bronchiolitis obliterans syndrome: utility of the new guidelines in single lung transplant recipients. J Heart Lung Transplant 2003;22: 427–432.
118. Cooper JD, Billingham M, Egan T, Hertz MI, Higenbottam T, Lynch J, Mauer J, Paradis I, Patterson GA, Smith C, et al.A working formulation for the standardization of nomenclature and for clinical staging of chronic dysfunction in lung allografts. International Society for Heart and Lung Transplantation. J Heart Lung Transplant 1993;12:713–716.
119. Estenne M, Maurer JR, Boehler A, Egan JJ, Frost A, Hertz M, Mallory GB, Snell GI, Yousem S. Bronchiolitis obliterans syndrome 2001: an update of the diagnostic criteria. J Heart Lung Transplant 2002;21:297–310.
120. Lama VN, Murray S, Mumford JA, Flaherty KR, Chang A, Toews GB, Peters-Golden M, Martinez FJ. Prognostic value of bronchiolitis obliterans syndrome stage 0-p in single-lung transplant recipients. Am J Respir Crit Care Med 2005;172:379–383.
121. Hachem RR, Chakinala MM, Yusen RD, Lynch JP, Aloush AA, Patterson GA, Trulock EP. The predictive value of bronchiolitis obliterans syndrome stage 0-p. Am J Respir Crit Care Med 2004;169:468–472.
122. Studer SM, Orens JB, Rosas I, Krishnan JA, Cope KA, Yang S, Conte JV, Becker PB, Risby TH. Patterns and significance of exhaled-breath biomarkers in lung transplant recipients with acute allograft rejection. J Heart Lung Transplant 2001;20:1158–1166.
123. Van Muylem A, Melot C, Antoine M, Knoop C, Estenne M. Role of pulmonary function in the detection of allograft dysfunction after heart-lung transplantation. Thorax 1997;52:643–647.
124. Lee ES, Gotway MB, Reddy GP, Golden JA, Keith FM, Webb WR. Early bronchiolitis obliterans following lung transplantation: accuracy of expiratory thin-section CT for diagnosis. Radiology 2000;216:472–477.
125. Siegel MJ, Bhalla S, Gutierrez FR, Hildebolt C, Sweet S. Post-lung transplantation bronchiolitis obliterans syndrome: usefulness of expiratory thin-section CT for diagnosis. Radiology 2001;220:455–462.
126. Bankier AA, Van Muylem A, Knoop C, Estenne M, Gevenois PA. Bronchiolitis obliterans syndrome in heart-lung transplant recipients: diagnosis with expiratory CT. Radiology 2001;218:533–539.
127. Reynaud-Gaubert M, Thomas P, Badier M, Cau P, Giudicelli R, Fuentes P. Early detection of airway involvement in obliterative bronchiolitis after lung transplantation. Functional and bronchoalveolar lavage cell findings. Am J Respir Crit Care Med 2000;161:1924–1929.
128. Zheng L, Walters EH, Ward C, et al. Airway neutrophilia in stable and bronchiolitis obliterans syndrome patients following lung transplantation. Thorax 2000;55:53–59.
129. DiGiovine B, Lynch JP, 3rd, Martinez FJ, et al. Bronchoalveolar lavage neutrophilia is associated with obliterative bronchiolitis after lung transplantation: role of IL-8. J Immunol 1996;157:4194–4202.
130. Slebos DJ, Postma DS, Koeter GH, Van Der Bij W, Boezen M, Kauffman HF. Bronchoalveolar lavage fluid characteristics in acute and chronic lung transplant rejection. J Heart Lung Transplant 2004;23:532–540.
131. Belperio JA, Keane MP, Burdick MD, et al. Critical role for CXCR3 chemokine biology in the pathogenesis of bronchiolitis obliterans syndrome. J Immunol 2002;169:1037–1049.
132. Belperio JA, Keane MP, Burdick MD, et al. Critical role for the chemokine MCP-1/CCR2 in the pathogenesis of bronchiolitis obliterans syndrome. J Clin Invest 2001;108:547–556.
133. Belperio JA, DiGiovine B, Keane MP, et al. Interleukin-1 receptor antagonist as a biomarker for bronchiolitis obliterans syndrome in lung transplant recipients. Transplantation 2002;73: 591–599.
134. Jackson CH, Sharples LD, McNeil K, Stewart S, Wallwork J. Acute and chronic onset of bronchiolitis obliterans syndrome (BOS): are they different entities? J Heart Lung Transplant 2002;21:658–666.

135. Tamm M, Sharples LD, Higenbottam TW, Stewart S, Wallwork J. Bronchiolitis obliterans syndrome in heart-lung transplantation: surveillance biopsies. Am J Respir Crit Care Med 1997;155:1705–1710.

136. Brugiere O, Pessione F, Thabut G, et al. Bronchiolitis obliterans syndrome after single-lung transplantation: impact of time to onset on functional pattern and survival. Chest 2002;121: 1883–1889.

137. Kesten S, Maidenberg A, Winton T, Maurer J. Treatment of presumed and proven acute rejection following six months of lung transplant survival. Am J Respir Crit Care Med 1995; 152:1321–1324.

138. Dusmet M, Maurer J, Winton T, Kesten S. Methotrexate can halt the progression of bronchiolitis obliterans syndrome in lung transplant recipients. J Heart Lung Transplant 1996; 15:948–954.

139. Verleden GM, Buyse B, Delcroix M, et al. Cyclophosphamide rescue therapy for chronic rejection after lung transplantation. J Heart Lung Transplant 1999;18:1139–1142.

140. Cahill BC, Somerville KT, Crompton JA, et al. Early experience with sirolimus in lung transplant recipients with chronic allograft rejection. J Heart Lung Transplant 2003;22:169–176.

141. Ussetti P, Carreno MC, de Pablo A, Gamez P, Varela A. Rapamycin and chronic lung rejection. J Heart Lung Transplant 2004;23:917–918.

142. Brock MV, Borja MC, Ferber L, et al. Induction therapy in lung transplantation: a prospective, controlled clinical trial comparing OKT3, anti-thymocyte globulin, and daclizumab. J Heart Lung Transplant 2001;20:1282–1290.

143. Garrity ER, Jr., Villanueva J, Bhorade SM, Husain AN, Vigneswaran WT. Low rate of acute lung allograft rejection after the use of daclizumab, an interleukin 2 receptor antibody. Transplantation 2001;71:773–777.

144. Fisher AJ, Rutherford RM, Bozzino J, Parry G, Dark JH, Corris PA. The safety and efficacy of total lymphoid irradiation in progressive bronchiolitis obliterans syndrome after lung transplantation. Am J Transplant 2005;5:537–543.

145. Salerno CT, Park SJ, Kreykes NS, Kulick DM, Savik K, Hertz MI, Bolman RM 3rd. Adjuvant treatment of refractory lung transplant rejection with extracorporeal photopheresis. J Thorac Cardiovasc Surg 1999;117:1063–1069.

146. Iacono AT, Johnson BA, Grgurich WF, Youssef JG, Corcoran TE, Seiler DA, Dauber JH, Smaldone GC, Zeevi A, Yousem SA, Fung JJ, Burckart GJ, McCurry KR, Griffith BP. A randomized trial of inhaled cyclosporine in lung-transplant recipients. N Engl J Med 2006;354:141–150.

147. Gerhardt SG, McDyer JF, Girgis RE, Conte JV, Yang SC, Orens JB. Maintenance azithromycin therapy for bronchiolitis obliterans syndrome: results of a pilot study. Am J Respir Crit Care Med 2003;168:121–125.

148. Yates B, Murphy DM, Forrest IA, et al. Azithromycin reverses airflow obstruction in established bronchiolitis obliterans syndrome. Am J Respir Crit Care Med 2005;172:772–775.

149. Verleden GM, Dupont LJ. Azithromycin therapy for patients with bronchiolitis obliterans syndrome after lung transplantation. Transplantation 2004;77:1465–1467.

150. Shitrit D, Bendayan D, Gidon S, Saute M, Bakal I, Kramer MR. Long-term azithromycin use for treatment of bronchiolitis obliterans syndrome in lung transplant recipients. J Heart Lung Transplant 2005;24:1440–1443.

151. Hartwig MG, Appel JZ, Davis RD. Antireflux surgery in the setting of lung transplantation: strategies for treating gastroesophageal reflux disease in a high-risk population. Thorac Surg Clin 2005;15:417–427.

152. Young LR, Hadjiliadis D, Davis RD, Palmer SM. Lung transplantation exacerbates gastroesophageal reflux disease. Chest 2003;124:1689–1693.

153. Davis RD, Jr., Lau CL, Eubanks S, et al. Improved lung allograft function after fundoplication in patients with gastroesophageal reflux disease undergoing lung transplantation. J Thorac Cardiovasc Surg 2003;125:533–542.

154. Sharma S, Nadrous HF, Peters SG, et al. Pulmonary complications in adult blood and marrow transplant recipients: autopsy findings. Chest 2005;128:1385–1392.

155. Chien JW, Martin PJ, Gooley TA, et al. Airflow obstruction after myeloablative allogeneic hematopoietic stem cell transplantation. Am J Respir Crit Care Med 2003;168:208–214.
156. Khalid M, Al Saghir A, Saleemi S, et al. Azithromycin in bronchiolitis obliterans complicating bone marrow transplantation: a preliminary study. Eur Respir J 2005;25:490–493.
157. St John RC, Gadek JE, Tutschka PJ, Kapoor N, Dorinsky PM. Analysis of airflow obstruction by bronchoalveolar lavage following bone marrow transplantation. Implications for pathogenesis and treatment. Chest 1990;98:600–607.
158. Dudek AZ, Mahaseth H, DeFor TE, Weisdorf DJ. Bronchiolitis obliterans in chronic graft-versus-host disease: analysis of risk factors and treatment outcomes. Biol Blood Marrow Transplant 2003;9:657–666.
159. Hayes-Jordan A, Benaim E, Richardson S, Joglar J, Srivastava DK, Bowman L, Shochat SJ. Open lung biopsy in pediatric bone marrow transplant patients. J Pediatr Surg 2002;37: 446–452.
160. Sanchez J, Torres A, Serrano J, Román J, Martín C, Pérula L, Martínez F, Gómez P. Long-term follow-up of immunosuppressive treatment for obstructive airways disease after allogeneic bone marrow transplantation. Bone Marrow Transplant 1997;20:403–408.
161. Ratjen F, Rjabko O, Kremens B. High-dose corticosteroid therapy for bronchiolitis obliterans after bone marrow transplantation in children. Bone Marrow Transplant 2005;36:135–138.
162. Fullmer JJ, Fan LL, Dishop MK, Rodgers C, Krance R. Successful treatment of bronchiolitis obliterans in a bone marrow transplant patient with tumor necrosis factor-alpha blockade. Pediatrics 2005;116:767–770.
163. Favaloro R, Bertolotti A, Gomez C, et al. Lung transplant at the Favaloro Foundation: a 13-year experience. Transplant Proc 2004;36:1689–1691.
164. Ishii T, Manabe A, Ebihara Y, et al. Improvement in bronchiolitis obliterans organizing pneumonia in a child after allogeneic bone marrow transplantation by a combination of oral prednisolone and low dose erythromycin. Bone Marrow Transplant 2000;26:907–910.
165. Palmas A, Tefferi A, Myers JL, et al. Late-onset noninfectious pulmonary complications after allogeneic bone marrow transplantation. Br J Haematol 1998;100:680–687.
166. Dodd JD, Muller NL. Bronchiolitis obliterans organizing pneumonia after bone marrow transplantation: high-resolution computed tomography findings in 4 patients. J Comput Assist Tomogr 2005;29:540–543.
167. Mathew P, Bozeman P, Krance RA, Brenner MK, Heslop HE. Bronchiolitis obliterans organizing pneumonia (BOOP) in children after allogeneic bone marrow transplantation. Bone Marrow Transplant 1994;13:221–223.

Chapter 7
Hypersensitivity Pneumonitis

Moisés Selman, Guillermo Carrillo, Carmen Navarro, and Miguel Gaxiola

Introduction

Hypersensitivity pneumonitis (HP), also known as extrinsic allergic alveolitis, is a complex syndrome of varying intensity, clinical presentation, and natural history [1,2]. Numerous provocative agents have been described around the world, including, mammalian and avian proteins, fungi, thermophilic bacteria, and certain small-molecular-weight chemical compounds (Table 7.1). Importantly, new HP antigens are being constantly described. For example, in the last decade evidence has accumulated supporting that mycobacterium avium complex (MAC), often from hot tub exposure, may provoke the disease [3,4]. Therefore, in the presence of acute respiratory illness or a patient with a clinical behavior of an interstitial lung disease, clinicians should always consider HP in the spectrum of the differential diagnosis and should carefully search for any potential source of HP-related antigens.

The incidence and prevalence of HP remain largely unknown. Much of the epidemiological information has been derived from studies of farmers and bird fanciers and primarily from acute cases. Both the prevalence and incidence of HP varies considerably around the world, depending upon disease definitions and diagnosis, intensity of exposure to offensive antigens, geographical and local conditions, cultural practices, and genetic risk factors. Farmer's lung disease is one of the most common forms of HP, affecting variable percentages of the farming population. For example, the mean annual incidence of farmer's lung among the entire farming population (standardised for age and sex to the total population in Finland in 1975) was 44 per 100,000 persons in farming [5]. However, more recent studies indicate that the incidence of farmer's lung is now in decline [6].

A study estimating the incidence of HP in the UK showed that between 1991 and 2003 the incident rate for this disorder was stable at approximately 0.9 cases per 100,000 person-years [7]. Data from a European survey suggest that HP constitutes 4–13% of all interstitial lung diseases [8]. In general, the prevalence of HP is difficult to estimate accurately because represents a group of syndromes with different causative agents, and because epidemiologic studies lack uniform diagnostic criteria. Overall, the prevalence and incidence of HP are low, in part because a number

R.P. Baughman et al. (eds.), *Pulmonary Arterial Hypertension and Interstitial Lung Diseases,*
© Humana Press, a part of Springer Science + Business Media, LLC 2009

Table 7.1 Identified Agents That Cause HP

Disease	Antigen	Source
Fungal and bacterial		
Farmer's lung	*Saccharopolyspora rectivir-gula, Thermoactinomyces vulgaris, Absidia corymbifera*	Moldy hay, grain, silage
Mushroom worker's lung	*Thermoactinomyces sacchari*	Moldy mushroom compost
Malt worker's lung	*Aspergillus fumigatus, Aspergillus clavus*	Moldy barley
Woodworker's lung	*Alternaria sp,* wood dust	Oak, cedar, and mahogany dust, pine and spruce pulp
Maple bark stripper's lung	*Cryptostroma corticale*	Moldy maple bark
Cheese washer's lung	*Penicillium caseii*	Moldy cheese
Sewage worker's lung	*Cephalosporium*	Sewer
Sequoiosis	*Pullularia*	Moldy sawdust
Stipatosis	*Aspergillus fumigatus*	Esparto fibers
Suberosis	*Penicillium frequentans, Aspergillus fumigatus*	Cork dust
Harwood lung	*Paecilomyces*	Hardwood processing plant
Bagassosis	*Thermoactinomyces sacchari*	Moldy sugarcane
Sauna taker's lung	*Aureobasidium sp, pullularia*	Contaminated sauna water
Ventilation/humidifier lung.	*Thermoactinomyces vulgaris, Thermoactinomyces sacchari, Thermoactinomyces candidus*	Contaminated forced-air systems; water reservoirs
Metal working fluid-associated HP	*Mycobacterium immunogenum*	Metal working fluids
Sax lung	*Candida albicans*	Saxophone
Hot-tub lung	*Mycobacterium avium complex*	Hot-tubs; swimming pools, whirlpools
Summer-type pneumonitis	*Trichosporon cutaneum*	Contaminated old houses
HP in peat moss processing plant workers	*Monocillium sp. Penicillium citreonigrum*	Peat moss processing plants
Animal proteins		
Pigeon breeder's disease	Avian droppings, feathers, serum	Parakeets, budgerigars, pigeons, chickens, turkeys
Furrier's lung	Animal-fur dust	Animal pelts
Animal handler's lung; Laboratory worker's lung	Rats, gerbils	Urine, serum, pelts proteins
Pituitary snuff taker's lung	Pork	Pituitary snuff
Chemical compounds		
Pauli's reagent alveolitis	Sodium diazobenzene sulfate	Laboratory reagent
Chemical worker's lung	Isocyanates; trimellitic anhydride	Polyurethane foams, spray paints, special glues.
Epoxy resin lung	Phthalic anhydride	heated epoxy resin
Pyrethrum pneumonitis	Pyrethrum	Insecticide

of individuals with mild HP are not detected and patients with subacute and chronic disease are misdiagnosed as having other type of interstitial lung disease.

It is well known that HP occurs more frequently in nonsmokers than in cigarette smokers under similar risk exposures [9–11]. However, when the disease occurs in smokers it seems to be characterised by an insidious and chronic presentation with a worse clinical outcome [12].

Pathogenic Mechanisms

The pathogenesis of HP is complex and probably involves the coexistence of genetic and/or environmental risk factors with the exposure to the offending HP antigen. The nature of the genetic predisposition is unknown, but susceptibility associated to the major histocompatibility complex (MHC) class II alleles has been reported [13]. Some other host processes may also contribute as a risk factor. In this context, it has been recently reported that female patients with HP show increased frequency of microchimerism, that is, the presence of circulating cells transferred from one genetically distinct individual to another [14]. In this study, fetal micro-chimeric cells also were found in bronchoalveolar lavage (BAL) and lung tissues of HP patients, demonstrating that these cells traffic to and from the lungs. However, the putative role of these microchimeric fetal cells in the HP lungs is presently unknown, although they seem to increase the severity of the disease. Viral infections involving common respiratory viruses, primarily Influenza A, and the exposure to a second inhalatory injury (i.e., pesticides) may also have a promoting effect enhancing the development of HP [15,16].

The mechanisms of hypersensitivity lung damage involve both humoral and cellular processes, depending on the clinical presentation. Inflammation in the acute episodes seems to be provoked by immune-complexes deposit, which may explain the 4- to 8-h late onset of symptoms after massive antigen inhalation. Supporting this concept are the findings of activated complement components, activated blood neutrophils, and BAL neutrophilia in patients with acute HP and in those studied few hours/days after antigen inhalation challenge [17–19].

In contrast, subacute and chronic HP appears to be mediated by an exaggerated T–cell-mediated response and, actually, a striking increase of T lymphocytes characterises this disorder. The mechanisms implicated in the T-cell alveolitis are not completely understood but appear to include increased T-cell recruitment and migration, increased proliferation in the local microenvironment, and decreased programmed cell death [20–24]. A recent global gene expression study identified a variety of genes typically associated with inflammation, T-cell activation, and immune responses in the lungs of patients with subacute/chronic disease [25]. Genes related to T-lymphocyte activation included Src-like-adaptor 2, CD2, components of the T-cell receptor complex (CD3-D and -E), and the alpha chain of CD8.

Likewise, MHC class II transactivator, the master regulator of MHC class II expression, and several genes encoding MHC class I and II molecules were also overexpressed. CXCL9 and CXCL10 chemokines involved in recruitment of activated T cells and natural killer cells and in Th1 immune response were up-regulated. CXCR4 and CCR5 and their ligands CCL5 and CCL4 were overexpressed as well, suggesting that the recruiting/homing program for lung lymphocytes involves multiple chemokines.

Clinical Behavior

The clinical features of the disease are usually similar, regardless of the type of the inhaled dust. In general, three overlapping clinical forms are recognised: acute, subacute, and chronic [1]. The nature of the antigen, as well as the intensity and frequency of antigen exposure influence the clinical presentation.

Acute HP

This form of HP usually follows a heavy exposure to an offending agent. Acute presentation is characterised by an abrupt onset of symptoms few hours after intermittent and intense antigen exposure. Patients present fever, chills, dyspnea, chest tightness, and dry or mildly productive cough. Removal from exposure to the provoking antigen results in improvement of symptoms within hours to days and complete resolution of clinical and radiographic findings within several weeks. However, the disease often recurs after the next inhalation of the causative antigen.

Occasionally, respiratory failure mimicking adult respiratory distress syndrome may occur, requiring intensive unit care management [26]. Acute HP behaves similar to an acute respiratory infection provoked by virus or mycoplasma [1]. In farmers, the differential diagnosis must include the organic dust toxic syndrome (ODTS) provoked by exposure to bacterial endotoxins and fungal toxins of moldy hay [27]. In contrast to patients with acute HP, patients with ODTS have no precipitins to antigens of molds, and usually present with normal clinical findings upon respiratory examination and chest radiographs. ODTS is usually self-limiting, with symptoms rarely exceeding 36 hours

Subacute HP

Subacute HP is characterised by progressive dyspnea and cough occurring during weeks or few months after continued exposure. Patients often display fever, fatigue, anorexia, and weight loss. Some improvement of symptoms is noticed if patients avoid further exposure, but takes longer than with the acute form of the disease (weeks to months), and usually pharmacological treatment is necessary.

Chronic HP

Chronic HP may exhibit different clinical behaviors [28–31]. One subgroup of patients evolves to interstitial lung fibrosis after recurrent acute episodes (chronic recurrent HP); other subgroup of patients presents slowly progressive chronic fibrotic disease with no history of acute/subacute episodes (chronic insidious HP), and finally a third subgroup may progress to a chronic obstructive lung disease. The reasons for these different outcomes (fibrosis versus emphysema) are unknown, but they may be related to the characteristics of the inhaled antigen, the type of exposure, cigarette smoking status, and the genetic background of the patient. Pulmonary fibrosis is the general outcome of chronic HP induced by avian antigens whereas emphysematous lung lesions are observed in farmers exposed to thermophilic bacteria and fungi.

Subacute HP as well as chronic recurrent and insidious HP may mimic virtually any interstitial lung disease and the diagnosis may be extremely difficult. Differential diagnosis of subacute HP includes some lung infections such as miliary tuberculosis or histoplasmosis, as well as noninfectious granulomatous lung disorders, including sarcoidosis. The Presence of large adenopathies, extra-thoracic involvement (peripheral lymph nodes, eyes skin, liver, and heart among others) hypercalciuria, and increased levels of serum angiotensin converting enzyme are frequent in sarcoidosis and virtually absent in HP. Also, several idiopathic interstitial pneumonias such as lymphoid interstitial pneumonia, cryptogenic organizing pneumonia, and idiopathic nonspecific interstitial pneumonia should be considered. Chronic HP (primarily the insidious form) may be misdiagnosed as idiopathic pulmonary fibrosis or other advanced fibrotic lung disorder if a careful history and specific studies are not carried out [28,29]. Tachypnea and bibasilar dry crackles, are common findings in any clinical presentation of HP. Patients with chronic insidious or recurrent HP may develop digital clubbing, pulmonary arterial hypertension, and even cor pulmonale [1,32].

Chest Imaging

The chest radiograph is used to confirm that the patient has some kind of interstitial lung disease. However, is generally nonspecific. Also, the sensitivity of chest radiographs for detecting HP seems to have steadily declined during the last decades [33], and patients with acute and occasionally mild subacute HP may exhibit normal chest x-ray results. When abnormal, chest radiographs show nodular opacities with ground-glass attenuation in acute/subacute presentations, whereas the chronic stages are characterised by a predominantly reticular pattern that may evolve to honeycombing changes.

Findings on High-Resolution Computed Tomography (HRCT)

Acute HP is characterised by a diffuse and hazy increase of parenchymal density (ground-glass attenuation) and occasionally by patchy or widespread air space consolidation [30]. Patients with subacute HP show areas of ground-glass opacities, small

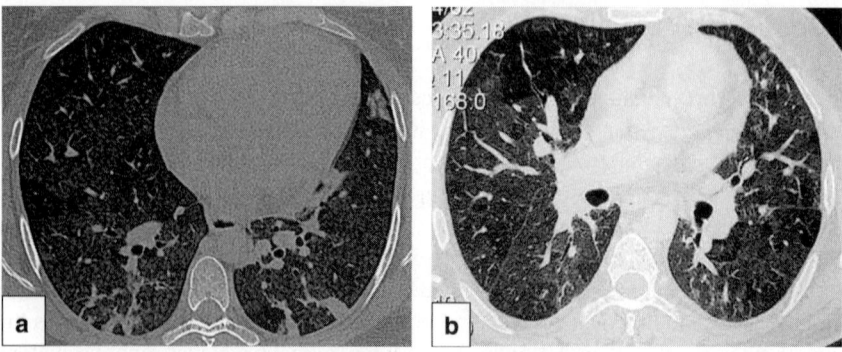

Fig. 7.1 **A** HRCT image showing bilateral poorly defined centrilobular nodules and ground-glass opacities in a HP patient with subacute presentation. **B** HRCT illustrates ground glass opacities and areas of decreased attenuation (mosaic pattern) that are typical findings in subacute disease

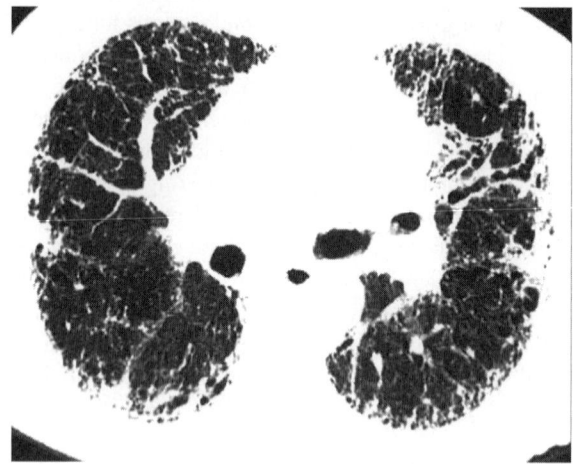

Fig. 7.2 HRCT scan of a patient with chronic HP. It can be observed bilateral reticular opacities, traction bronchiectasis, and subpleural microcysts. Idiopathic pulmonary fibrosis is the usual differential diagnosis

poorly defined centrilobular nodules, and mosaic attenuation (Figs. 7.1A and 7.1B) [34–36]. A CT scan obtained at the end of a patient's breath expiration is useful to detect patchy air trapping images. The micronodular pattern consists of poorly defined micronodules, usually of less than 5 mm in diameter, with a centrilobular distribution that affect both the central and peripheral portions of the lung.

Chronic fibrotic HP is characterised by the presence of reticular opacities superimposed on findings of subacute HP. Reticulation may evolve to honeycombing, mainly in chronic patients that show slowly progressive (insidious) disease (Fig. 7.2) [28,37]. In these cases, the disease may mimic idiopathic pulmonary fibrosis. Patients with chronic farmer's lung more frequently exhibit emphysematous changes than interstitial fibrosis [30,31].

Physiological Abnormalities

The main purpose of the pulmonary function tests is to determine the severity of the lung impairment. HP is characterised by a restrictive ventilatory defect with a reduction of forced vital capacity and total lung capacity [38]. The static expiratory pressure-volume curve is downward and rightward shifted of the normal curve, showing a decrease in lung compliance over the entire range of the reduced inspiratory capacity [39]. However, these changes are neither specific nor diagnostic for HP because similar abnormalities are revealed in most interstitial lung diseases.

Patients display impaired gas exchange characterised by hypoxemia. which usually worsens with exercise, and increased alveolar-arterial oxygen gradient $[P(A-a)O_2]$. Patients with mild disease or in the early stages may present normoxemia at rest, but exercise always reveals hypoxemia. Diffusing capacity of carbon monoxide (DL_{CO}) is typically reduced and is a good predictor of arterial oxygen desaturation during exercise.

Some degree of obstruction of the peripheral airways, as suggested by a decrease in the maximum to mid-flow rates and in the ratio of dynamic to static lung compliance, may be present as the result of bronchiolitis [40]. However, the obstruction of small airways usually is not detected with the use of functional tests [41]. However, in chronic farmer's lung, functional defects reflecting airways obstruction and emphysematous lesions can be noticed [31].

The correlation between pulmonary functional abnormality and the severity or prognosis of HP is poor. Patients with a severe decrease in lung volume and DL_{CO} may recover fully, whereas others with relatively mild functional abnormalities at the onset of disease may develop progressive pulmonary fibrosis or airway obstruction and emphysematous changes.

Hemodynamic Measurements

Studies in which authors examine the effect of lung inflammation/fibrosis on pulmonary arterial vessels in HP are scanty and, actually, few data exist (mostly from case reports) characterizing hemodynamics and cardiac function in this population. In most of the case reports, a marked pulmonary arterial hypertension (PAH) has been found in acute/subacute patients, where pulmonary embolism has been suspected [42–45]. In a familial case of HP that involved the mother and two children, the index case, an 8-year-old girl, was diagnosed as primary pulmonary arterial hypertension [46]. In this patient, echocardiography revealed enlarged right heart chambers, moderate tricuspid regurgitation, and increased pulmonary artery pressure (80 mmHg) in an otherwise-nondiseased heart. In general, in these reported cases, the pulmonary hypertension and concomitant right ventricular dilatation have been resolved after corticosteroid treatment for the HP.

In an old study dealing with 10 patients with HP that was performed with right heart catheterization, it was found that all patients had PAH and increased pulmonary arterial resistance [47]. Abnormal pulmonary artery diastolic pressure/pulmonary wedge pressure difference was noticed in most of the patients. Hemodynamic abnormalities correlated with arterial oxygen saturation and furthermore, a significant improvement was observed after oxygen breathing. Interestingly, all patients showed vascular abnormalities on lung tissues. Most of them displayed medial hypertrophy in arteries and arterioles, whereas in some of them cellular intimal proliferation in the smallest muscular arteries and intimal fibrosis was also seen. The study was performed in Mexico City at 2,240 meters altitude, and the authors concluded that alveolar hypoxia produced by HP presumably enhanced by living at a high altitude provoke pulmonary hypertension. Other studies examining with the histopathologic changes in HP have also reported vascular abnormalities, including intimal hyperplasia and some muscle hypertrophy in chronic cases [48].

We have recently reviewed 87 patients with chronic HP in which an echocardiography was performed as part of their clinical evaluation. One-third of the patients exhibited increased pulmonary artery systolic pressure (Fig. 7.3). Greater defect in gas exchange was the only parameter that correlated with the presence of PAH (Table 7.2). Alveolar hypoxia may lead to vasoconstriction of small pulmonary arteries (hypoxic pulmonary hypertension) and right heart failure. Hypoxic pulmonary vasoconstriction contributes to ventilation–perfusion matching in the lung by

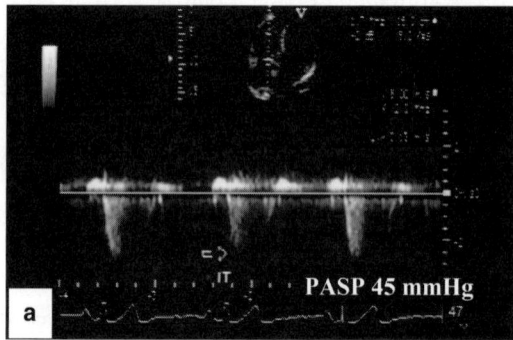

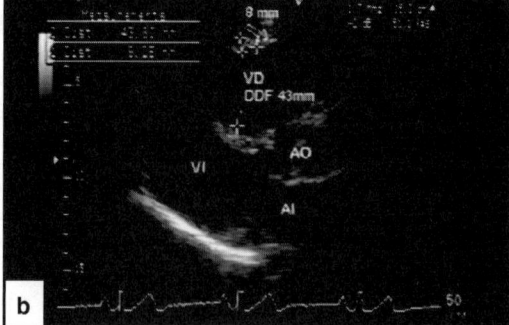

Fig. 7.3 Echocardiography in HP patients showing tricuspid insufficiency and increased pulmonary artery systolic pressure (**A**) and dilation and hypertrophy of right ventricle (**B**) (*See Color Plates*)

Table 7.2 Differences in gas exchange between HP patients with or without pulmonary hypertension.

	Without PAH ($n = 57$)	With PAH ($n = 30$)	p value
PaO$_2$ (mmHg)	50 ± 10	45 ± 9	0.03
Rest SpO$_2$ %	85 ± 7	80 ± 9	0.01
PASP	25 ± 4.7	51 ± 18.3	0.0001

PaO$_2$, arterial pressure of oxygen; SpO$_2$, pulse oximetric saturation; PASP, pulmonary artery systolic pressure

diverting blood flow to oxygen-rich areas. With prolonged hypoxia, small pulmonary arteries suffer a process described as pulmonary vascular remodeling, characterised primarily by thickening of the smooth vascular layer with neointima formation, medial thickening, inflammatory cell recruitment, and endothelial dysfunction. Both hypoxic vasoconstriction and architectural remodeling contribute to the development of progressive pulmonary hypertension.

It is important to take into account however, that our study was performed with echocardiography that compared with right heart catheterisation, may give an inaccurate measurement of systolic pulmonary artery pressure, mainly in patients with advanced lung disease, which leads to considerable overdiagnoses of pulmonary hypertension [49].

Diagnostic Appraisal and Additional Tools for Difficult Cases

In general, the criteria for HP diagnosis should include a high index of suspicion by the clinician when dealing with an interstitial lung disease. In any case of an acute respiratory illness, or a subacute/chronic ILD, clinicians should always consider HP in the spectrum of the differential diagnosis and should carefully search for any potential source of HP-related antigens. Although the disease seems to be less frequent in children, it should be considered in any child with recurrent or unexplained respiratory symptoms [50,51].

A key consideration in acute HP is the important improvement of a flu-like syndrome after removing the patient from the suspected environment, and worsening after re-exposure. Similar improvement although less dramatic can be also observed in the subacute form.

In a multicenter study that included a cohort of 400 patients (116 with HP and 284 with other interstitial lung disease), 6 significant clinical predictors of HP were identified [52]: (1) exposure to a known offending antigen, (2) positive precipitating antibodies to the offending antigen, (3) recurrent episodes of symptoms, (4) inspiratory crackles on physical examination, (5) symptoms occurring 4 to 8 hours after exposure, (6), and weight loss.

As mentioned, HRCT plays a central role for diagnosis. The acute form is characterised by ground glass attenuation and confluent opacities. The subacute form is distinguished by centrilobular nodules, areas of ground-glass attenuation, a mosaic perfusion pattern, and air trapping on expiratory imaging. The chronic phase is characterised by irregular reticular opacities superimposed to some subacute changes and with associated architectural distortion. The following subsections detail other important tests to evaluate patients with suspected HP:

Specific Antibodies

Precipitating IgG antibodies against the offending antigens can be identified in the patient's serum. However, a percent of exposed but asymptomatic individuals (mostly with a high degree of exposure) may also have positive serum precipitins [53–56]. Perhaps more important from the clinical point of view is that in a number of patients with chronic insidious HP, circulating specific antibodies are not detected [28]. Therefore, the absence of serum precipitins does not rule out HP, whereas the presence of them does not rule in. Ideally, it will be better to obtain a sample of the suspected causative agent from the original source and test it against the patient's blood.

BAL

BAL may give important supportive evidence for diagnosis of HP because it is a highly sensitive tool to detect the alveolitis [1,57–59]. The disease (in any of its clinical presentations) is characterised by a remarkable increment of lymphocytes, usually greater than 30% and often exceeding 50% of the inflammatory cells recovered (Fig. 7.4). However, as mentioned for the presence of specific antibodies, the presence of an alveolar lymphocytosis by itself does not establish the diagnosis because asymptomatic, exposed individuals can also have increased numbers of lymphocytes in their BAL [60]. Also, similar levels can be found in infectious and noninfectious granulomatous diseases, such as sarcoidosis, berylliosis, or miliary tuberculosis.

It is the general belief that the main lymphocyte subset that increases is the CD8+ with the subsequent decrease of BAL CD4+/CD8+ ratio to less than 1.0 [61]. However, a number of studies have found that CD4+ T cells are increased with the consequent increased CD4+/CD8+ ratio [62,63]. Several circumstances seem to explain this variability, including the clinical form (acute, subacute or chronic), cigarette smoking habit, type/dose of inhaled antigen, and the time elapsed since antigen exposure. A predominant increase of CD8+ seems to occur in nonsmokers with acute/subacute HP, whereas an increase of CD4+ is frequently found in smokers or those with chronic/fibrotic forms of the disease.

BAL neutrophils are usually increased in acute cases and after recent antigen exposure [64]. Therefore, an increase in BAL lymphocytes and neutrophils in a patient with an acute respiratory syndrome is strongly indicative of HP. Also, a modest but significant increase of neutrophils is detected in advanced disease [65].

Several studies have reported a modest but significant increase of plasma cells mainly after recent exposure [66]. This finding, together with the increase in

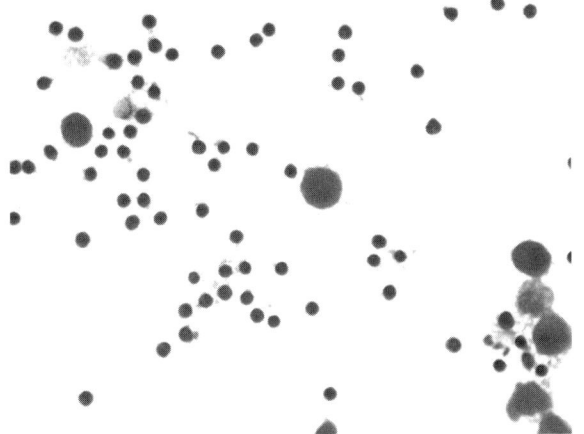

Fig. 7.4 BAL from a patient with subacute HP. Most of the lavaged cells are lymphocytes (hematoxylin & eosin [H&E], original magnification ×20) (*See Color Plates*)

T lymphocytes, may help to distinguish HP from others ILD [67]. Also, a small but significant increase of mast cells has been reported in HP [68,69].

Antigen-Induced Lymphocyte Proliferation

In vitro proliferation of peripheral and bronchoalveolar lymphocytes to avian antigens has been assayed for diagnostic and research purposes [28,70]. Importantly, this test resulted to be positive in more than 90% of the recurrent and insidious cases of chronic pigeon breeder's disease where the presence of circulating antibodies may be negative [28]. Experiments also demonstrated that a positive stimulation index was usually 2.0 or greater.

Lung Biopsy

Histopathological confirmation of the diagnosis is required in a number of subacute and chronic cases. It is critical that the pathologist is informed when HP is being considered; the findings are often subtle and must be interpreted with knowledge of the clinical presentation. This is particularly important because we now know that a relatively large number of patients with subacute or chronic HP may exhibit a different histological pattern, including nonspecific interstitial pneumonia [71] cryptogenic organizing pneumonia, or even usual interstitial pneumonia-like changes.

Classical histopathologic findings include small, poorly formed noncaseating bronchiolocentric granulomas (Fig. 7.5A and 7.5B) [72]. These poorly defined aggregates of epithelioid macrophages are often associated with multinucleated

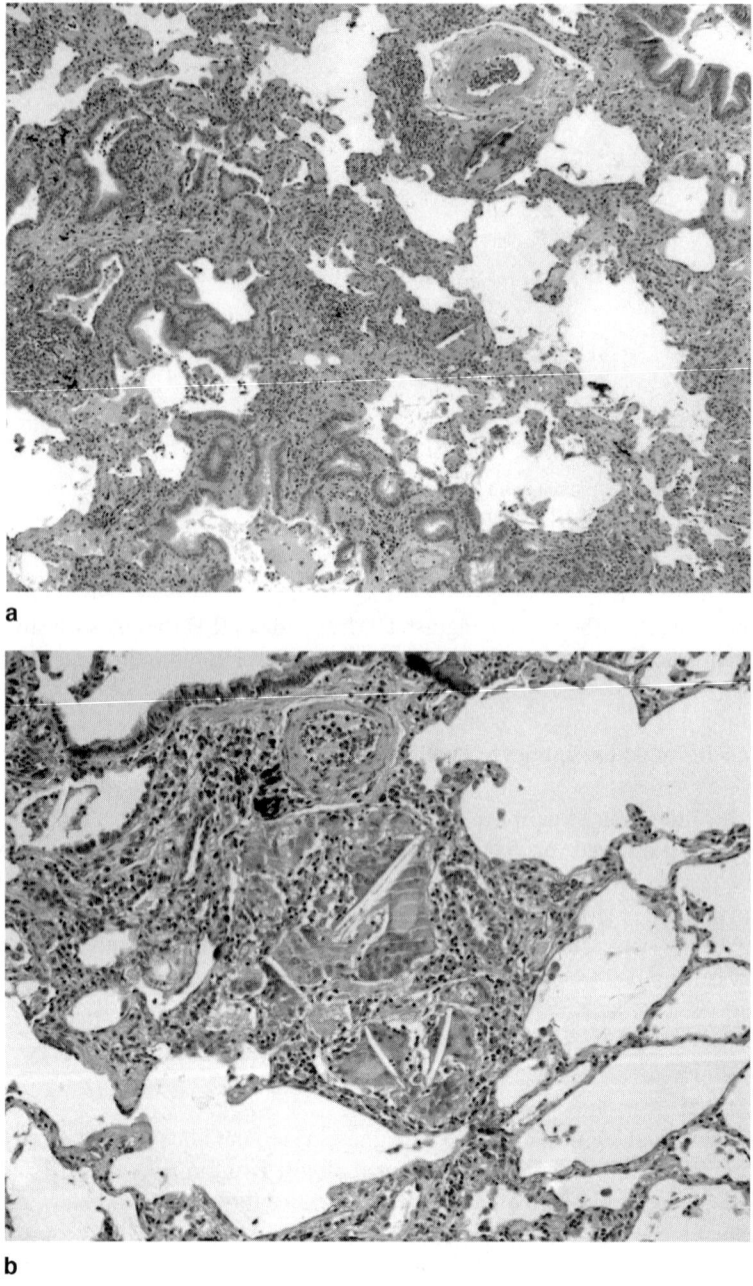

a

b

Fig. 7.5 **A** Photomicrograph of histopathologic specimen of a patient with subacute hypersensitivity pneumonitis showing, diffuse, chronic lymphocytic inflammatory infiltrate (H&E ×10X). **B** Another patient with subacute disease showing a granulomatous lesion with several multinucleated giant cells (H&E, ×40) (*See Color Plates*)

giant cells. There is also a patchy mononuclear cell infiltration (predominantly lymphocytes and plasma cells) of the alveolar walls, typically in a bronchiolocentric distribution. Bronchiolar abnormalities are usually present, although they may differ according with the type of HP. Thus, in farmer's lung, it has been described proliferative bronchiolitis obliterans [73], whereas in pigeon breeder's disease, peribronchiolar inflammation/fibrosis with smooth muscle hypertrophy and extrinsic narrowing of the small airways are usually found [74]. Occasionally, classic bronchiolitis obliterans organizing pneumonia -like lesions are described [75,76].

The chronic stage is characterised by variable degrees of interstitial fibrosis (Fig. 7.6A and 7.6B). In these cases, the presence of giant cells, poorly formed granulomas, or inflammatory features of subacute HP may corroborate the diagnosis of HP [28,29,77]. It has been recently proposed that three different patterns of fibrosis may occur: (1) predominantly peripheral fibrosis in a patchy pattern with architectural distortion and fibroblast foci resembling usual interstitial pneumonia; (2) temporal and geographic homogeneous interstitial fibrosis resembling fibrotic nonspecific interstitial pneumonia; and (3) irregular peribronchiolar fibrosis [78]. Other features of chronic HP are alveolar epithelial cell hyperplasia, and thickened arterioles [79].

Inhalation Challenge Test

Re-exposure of the patients to the environment of the suspected agent may be recommended. Inhalation challenge in the hospital is not generally performed because lack of standardised antigens, and limited access to a specialised setting to conduct the study. A positive challenge is characterised by fever, malaise, headache, peripheral and BAL neutrophilia, and decrease of forced vital capacity and/or oxygen saturation 8–12h after exposure [70,80,81]. Inhalation challenge must be rigorously controlled to avoid an exaggerated reaction. In addition, the patient should be monitored closely for at least 24 h. Occasionally, the patient may present a two-stage reaction with an immediate, transient wheezing and a decrease in the Forced expiratory volume in one second, which is followed in 4–6h by decrease in forced vital capacity, fever, and leukocytosis. In our experience, false-positive results are obtained in approximately 15% of patients with other ILD but not in avian antigen exposed subjects, suggesting that provocation test can identify patients with HP in the majority of the cases [80].

Treatment and Prognosis

Early diagnosis and identification and avoidance of the inciting antigen exposure are vital in the management of HP. In acute form, avoidance alone may be sufficient intervention. In a study, no recurrence of summer-type HP was noticed when the colonization by *Trichosporon cutaneum*, the causative agent, was eliminated from

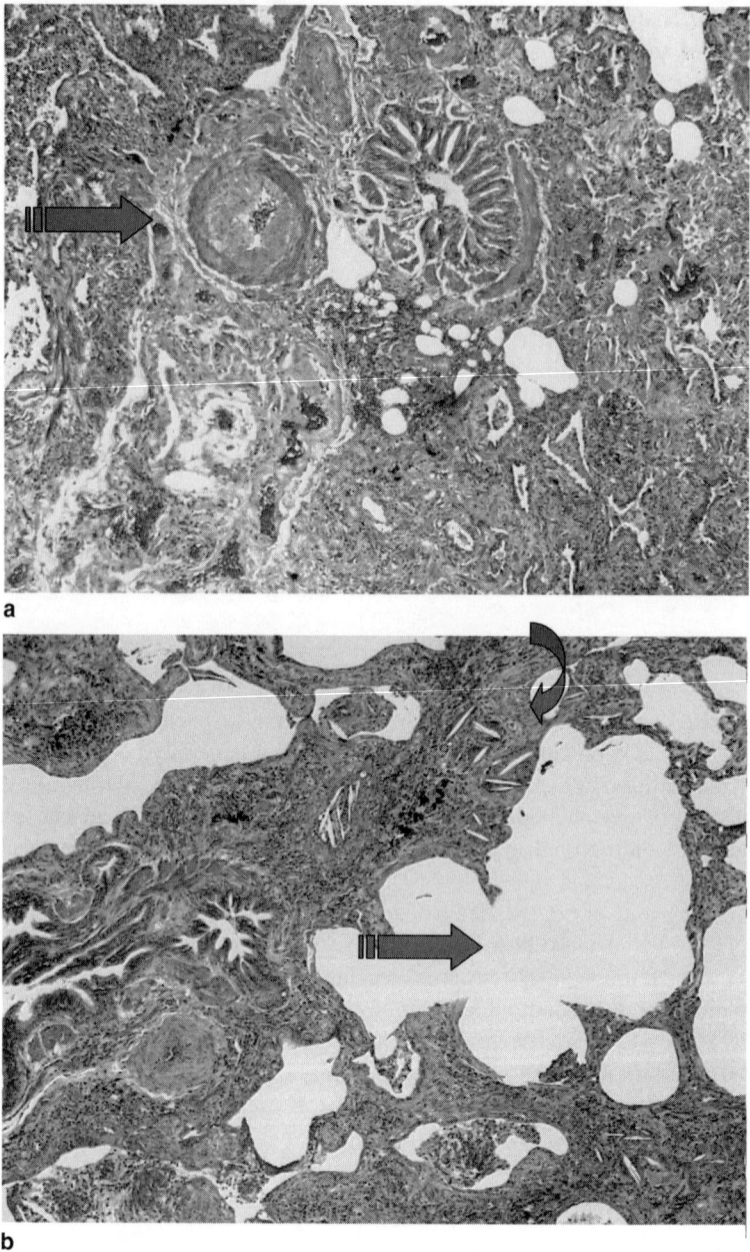

a

b

Fig. 7.6 Photomicrographs of histopathologic samples from two patients with (**A**) chronic HP showing collagen deposit (Masson's thrichrome, ×10) and (**B**) honeycomb changes (see arrow, H&E, ×10). It can be noticed the vascular remodeling (arrow in A). In **B**, There is moderate inflammatory infiltrate and a small granuloma (curved arrow). (*See Color Plates*)

the domestic environment. By contrast, recurrence was observed in all patients who resided in homes that were not cleaned or in homes where cleaning was not adequate [82]. In occupationally exposed individuals, the risk of HP can be reduced by adapting modern practices and conditions that reduce the content of causative antigens. Nevertheless, in chronic fibrotic HP patients, subsequent antigen avoidance may not reverse the disease, and some of them show progressive worsening and eventually die from the disease. Prednisone is indicated in subacute/chronic presentations, although long-term efficacy of these agents has yet to be determined. An optional approach consists of 0.5 mg per kg per day of prednisone for a month, followed by a gradual reduction until a maintenance dose of 10 to 15 mg per day is reached. Prednisone is discontinued when the patient is considered to be healed (or after a substantial improvement of symptoms and functional abnormalities) or when there is no clinical and/or functional response. Inhaled corticosteroids have been suggested for acute/subacute cases but long-term experience is scanty. Because pulmonary hypertension may negatively influence the outcome, treatment with antihypertensive drugs such as sildenafil or iloprost may be considered on individual basis.

The prognosis of this disease for patients displaying the acute and subacute presentations is favorable (in the absence of further exposure), and most patients heal or display a significant improvement with some residual respiratory functional abnormalities remaining. In contrast, patients with chronic HP, primarily those with pigeon breeder's disease, may evolve to interstitial fibrosis, showing a high rate of mortality with median survivals of 5 and 7 years, respectively [29,83]. Patients with farmer's lung, mainly those that experience recurrent acute attacks, develop more often a syndrome similar to chronic obstructive pulmonary disease with airflow obstruction and emphysema, but survival data are unavailable [84,85].

References

1. Selman M. Hypersensitivity pneumonitis: a multifaceted deceiving disorder. Clin Chest Med 2004;25:531–547.
2. Fink JN, Ortega HG, Reynolds HY, Cormier YF, Fan LL, Franks TJ, Kreiss K, Kunkel S, Lynch D, Quirce S, Rose C, Schleimer RP, Schuyler MR, Selman M, Trout D, Yoshizawa Y. Needs and opportunities for research in hypersensitivity pneumonitis. Am J Respir Crit Care Med 2005;171:792–798.
3. Marras TK, Wallace RJ Jr, Koth LL, Stulbarg MS, Cowl CT, Daley CL. Hypersensitivity pneumonitis reaction to Mycobacterium avium in household water. Chest 2005;127: 664–671.
4. Martinez S, McAdams HP, Batchu CS. The many faces of pulmonary nontuberculous mycobacterial infection. AJR Am J Roentgenol 2007;189:177–186.
5. Terho EO, Heinonen OP, Lammi S, Laukkanen V. Incidence of clinically confirmed farmer's lung in Finland and its relation to meteorological factors. Eur J Respir Dis Suppl 1987; 152:47–56.
6. Arya A, Roychoudhury K, Bredin CP. Farmer's lung is now in decline. Ir Med J 2006;99: 203–205.

7. Solaymani-Dodaran M, West J, Smith C, Hubbard R. Extrinsic allergic alveolitis: incidence and mortality in the general population. QJM 2007;100:233–237.

8. Thomeer MJ, Costabe U, Rizzato G, Poletti V, Demedts M. Comparison of registries of interstitial lung diseases in three European countries. Eur Respir J Suppl 2001;32:114s–118s.

9. Arima K, Ando M, Ito K, Sakata T, Yamaguchi T, Araki S, Futatsuka M. Effect of cigarette smoking on prevalence of summer-type hypersensitivity pneumonitis caused by Trichosporon cutaneum. Arch Environ Health 1992;47:274–278.

10. Cormier Y, Israël-Assayag E, Bédard G, Duchaine C. Hypersensitivity pneumonitis in peat moss processing plant workers. Am J Respir Crit Care Med 1998;158:412–417.

11. Dalphin JC, Debieuvre D, Pernet D, Maheu MF, Polio JC, Toson B, Dubiez A, Monnet E, Laplante JJ, Depierre A. Prevalence and risk factors for chronic bronchitis and farmer's lung in French dairy farmers. Br J Ind Med 1993;50:941–944.

12. Ohtsuka Y, Munakata M, Tanimura K, Ukita H, Kusaka H, Masaki Y, Doi I, Ohe M, Amishima M, Homma Y, et al. Smoking promotes insidious and chronic farmer's lung disease, and deteriorates the clinical outcome. Intern Med 1995;34:966–971.

13. Camarena A, Juárez A, Mejía M, Estrada A, Carrillo G, Falfán R, Zuñiga J, Navarro C, Granados J, Selman M. Major histocompatibility complex and tumor necrosis factor-alpha polymorphisms in pigeon breeder's disease. Am J Respir Crit Care Med 2001;163: 1528–1533.

14. Bustos ML, Frías S, Ramos S, Estrada A, Arreola JL, Mendoza F, Gaxiola M, Salcedo M, Pardo A, Selman M. Local and circulating microchimerism is associated with hypersensitivity pneumonitis. Am J Respir Crit Care Med 2007;176:90–95.

15. Cormier Y, Samson N, Israel-Assayag E. Viral infection enhances the response to Saccharopolyspora rectivirgula in mice prechallenged with this farmer's lung antigen. Lung 1996;174:399–407.

16. Hoppin JA, Umbach DM, Kullman GJ, Henneberger PK, London SJ, Alavanja MC, Sandler DP. Pesticides and other agricultural factors associated with self-reported farmer's lung among farm residents in the Agricultural Health Study. Occup Environ Med 2007;64:334–341.

17. Fournier E, Tonnel AB, Gosset P, Wallaert B, Ameisen JC, Voisin C. Early neutrophil alveolitis after antigen inhalation in hypersensitivity pneumonitis. Chest 1985;88:563–566.

18. Yoshizawa Y, Nomura A, Ohdama S, Tanaka M, Morinari H, Hasegawa S. The significance of complement activation in the pathogenesis of hypersensitivity pneumonitis; sequential changes of complement components and chemotactic activities in bronchoalveolar lavage fluids. Int Arch Allergy Appl Immunol 1988;87:417–423.

19. Vogelmeier C, Krombach F, Munzing S, Konig G, Mazur G, Beinert T, Fruhmann G. Activation of blood neutrophils in acute episodes of farmer's lung. Am Rev Respir Dis. 1993;148:396–400.

20. Laflamme C, Israel-Assayag E, Cormier Y. Apoptosis of bronchoalveolar lavage lymphocytes in hypersensitivity pneumonitis. Eur Respir J 2003;21:225–231.

21. Ohtsuka M, Yoshizawa Y, Naitou T, Yano H, Sato T, Hasegawa S. The motility of lung lymphocytes in hypersensitivity pneumonitis and sarcoidosis. Am J Respir Crit Care Med 1994; 149:455–459.

22. Dakhama A, Israel-Assayag E, Cormier Y. Role of interleukin-2 in the development and persistence of lymphocytic alveolitis in farmer's lung. Eur Respir J 1998;11:1281–1286.

23. Trentin L, Migone N, Zambello R, di Celle PF, Aina F, Feruglio C, Bulian P, Masciarelli M, Agostini C, Cipriani A, Semenzato G. Mechanisms accounting for lymphocytic alveolitis in hypersensitivity pneumonitis. J Immunol 1990;145:2147–2154.

24. Dakhama A, Israel-Assayag E, Cormier Y. Altered immunosuppressive activity of alveolar macrophages in farmer's lung disease. Eur Respir J 1996;9:1456–1462.

25. Selman M, Pardo A, Barrera L, Estrada A, Watson SR, Wilson K, Aziz N, Kaminski N, Zlotnik A. Gene expression profiles distinguish idiopathic pulmonary fibrosis from hypersensitivity pneumonitis. Am J Respir Crit Care Med. 2006 Jan 15;173:188–198.

26. Da Broi U, Orefice U, Cahalin C, Bonfreschi V, Cason L. ARDS after double extrinsic exposure hypersensitivity pneumonitis. Intensive Care Med 1999;25:755–757.

27. Seifert SA, Von Essen S, Jacobitz K, Crouch R, Lintner CP. Organic dust toxic syndrome: a review. J Toxicol Clin Toxicol 2003;41:185–193.
28. Ohtani Y, Saiki S, Sumi Y, Inase N, Miyake S, Costabel U, Yoshizawa Y. Clinical features of recurrent and insidious chronic bird fancier's lung. Ann Allergy Asthma Immunol 2003;90: 604–610.
29. Pérez-Padilla R, Salas J, Chapela R, Sánchez M, Carrillo G, Pérez R, Sansores R, Gaxiola M, Selman M. Mortality in Mexican patients with chronic pigeon breeders lung compared to those with usual interstitial pneumonia. Am Rev Respir Dis 1993;148:49–53.
30. Cormier Y, Brown M, Worthy S, Racine G, Muller NL. High-resolution computed tomographic characteristics in acute farmer's lung and in its follow-up. Eur Respir J 2000;16: 56–60.
31. Erkinjuntti-Pekkanen R, Rytkonen H, Kokkarinen JI, Tukiainen HO, Partanen K, Terho EO. Long-term risk of emphysema in patients with farmer's lung and matched control farmers. Am J Respir Crit Care Med 1998;158:662–665.
32. Sansores R, Salas J, Chapela R, Barquin N, Selman M. Clubbing in hypersensitivity pneumonitis. Its prevalence and possible prognostic role. Arch Intern Med 1990;150:1849–1851.
33. Hodgson MJ, Parkinson DK, Karpf M. Chest x-rays in hypersensitivity pneumonitis: a metaanalysis of secular trend. Am J Ind Med 1989;16:5–53.
34. Glazer CS, Rose CS, Lynch DA. Clinical and radiologic manifestations of hypersensitivity pneumonitis. J Thorac Imaging 2002;17:261–272.
35. Small JH, Flower CD, Traill ZC, Gleeson FV. Air-trapping in extrinsic allergic alveolitis on computed tomography. Clin Radiol 1996;51:684–688.
36. Silva CI, Churg A, Muller NL. Hypersensitivity pneumonitis: spectrum of high-resolution CT and pathologic findings. AJR Am J Roentgenol 2007;188:334–344.
37. Akira M. High-resolution CT in the evaluation of occupational and environmental disease. Radiol Clin N Am 2002;40:43–59.
38. Du Wayne Schmidt C, Jensen RL, Christensen LT, Crapo RO, Davis JJ. Longitudinal pulmonary function changes in pigeon breeders. Chest 1988;93:359–363.
39. Sansores R, Pérez-Padilla R, Pare P, Selman M. Exponential analysis of the lung pressure-volume curve in patients with chronic pigeon breeder's lung. Chest 1992;101:1352–1356.
40. Pérez J, Selman M, Rubio H, Ocaña H, Chapela R. Relationship between lung inflammation or fibrosis and frequency dependence of compliance in interstitial pulmonary diseases. Respiration 1987;52:254–262.
41. Pérez-Padilla R, Gaxiola M, Salas J, Mejía M, Ramos C, Selman M. Bronchiolitis in chronic pigeon breeder's disease. Morphologic evidence of a spectrum of small airway lesions in hypersensitivity pneumonitis induced by avian antigens. Chest 1996;110:371–377.
42. McKeown PF, Walsh SJ, Menown IB. Images in cardiology: an unusual case of right ventricular dilatation. Heart 2005;91:1147.
43. Krasniuk EP, Petrova IS, Pilinskii VV. Exogenous allergic alveolitis in workers engaged in the manufacture of pepsin. Lik Sprava 2001;(4):168–71.
44. Gainet M, Chaudemanche H, Westeel V, Lounici A, Dubiez A, Depierre A, Dalphin JC. A misleading form of hypersensitivity pneumonitis. Rev Mal Respir 2000;17:987–989.
45. Ostergaard JR. Reversible pulmonary arterial hypertension in a 6-year-old girl with extrinsic allergic alveolitis. Acta Paediatr Scand 1989;78:145–148.
46. Ceviz N, Kaynar H, Olgun H, Onbas O, Misirligil Z. Pigeon breeder's lung in childhood: is family screening necessary? Pediatr Pulmonol 2006;41:279–282.
47. Lupi-Herrera E, Sandoval J, Bialostozky D, Seoane M, Martinez ML, Bonetti PF, Reyes P, Barrios R. Extrinsic allergic alveolitis caused by pigeon breeding at a high altitude (2,240 meters). Hemodynamic behavior of pulmonary circulation. Am Rev Respir Dis 1981;124:602–607.
48. Seal RM, Hapke EJ, Thomas GO, Meek JC, Hayes M. The pathology of the acute and chronic stages of farmer's lung. Thorax 1968;23:469–489.
49. Arcasoy SM, Christie JD, Ferrari VA, Sutton MS, Zisman DA, Blumenthal NP, Pochettino A, Kotloff RM. Echocardiographic assessment of pulmonary hypertension in patients with advanced lung disease. Am J Respir Crit Care Med 2003;167:735–740.

50. Nacar N, Kiper N, Yalcin E, Dogru D, Dilber E, Ozcelik U, Misirligil Z. Hypersensitivity pneumonitis in children: pigeon breeder's disease. Ann Trop Paediatr 2004;24:349–355.
51. Stauffer Ettlin M, Pache JC, Renevey F, Hanquinet-Ginter S, Guinand S, Barazzone Argiroffo C. Bird breeder's disease: a rare diagnosis in young children. Eur J Pediatr 2006;165:55–61.
52. Lacasse Y, Selman M, Costabel U, Dalphin JC, Ando M, Morell F, Erkinjuntti-Pekkanen R, Muller N, Colby TV, Schuyler M, Cormier Y. Clinical diagnosis of hypersensitivity pneumonitis. Am J Respir Crit Care Med 2003;168:952–958.
53. Hébert J, Beaudoin J, Laviolette M, Beaudoin R, Bélanger J, Cormier Y. Absence of correlation between the degree of alveolitis and antibody levels to Micropolysporum faeni. Clin Exp Immunol 1985;60:572–578.
54. Pinon JM, Geers R, Lepan H, Pailler S. Immunodetection by enzyme-linked immuno-filtration assay (ELIFA) of IgG, IgM, IgA and IgE antibodies in bird breeder's disease. Eur J Respir Dis 1987;71:164–169.
55. Fink JN. Epidemiologic aspects of hypersensitivity pneumonitis. Monogr Allergy 1987;21:59–69.
56. Dalphin JC, Toson B, Monnet E, Pernet D, Dubiez A, Laplante JJ, Aiache JM, Depierre A. Farmer's lung precipitins in Doubs (a department of France): prevalence and diagnostic value. Allergy 1994;49:744–750.
57. Welker L, Jörres RA, Costabel U, Magnussen H. Predictive value of BAL cell differentials in the diagnosis of interstitial lung diseases. Eur Respir J 2004;24:1000–1006.
58. Cormier Y, Bélanger J, LeBlanc P, Laviolette M. Bronchoalveolar lavage in farmers' lung disease: diagnostic and physiological significance. Br J Ind Med 1986;43:401–405.
59. Selman M, Pardo A, Barrera L, Estrada A, Watson SR, Wilson K, Aziz N, Kaminski N, Zlotnik A. Gene expression profiles distinguish idiopathic pulmonary fibrosis from hypersensitivity pneumonitis. Am J Respir Crit Care Med 2006;173:188–198.
60. Cormier Y, Belanger J, Laviolette M. Persistent bronchoalveolar lymphocytosis in asymptomatic farmers. Am Rev Respir Dis 1986;133:843–847.
61. Semenzato G. Immunology of interstitial lung diseases: cellular events taking place in the lung of sarcoidosis, hypersensitivity pneumonitis and HIV infection. Eur Respir J 1991;4: 94–102.
62. Murayama J, Yoshizawa Y, Ohtsuka M, Hasegawa S. Lung fibrosis in hypersensitivity pneumonitis. Association with CD4+ but not CD8+ cell dominant alveolitis and insidious onset. Chest 1993;104:38–43.
63. Ando M, Konishi K, Yoneda R, Tamura M. Difference in the phenotypes of bronchoalveolar lavage lymphocytes in patients with summer-type hypersensitivity pneumonitis, farmer's lung, ventilation pneumonitis, and bird fancier's lung: report of a nationwide epidemiologic study in Japan. J Allergy Clin Immunol. 1991;87:1002–1009.
64. Drent M, van Velzen-Blad H, Diamant M, Wagenaar SS, Hoogsteden HC, van den Bosch JM. Bronchoalveolar lavage in extrinsic allergic alveolitis: effect of time elapsed since antigen exposure. Eur Respir J 1993;6:1276–1281.
65. Pardo A, Barrios R, Gaxiola M, Segura-Valdez L, Carrillo G, Estrada A, Mejía M, Selman M. Increase of lung neutrophils in hypersensitivity pneumonitis is associated with lung fibrosis. Am J Respir Crit Care Med 2000;161:1698–1704.
66. Drent M, Velzen-Blad H, Diamant M, Wagenaar SS, Donckerwolck-Bogaert M, van den Bosch JM. Differential diagnostic value of plasma cells in bronchoalveolar lavage fluid. Chest 1993;103:1720–1724.
67. Drent M, Wagenaar SjSc, Velzen-Blad H, Mulder PG, Hoogsteden HC, van den Bosch JM. Relationship between plasma cell levels and profile of bronchoalveolar lavage fluid in patients with subacute extrinsic allergic alveolitis. Thorax 1993;48:835–839.
68. Laviolette M, Cormier Y, Loiseau A, Soler P, Leblanc P, Hance AJ. Bronchoalveolar mast cells in normal farmers and subjects with farmer's lung. Diagnostic, prognostic, and physiologic significance. Am Rev Respir Dis 1991;144:855–860.
69. Miadonna A, Pesci A, Tedeschi A, Bertorelli G, Arquati M, Olivieri D. Mast cell and histamine involvement in farmer's lung disease. Chest 1994;105:1184–1189.

70. Ohtani Y, Kojima K, Sumi Y, Sawada M, Inase N, Miyake S, Yoshizawa Y. Inhalation provocation tests in chronic bird fancier's lung. Chest 2000;118:1382–1389.
71. Vourlekis JS, Schwarz MI, Cool CD, Tuder RM, King TE, Brown KK. Nonspecific interstitial pneumonitis as the sole histologic expression of hypersensitivity pneumonitis. Am J Med 2002;112:490–493.
72. Coleman A, Colby TV. Histologic diagnosis of extrinsic allergic alveolitis. Am J Surg Pathol 1988;12:514–518.
73. Reyes CN, Wenzel FJ, Lawton BR, Emanuel DA. The pulmonary pathology of farmer's lung disease. Chest 1982;81:142–146.
74. Pérez-Padilla R, Gaxiola M, Salas J, Mejía M, Ramos C, Selman M. Bronchiolitis in chronic pigeon breeder's disease. Morphological evidence of a spectrum of small airway lesions in hypersensitivity pneumonitis induced by avian antigens. Chest 1996;110:371–377.
75. Ohtani Y, Saiki S, Kitaichi M, Usui Y, Inase N, Costabel U, Yoshizawa Y. Chronic bird fancier's lung: histopathological and clinical correlation. An application of the 2002 ATS/ERS consensus classification of the idiopathic interstitial pneumonias. Thorax 2005;60:665–671.
76. Herraez I, Gutierrez M, Alonso N, Allende J. Hypersensitivity pneumonitis producing a BOOP-like reaction: HRCT/pathologic correlation. J Thorac Imaging 2002;17:81–83.
77. Hayakawa H, Shirai M, Sato A, Yoshizawa Y, Todate A, Imokawa S, Suda T, Chida K, Tamura R, Ishihara K, Saiki S, Ando M. Clinicopathological features of chronic hypersensitivity pneumonitis. Respirology 2002;7:359–364.
78. Churg A, Muller NL, Flint J, Wright JL. Chronic hypersensitivity pneumonitis. Am J Surg Pathol 2006;30:201–208.
79. Khalil N, Churg A, Muller N, O'Connor R. Environmental, inhaled and ingested causes of pulmonary fibrosis. Toxicol Pathol 2007;35:86–96.
80. Ramirez-Venegas A, Sansores RH, Pérez-Padilla R, Carrillo G, Selman M. Utility of a provocation test for diagnosis of chronic pigeon breeder's disease. Am J Respir Crit Care Med 1998;158:862–869.
81. Reynolds SP, Jones KP, Edwards JH, Davies BH. Inhalation challenge in pigeon breeder's disease: BAL fluid changes after 6 hours. Eur Respir J 1993;6:467–476.
82. Yoshida K, Ando M, Sakata T, Araki S. Prevention of summer-type hypersensitivity pneumonitis: effect of elimination of *Trichosporon cutaneum* from the patient's homes. Arch Environ Health 1989;44:317–322.
83. Vourlekis JS, Schwarz MI, Cherniack RM, Curran-Everett D, Cool CD, Tuder RM, King TE Jr, Brown KK. The effect of pulmonary fibrosis on survival in patients with hypersensitivity pneumonitis. Am J Med 2004;116:662–668.
84. Cormier Y, Bélanger J. Long-term physiologic outcome after acute farmer's lung. Chest 1985;87:796–800.
85. Erkinjuntti-Pekkanen R, Rytkonen H, Kokkarinen JI, Tukiainen HO, Partanen K, Terho EO. Long-term risk of emphysema in patients with farmer's lung and matched control farmers. Am J Respir Crit Care Med 1998;158:662–665.

Chapter 8
Connective Tissue Disease and Vasculitis-Associated Interstitial Lung Disease

Alan N. Brown and Charlie Strange

Introduction

Connective tissue diseases (CTDs) remain among the most difficult causes of interstitial lung diseases (ILDs) to correctly diagnose and treat. Part of the difficulty occurs because the symptoms of cough, dyspnea, and exercise limitation are common to all of the ILDs. Therefore, consideration of other factors that define the systemic illness becomes important. Unfortunately, CTDs can involve every organ in the body; therefore, a working knowledge of all of internal medicine becomes important in this set of diseases.

All of the CTDs are characterized by evidence of vascular injury, autoimmunity, tissue inflammation, and organ dysfunction. Some of these diseases have more inflammatory vascular disease than others. In this chapter, we will discuss the CTDs that have prominent pulmonary presentations, and separately discuss the antineutrophil cytoplasmic antibody (ANCA)-associated vasculitides Wegener's granulomatosis and microscopic polyangiitis. A comprehensive discussion of the lung vasculature is not included in this chapter.

CTDs and the Lung

Many of the CTD have pulmonary presentations. The lungs may be the primary site of initial clinical symptoms, may have an occult involvement at any time during the disease process, and may develop symptomatic pathology after many years. The pulmonary presentations are distinct to each individual CTD. Therefore, this chapter will discuss the pulmonary manifestations within the context of the diseases. Although ILD is common to all of the diseases, a working knowledge of the other causes of dyspnea becomes important to understand when following an individual patient who is not responding well to therapy.

R.P. Baughman et al. (eds.), *Pulmonary Arterial Hypertension and Interstitial Lung Diseases,*
© Humana Press, a part of Springer Science + Business Media, LLC 2009

Rheumatoid Arthritis (RA)

The most common ILD associated with CTD occurs with RA. RA affects up to 1% of the population and is three times more common in women than in men; the peak age of onset is in the third to fifth decades of life but can occur at any age. The hallmark presentation is symmetrical polyarthritis of unknown etiology. The diagnosis of RA is established by the American College of Rheumatology criteria (Table 8.1) [1]. The majority of extra-articular manifestations of RA occur in a population of rheumatoid factor (RF) or anti-cyclic citullinated peptide (anti-CCP) positive patients.

One of the more recent diagnostic tests for RA is a serum assay for anti-CCP. This antibody recognizes a binding domain on citrullinated extracellular fibrin on the rheumatoid synovium, and current research has defined a pathogenic role of this protein in RA [2]. Anti-CCP appears to have a marginally greater sensitivity and specificity for RA than RF and, thus, may supplant or supplement serum testing.

The prevalence of interstitial lung disease in RA is dependent on the diagnostic test administered to search for the disease. Pathologically, open lung biopsies have shown usual interstitial pneumonia (UIP) in the majority of cases [3]. Because UIP is also the pathology of idiopathic pulmonary fibrosis (IPF), a clinical joint evaluation is appropriate in all patients with IPF.

Pulmonary fibrosis can be the presenting manifestation of RA. Joint disease can be clinically silent for up to 2 years while the disease progresses. Furthermore, the diagnosis of RA is complicated by the nonspecific nature of RF, because this assay is above the upper limits of normal in 36% of patients with IPF [4]. Therefore, IPF patients with a positive RF should receive further testing to include hand and feet radiographs, as well as anti-CCP antibody titers.

The ILD of RA should be distinguished from rheumatoid nodules. Rheumatoid nodules in the lung are often multiple and can occur as a myriad of small ill defined infiltrates on the chest computed tomography [5]. Rheumatoid nodules usually grow when rheumatoid disease activity is active. Growth is suppressed, and most nodules regress to some degree on adequate levels of disease modifying drugs. However, therapy with methotrexate does not always cause regression of rheumatoid nodules [6]. Because RA is associated with an increased risk of malignancy,

Table 8.1 Diagnostic Criteria for RA [1]*

1. Morning stiffness in and around joints lasting at least 1 h before maximal improvement for 6 weeks
2. Soft-tissue swelling (arthritis) of three or more joint areas observed by a physician present for 6 weeks
3. Swelling (arthritis) of the proximal interphalangeal, metacarpophalangeal, or wrist joints present for 6 weeks
4. Symmetric joint swelling present for 6 weeks.
5. Rheumatoid nodules
6. The presence of rheumatoid factor
7. Radiographic erosions and/or periarticular osteopenia in hand and/or wrist joints

*Four of the seven findings must be present.

serial examination of nodules should define that these regress at the same degree. The possibility of lung cancer should be entertained when one nodule grows while others regress in size.

Other pulmonary manifestations of RA (Table 8.2) include arthritis of the cricoarytenoid joint that causes upper airway obstruction from bilateral vocal cord paresis, pleural effusions, airways disease, organizing pneumonia, and acute presentations of diffuse alveolar damage [7]. In addition, the toxicity of medications such as methotrexate should be considered. Pleural effusions are neutrophilic exudates with a characteristically low glucose and pH. These can lead to trapped lung, a condition in which the pleura is thickened and inelastic, leading to dyspnea from inadequate lung excursion.

Airway diseases associated with RA remain among the most difficult manifestations to accurately diagnose and treat. Pathologically, an inflammatory infiltrate of small airway walls can lead to airway narrowing, air trapping, and small airway closure (bronchiolitis obliterans). More proximal airways can become injured, resulting in bronchiolectasis or bronchiectasis that subsequently may become colonized with unusual pathogens. In the setting of immunosuppressants for RA, these airway pathogens may become a source of symptoms. An organizing pneumonia may be present with the organizing airways disease that defines the disease bronchiolitis obliterans organizing pneumonia. When this disease is idiopathic, the terminology changes to cryptogenic organizing pneumonia [8].

Rarely, a more acute presentation of RA may involve the lung. These individuals present with the abrupt onset of fever and dyspnea, diffuse alveolar infiltrates on radiography, and hypoxemia. The pathology of this presentation is diffuse alveolar damage [9], the same pathology as seen in the acute respiratory distress syndrome (ARDS). This syndrome may be subtly different from ARDS on biopsy with a more active vascular inflammatory infiltrate that helps define this as a variant of rheumatoid vasculitis.

To date, there is no randomized study that proves that treatment of the lung disease independent of the activity of joint disease leads to improved pulmonary

Table 8.2 Manifestations of RA Causing Dyspnea

ILD	UIP
	NSIP
	Cryptogenic organizing pneumonia
	Apical fibrobullous disease
Airway disease	Bronchiolitis obliterans
	Follicular bronchiolitis
	Bronchiectasis
Pleural disease	Pleural effusion
	Pleural fibrosis causing trapped lung
Acute lung injury	Diffuse alveolar damage
	Pulmonary hemorrhage with capillaritis
Parenchymal lung nodules	Rheumatoid nodule (cavitary or noncavitary)
Upper airway obstruction	Tracheal rheumatoid nodules
	Arthritis of the cricoarytenoid joint causing vocal cord paresis
	Vasculitis of the recurrent laryngeal nerve

outcomes. However, because lung disease can precede and cause more symptoms than joint disease when present, many physicians will transition patients to tumour necrosis factor inhibitors, which are the most effective disease-modifying drugs when RA lung manifestations are present. Successful treatment of ILD has been reported with corticosteroids, methotrexate, azathioprine, cyclosporine [10], cyclo-phosphamide, and tumor necrosis factor inhibitors. It remains unknown whether any aspects of UIP improve; however, inflammatory lesions in the lungs of RA patients with progressive lung disease may improve. Therefore, the typical response of aggressive therapy for RA ILD is stabilization of lung function decline, regression of any lung nodules present, improved joint symptoms and exercise tolerance, and improved quality of life. Although a nonspecific test, the Westergren sedimentation rate is used by some practitioners to follow rheumatoid disease activity.

Systemic Sclerosis (SSc)

SSc is a CTD characterized by abnormalities of the skin (scleroderma). The American College of Rheumatology provides a case definition and subset differentiation on skin findings that include a diffuse cutaneous variant and a limited cutaneous (CREST) variant (Table 8.3). However, the excess mortality in this disease is defined by systemic organ involvement that often causes dyspnea from pulmonary or cardiac involvement.

SSc is a rare disease with an incidence of 1–2 cases per 100,000 individuals yearly and a US prevalence of 26 cases per 100,000 population [11]. A female predominance of 6–8:1 is similar to other CTD, although men who are affected tend to experience more severe disease. Raynaud's phenomenon is almost universal and is usually the first symptom of disease.

The pathogenesis of SSc remains unknown and is the focus of active research. Pathologic studies have documented proliferative and obliterative vascular change, particularly of small blood vessels as part of disease pathogenesis. The most obvious clinical disease apparent to a pulmonary clinician is pulmonary arterial

Table 8.3 Findings of SS Variants

	Diffuse cutaneous	Limited cutaneous (CREST variant)
Skin findings	Diffuse	Limited to hands to the elbows, feet to the knees, and face
Percent female	>70%	>90%
Raynaud phenomenon	Yes, short duration	Yes, long duration
Nailfold Capillaries	Dropout, dilated loops	Dilated loops
ANA	Positive, Anti-Scl-70 in ~30%	Positive, Anti-centromere in ~75%
HLA	DR5	DR1;DR4 and DRw8
Common organ manifestations	Lung, esophagus, heart, kidney, small bowel	Lung, pulmonary arterioles, systemic calcinosis, esophagus, diffuse telangiectasias.
10-year survival	70%	95%

hypertension, although the extent that abnormal vascular disease leads to the changes in esophageal dysmotility, pulmonary fibrosis, renal vascular disease, and cardiac and skin fibrosis remains unknown.

Autoimmunity is likely important in disease pathogenesis. Antinuclear antibodies (ANAs) are positive in >95% of patients and is often in high titer. Antibodies associated with topoisomerase (Scl-70), as well as a variety of other antigens have been described. Scl-70 antibodies, although present in a minority of diffuse cutaneous SSc patients are associated with the presence of lung disease [12].

Genetic factors have been implicated in disease pathogenesis. HLA alleles are among the most common risk factors, although different ethnic populations have different alleles that place them at risk. In short, the strongest risk factor for the development of SSc is a family history of SSc, although the absolute risk for any family member remains quite low [11]. The role of abnormal collagen deposition from the myofibroblast, a cell with smooth muscle and fibroblast features, is in active study. These cells found in skin and lung have dysregulated collagen turnover.

Pulmonary involvement is common in SSc, with approximately equal distribution of pulmonary hypertension and ILD. The authors of some series suggest that ILD is present in 60% of SSc patients at presentation and in 80% of SSc patients when followed serially [13]. The type of ILD is pathologically nonspecific interstitial pneumonitis (NSIP) more commonly than UIP [14]. High-resolution computed tomography (HRCT) of the lung often defines the extent of disease and can be graded as limited ILD (<10% of the lung involved) and extensive ILD (>30% of the lung involved), since the group of patients with extensive disease is most likely to progress [15]. Spirometry is also useful to grade the severity of disease showing restriction. A forced vital capacity (FVC) <70% suggests a patient is at risk of further ILD progression [16].

Rarely, lung disease can occur before the development of other systemic manifestations of disease. "SSc sine scleroderma" is defined by manifestations of organ involvement prior to skin thickening [17]. Therefore, an appropriate screening for connective tissue disease in an ILD evaluation requires a complete review of systems focusing on skin, joint and esophageal symptoms.

Much work has focused on whether biomarkers, bronchoalveolar lavage cellularity, or specific HRCT patterns such as ground glass opacity make a difference in disease progression. Some biomarkers hold promise in lung disease diagnosis. Serum levels of surfactant proteins A and D are increased in SSc patients with lung disease. KL-6, a mucin-like glycoprotein expressed on type II pneumocytes also is increased in individuals with ILD. Whether these biomarkers define a therapy responsive population remains to be determined.

Recent large studies have suggested that HRCT fibrosis but not ground glass opacity or the BAL characteristics are helpful in defining a population who will subsequently progress or respond to specific therapy for ILD [15]. The ILD is typically subpleural in a circumferential pattern beginning in the lower lobes. Ground glass opacity, particularly if associated with traction bronchiectasis, suggests a fibrotic area of the lung parenchyma. However, it is the reticular extent of disease that is most associated with functional impairment [18].

Bronchoalveolar lavage (BAL) has been used to assess the cellularity of the lower airways in SSc ILD finding that abnormal polymorphonuclear leukocyte percentages >3% and/or eosinophil percentages >2% are associated with more advanced disease [19]. Whether BAL cellularity predicts the subsequent ILD course remains much less clear. Although patients with excess BAL cellularity appeared more likely to respond to cyclophosphamide in some studies, a larger prospective randomized study failed to show that difference [20]. Because HRCT is easier to obtain than BAL, subsequent staging systems for the extent of ILD will not likely use BAL [16].

Treatment of SSc ILD remains controversial. The Scleroderma Lung Study was a large randomized controlled trial comparing cyclophosphamide to placebo in SSc ILD of onset <7 years from the first non-Raynaud's manifestation. The baseline adjusted FVC declined less in 1 year in the oral cyclophosphamide arm compared with placebo, although the absolute difference of FVC decline was within the minimal clinically significant change for FVC. Associated improvements in dyspnea, skin scores, and quality of life were also seen at the endpoint of 1 year [15]. Unfortunately, after stopping cyclophosphamide at 1 year, the benefits were not sustained at 24 months [21]. A study with similar design using intravenous cyclophosphamide produced similar results [22].

Other drugs have been tried without efficacy in SSc. The most promising drug for being a less toxic alternative to cyclophosphamide is mycophenolate mofetil. Numerous case series have been performed, with sometimes dramatic improvement found in HRCT and FVC results [23,24]. Prospective randomized studies are pending.

Although severe esophageal dysmotility is common in patients with SSc, the impact of aspiration on lung disease is confirmed in a minority of patients. The severity of lung disease does not correlate closely with the severity of esophageal disease, as measured by the propensity for reflux [25]. However, most patients should be treated with proton pump inhibitors for life to avoid the complications of chronic acid reflux, including Barrett's esophagus and malignancy.

Lung cancer occurs with increased frequency in patients with SSc, and any nodules should be aggressively managed because there is not a nodular form of SSc in the thorax. Organizing pneumonia is occasionally observed; this will often respond to corticosteroid therapy. However, corticosteroids are associated with increased incidence of SSc renal crisis. Whether the corticosteroid risk still holds with concomitant angiotensin-converting enzyme inhibitor treatment has not been assessed. Finally, a rare obstructive lung disease has been noted.

Pulmonary vascular abnormalities in the absence of ILD may occur in up to 30% of patients with limited cutaneous scleroderma (CREST variant). The pulmonary vascular disease is characterised by medial and intimal proliferation with vascular dropout when the vascular lumen is small [26]. Plexiform lesions can be seen. This form of pulmonary arterial hypertension (PAH) accounts for up to 50% of the cases of PAH seen in some referral centers.

A more complicated disease occurs when pulmonary hypertension is associated with ILD or smoking-related emphysema. In these conditions, some of the loss of vasculature is caused by the absence of functional vessels, whereas other patients may have some element of hypoxemia associated vasoconstriction. Therapy in these cases requires careful treatment to assure that worsened ventilation perfusion matching does not occur if pulmonary vasodilators are given [27]. Prostacyclins, endothelin receptor antagonists, and phosphodiesterase inhibitors have been successful in improving functional capacity and mortality in SSc PAH.

One of the consequences of treatment for pulmonary hypertension is the possibility of pulmonary oedema. Veno-occlusive disease and capillary hemangiomatosis have both been reported in patients with scleroderma [28]. However, fibrosis of the heart is also a common finding in patients presenting with this disease [29]. Unrecognized diastolic dysfunction may produce dyspnea, pulmonary hypertension, and right heart failure. Cardiac catheterization is necessary to define proper therapy in the majority of patients.

Pleural disease is uncommon in SSc occurring in <10% of patients over the lifetime of disease [30]. Overlap syndromes with other features suggestive of SLE are seen in some individuals. Pleural and pericardial effusions are occasionally large enough that drainage will improve outcome. Pneumothorax is seen rarely in ILD.

Bronchogenic carcinoma and other cancers are increased in frequency in SSc and frequently occur in nonsmokers. Because SSc does not have a nodular clinical presentation, diagnostic work for opportunistic infections or cancer should occur for most lung nodules.

Gastrointestinal involvement in patients with SSc is nearly universal. Esophageal dysmotility can lead to aspiration, although most studies suggest that aspiration does not influence the incidence or severity of ILD. Nevertheless, pulmonary infections are increased in studies in which the authors use BAL and failure to thrive may occasionally be improved by the administration of antibiotics for occult pulmonary infection. Abdominal distention can impact lung function and is sometimes improved with promotility agents because the small bowel is also affected with a dysmotility syndrome. Bacterial overgrowth, alternating diarrhea and constipation, and bloating are sometimes improved by courses of nonabsorbable antibiotics that limit bacterial overgrowth. Another treatable condition that can contribute to dyspnea is an inflammatory myositis that can occur in overlap from polymyositis/dermatomyositis (PM/DM) or independently. Muscle weakness is improved with small doses of corticosteroids.

PM/DM

The idiopathic inflammatory myopathies are a group of diseases that are characterized by muscle injury on biopsy and variable degrees of autoantibody production. Some of the idiopathic inflammatory myopathies such as inclusion body myositis do not have associated lung disease. However, the most common of these diseases, polymyositis, is an autoimmune disease that often involves the lung. When associated with skin disease, this disease is called dermatomyositis. A rare form of amyopathic dermatomyositis may exist in which the classic skin presentation does not have clinical or laboratory evidence of muscle injury present. Therefore, for purposes of this review, polymyositis and dermatomyositis (i.e., PM/DM) in all of its forms will be discussed as a single disease.

PM/DM is still diagnosed by the classic criteria of Peters and Bohm (Table 8.4), although other diagnostic criteria are being evaluated that involve improved use of the many new autoantibodies found in this idiopathic inflammatory myopathy (Table 8.5). Unfortunately, many of the acute clinical pulmonary presentations reviewed below will not meet classic diagnostic criteria. Therefore, a high index of suspicion is needed when clinical weakness is part of a pulmonary presentation with an undiagnosed diffuse lung disease.

In characterising the autoantibodies involved with muscle injury, a group of antibodies against transfer RNA synthetases were found. The first of these with clinical importance was named Jo-1. The Jo-1 antibody-associated antisynthetase syndrome was described as a subgroup of PM/DM with a high incidence of associated lung injury. Subsequently, other antibodies have been described that can be obtained from many laboratories in the form of myositis antibody panels.

The clinical presentation of patients with PM/DM is heterogeneous. Muscle weakness is a consistent feature of disease, but often it is discounted with a more prominent pulmonary presentation. Muscle weakness occurs in all striated muscle and therefore may occur in pharyngeal and upper esophageal musculature, which may complicate the risk of aspiration-associated lung disease. Diaphragmatic dysfunction may also occur from muscle weakness.

A common DM/PM presentation occurs when a patient is in the intensive care unit. Some case series suggest that up to 50% of patients may present with an acute to subacute presentation that clinically is similar to ARDS. The pathology of that presentation is diffuse alveolar damage, and no comparative treatment trials have been performed. Patients usually have a history of arthralgias and weakness that can be easily overlooked given the severity of pulmonary disease. Treatment with high-dose corticosteroids is associated with improvement that is sufficient enough to recover from acute respiratory failure in half of affected individuals. Most survivors have severe residual impairment of lung function.

Table 8.4 Diagnostic Criteria for PM/(DM [68,69]

1. Progressive proximal symmetrical weakness
2. Elevated muscle enzyme levels
3. Abnormal findings on electromyogram consistent with myopathy
4. Abnormal findings from muscle biopsy with myositis
5. Compatible cutaneous disease (defines dermatomyositis)

Definite PM = first four are present; probable PM = three of first four are present; possible PM = two of first four are present.
Definite DM = presence of rash + three other criteria; probable DM = presence of rash + two other; possible DM = presence of rash + one other criterion.

Table 8.5 Myositis-Specific Autoantibodies Found in Some Individuals With Myositis

Myositis-specific autoantibody	Antigen	Frequency in adult PM/DM	Comments
Jo-1	Histidyl-tRNA synthetase	20–30%	May be present in ILD before muscle symptoms begin
PL-7	Threonyl-tRNA synthetase	~3%	
PL-12	Alanyl-tRNA synthetase	~3%	
EJ	Glycyl-tRNA synthetase	~2%	
OJ	Isoleucyl-tRNA synthetase	~2%	
KS	Asparaginyl-tRNA synthetase	Rare	
Zo	Phenylalanyl-tRNA synthetase	Rare	
	Leucyl-tRNA synthetase	<1%	
	Lysyl-tRNA synthetase	<1%	
	GLUPRO-tRNA synthetase	<1%	
SRP	Signal recognition particle		
155/140	Transcriptional intermediary factor 1γ	20–30%	Low incidence of ILD; greater frequency in cancer associated PM/DM
U1-RNP	70-kDa polypeptide		
U3-RNP	34-kDa protein in U3-RNP particle		
Anti-Fibrillarin			
Ku	60- to 70- and 80- to 86-kDa proteins		
PM-Scl	PM-Scl proteins	~5%	Seen in overlap syndrome with Systemic Sclerosis
Mi-2	Nuclear helicase Mi-2	15–25%	Fulminant myositis; poor treatment responsiveness; increased in African American females

Ab, antibody; kDa, kilodalton.

Systemic Lupus Erythematosus (SLE)

SLE is a systemic autoimmune disease with the capacity to affect every organ system in the body. The etiology is unknown, although hormonal, racial, genetic, and environmental factors have been implicated. SLE is primarily a disease of young women, with a female-to-male ratio of 9:1. Black and Hispanic subjects are affected more commonly than are white subjects; the prevalence varies worldwide and is approximately 1 case per 2,000 people in the USA. Antinuclear antibodies are present in the serum of virtually every patient with SLE, whereas antibodies to the Smith antigen and double-stranded DNA are more specific for the diagnosis. Classification criteria have been established by the American College of Radiology (Table 8.6); the presence of 4 of the 11 criteria is sufficient to establish the diagnosis.

Table 8.6 1982 Revised Diagnostic Criteria for SLE [70]

- Serositis: pleurisy, pericarditis
- Oral ulcers: oral or nasopharyngeal, usually painless
- Arthritis: nonerosive peripheral polyarthritis
- Photosensitivity
- Blood disorders: leukopenia, lymphopenia, thrombocytopenia, Coombs-positive anemia
- Renal involvement: proteinuria or cellular casts
- ANAs
- Immunologic phenomena - lupus erythematosus cells; anti–double-stranded DNA; anti-Smith antibodies; antiphospholipid antibodies
- Neurologic disorder: seizures or psychosis
- Malar rash
- Discoid rash

In most cases, the diagnosis of SLE is made when four or more of the criteria have occurred at some time.

Pleuritis is the most common pulmonary manifestation in SLE, and occurs at some point in the disease course in approximately 50% of patients. Autopsy studies have shown the presence of pleural effusions in about two-thirds of patients [31]. The pathogenesis of pleural effusions in SLE is likely immune complex deposition, as low concentrations of complement and evidence of complement fixation are present in the pleural fluid [32]. Pleural fluid analysis shows an exudative effusion. The presence of LE cells is diagnostic of SLE, but this test is now largely obsolete. ANAs are commonly found in pleural fluid, but are not specific for SLE and need not be routinely obtained [33]. The treatment of pleuritis in SLE includes nonsteroidal anti-inflammatory drugs or corticosteroids (usually no more than 10 to 20 mg of prednisone equivalent daily); hydroxychloroquine is effective for long-term treatment.

Acute lupus pneumonitis is an uncommon pulmonary manifestation of SLE, with a prevalence of <10% [34]. The typical presentation is an acute onset of fever, cough, and dyspnea; diffuse alveolar infiltrates are seen on chest radiographs. An infectious process must be excluded. Acute lupus pneumonitis is often observed in the setting of other manifestations of active lupus and hence concomitant immunosuppression is common. BAL may be useful in this regard and may also help differentiate acute lupus pneumonitis from alveolar hemorrhage. The lavage fluid in pneumonitis shows increased numbers of red blood cells but not frankly hemorrhagic fluid [35]. The prognosis in patients is poor, with mortality rates approaching 50% [36]. Treatment includes high doses of corticosteroids; in addition, concomitant therapy with azathioprine or cyclophosphamide should be considered [37].

The shrinking lung syndrome is a rare complication of SLE characterised by progressive dyspnea, decreased lung volumes, and often a restrictive pattern on pulmonary function testing. The prevalence of this condition is uncertain, and has been reported to be rare (49 reported cases) [38] to fairly common (23% in one series.) [39]. The underlying pathogenesis is likewise not well defined; diaphragmatic myopathy, myositis, and muscle fibrosis as well as phrenic nerve lesions have all been implicated. Treatment of this condition includes moderate to high (30–60 mg of prednisone daily) doses of corticosteroids, theophylline, β-agonists, or immunosuppressive agents [40].

Alveolar hemorrhage is an abrupt and potentially devastating consequence of SLE. In one large case series, the prevalence was 3.7% for all hospital admissions related to SLE, with a mortality rate of 53% [41]. An acute presentation with cough, dyspnea, and hemoptysis is most common, although the absence of hemoptysis does not exclude the diagnosis. Laboratory studies may show anemia, and diffuse alveolar infiltrates are seen on chest radiography. BAL with return of bloody lavage fluid is diagnostic; cultures should be obtained to rule out infection as an inciting event. The pathogenesis is uncertain but likely involves pulmonary capillaritis. No randomized trials are available to guide therapy. Clinical experience suggests the most effective therapy is plasmapheresis combined with pulse-dose corticosteroids and cyclophosphamide [42].

Chronic interstitial lung disease is uncommon in SLE as compared with that encountered in RA, SSc, and PM/DM, although the clinical presentation is similar. The prevalence of chronic ILD has been reported to be from 3% to 8% in various studies [34], and its management is similar to that of ILD in other CTDs.

Pulmonary hypertension occurs in up to 14% of patients with SLE, and the clinical characteristics are similar to those in idiopathic PAH. However, the prognosis is significantly worse in SLE-associated pulmonary hypertension, with 5-year survival rates as low as 16.8% [43]. Its management is similar to that of idiopathic PAH.

Sjögren Syndrome (SS)

SS is an autoimmune disorder characterised by a lymphocytic infiltration of exocrine glands. The hallmark of this disorder is the sicca complex, characterised by dry eyes (keratoconjunctivitis sicca or xerophthalmia) and dry mouth (xerostomia.) However, extraglandular organs are also involved, and the disease has the capacity to affect multiple organ systems. SS may occur as a primary autoimmune disorder (primary SS or Sjögren disease) or as a constellation of symptoms associated with another autoimmune disorder such as RA, SLE, PM/DM, or SSc (secondary SS).

A wide variation in the frequency of respiratory tract involvement in SS has been reported; ranging from 9% to 75% [44]. The clinical spectrum of pulmonary tract involvement in SS ranges from xerotrachea (often resulting in a chronic cough) to bronchiolar disease, interstitial pneumonitis, ILD, and lymphoma.

Lymphocytic bronchiolitis is frequently present and may progress to a lymphocytic interstitial pneumonitis (LIP) [45]. The association of LIP and SS is well established with SS associated with 25% of the reported cases of LIP [46]. Lung cysts are a common finding in patients with LIP [47]; other pulmonary findings include ground glass opacities, centrilobular nodules, interstitial thickening, and lymphadenopathy [48].

In addition to LIP, a wide variety of histologic findings has been described in SS-associated ILD. NSIP has been reported to be the most common histologic subtype [49]. NSIP, organizing pneumonia, UIP, primary pulmonary lymphoma, and amyloidosis were each reported in one case series [44]. Lymphoma may be of the mucosal-associated lymphoid tissue type [50]. Corticosteroid and immunosuppressive therapy is commonly used in the treatment of SS-associated ILD, but optimal treatment has yet to be defined.

Wegener Granulomatosis (WG)

WG is a systemic vasculitis with the capacity to affect virtually every organ system in the body; the respiratory tract and kidneys are most commonly involved. WG may occur at any age, and occurs with equal frequency in men and women. The pathologic hallmark is a granulomatous vasculitis of small and medium arteries, although venules and large arteries may also be involved. Extravascular granulomatous inflammation of the upper and lower respiratory tract is also frequently seen [51]. The pathogenesis of the disease is unknown, although a strong association with the presence of ANCAs is recognized. The finding of ANCA in other forms of systemic vasculitis, including microscopic polyangiitis [52] and Churg-Strauss syndrome, suggests the possibility of a pathologic role for these antibodies. As a result of this finding, these disease entities are often considered part of a clinical spectrum of ANCA-associated vasculitides [53].

The presenting manifestations of WG are protean and commonly include constitutional symptoms such as fever, night sweats, and weight loss. Ocular, skin, and musculoskeletal manifestations are frequently encountered [54]. Up to 80% of patients will develop renal disease at some point in the disease course [51] A somewhat-artificial differentiation between "limited" WG (i.e., involving only the upper respiratory tract) and "diffuse" WG is often described. However, whether there are actual phenotypic differences in the limited and diffuse forms of WG is not well understood [55]. A predominance of pulmonary findings is a common presentation of WG [56]. Clinical manifestations of WG involving the respiratory tract include tracheal stenosis, diffuse alveolar hemorrhage, pulmonary nodules (solitary or multiple), cavitary lesions, and interstitial lung disease [57].

In the clinical setting of a pulmonary vasculitis, the diagnosis of WG is suggested by the presence of circulating ANCA. Virtually all patients with active WG have ANCA [58], but it remains unclear as to whether the presence of ANCA is a marker for disease activity [59]. In WG, ANCA are most commonly of the cytoplasmic staining pattern (c-ANCA); this is usually due to antibodies directed against proteinase-3 (anti PR-3) [53].

Aggressive therapy is indicated in the treatment of WG; a 90% mortality rate at 2 years is found in patients with untreated diffuse WG, most often the result of pulmonary disease or renal failure. The combination of oral cyclophosphamide and glucocorticoids to induce remission is the best-studied regimen [51]. A regimen of induction of remission with cyclophosphamide and maintenance of remission with azathioprine has been described and may have less toxic side effects [60]. Treatment with the tumour necrosis factor inhibitor etanercept was not effective in one trial and may have been associated with increased morbidity [61]. Rituximab, a monoclonal antibody directed against CD-20, has been reported to be effective in the management of refractory WG [62]. In general, limited WG carries a more favorable prognosis, and therapy might be include the use of less toxic immunosuppressants such as methotrexate, azathioprine, and/or corticosteroids [63].

Microscopic Polyangiitis (MPA)

MPA [52] is an ANCA-associated vasculitis affecting small vessels (capillaries, venules, arterioles). Histopathologically, a necrotizing vasculitis without immune complex deposition is seen. Similar to WG, the pathogenesis of MPA is unknown, although a strong association with ANCA is also found. Unlike WG, granuloma formation or granulomatous vasculitis are not features of MPA.

The presenting manifestations of MPA are not as varied as those seen in WG. Constitutional symptoms are quite common, and a rapidly progressive glomerulonephritis is seen in the vast majority of patients. Pulmonary manifestations, most commonly diffuse alveolar hemorrhage, are seen in approximately 25% of patients. Skin, joint, and neurologic findings are frequently seen [64].

Like WG, ANCA are a central feature of the diagnosis of MPA. In the latter, ANCA usually present with a perinuclear staining pattern (p-ANCA) indicating the presence of antibodies to myeloperoxidase (anti-MPO.) The presence of p-ANCA and anti-MPO in MPA are not as sensitive or specific as are c-ANCA and antiPR-3 [65]. ANCA have been reported to have a direct pathologic role in the pathogenesis of MPA [66]. In general, the therapy of MPA mirrors that of WG. A "limited" form such as has been described in WG is not usually seen in MPA. Aggressive corticosteroid therapy, cyclophosphamide, rituximab, and plasma exchange therapy have all been used in the treatment of MPA [67].

Summary

The connective tissue diseases cause a variety of diseases within the chest. Successful management depends on accurate diagnosis of the CTD and the specific chest manifestation. Management of the lung disease is usually by immunosuppressive medications after infection and drug toxicity has been excluded. The immune modulating drugs should be chosen on the basis of what is known about the treatment responsiveness of each CTD entity. Collaboration between rheumatologists and pulmonologists is important to achieve desired outcomes.

References

1. Arnett FC, Edworthy SM, Bloch DA, McShane DJ, Fries JF, Cooper NS, Healey LA, Kaplan SR, Liang MH, Luthra HS, et al. The American Rheumatism Association 1987 revised criteria for the classification of rheumatoid arthritis. Arthritis Rheum 1988;31:315–324.

2. Liao KP, Batra KL, Chibnik L, et al. Anti-CCP revised criteria for the classification of rheumatoid arthritis. Ann Rheum Dis 2008 epublished.
3. Lee HK, Kim DS, Yoo B, Seo JB, Rho JY, Colby TV, Kitaichi M. Histopathologic pattern and clinical features of rheumatoid arthritis-associated interstitial lung disease. Chest 2005;127: 2019–2027.
4. Haslam PL, Thompson B, Mohammed I, Townsend PJ, Hodson ME, Holborow EJ, Turner-Warwick M. Circulating immune complexes in patients with cryptogenic fibrosing alveolitis. Clin Exp Immunol 1979;37:381–390.
5. Ippolito JA, Palmer L, Spector S, Kane PB, Gorevic PD. Bronchiolitis obliterans organizing pneumonia and rheumatoid arthritis. Semin Arthritis Rheum 1993;23:70–78.
6. Kerstens PJ, Boerbooms AM, Jeurissen ME, Fast JH, Assmann KJ, van de Putte LB. Accelerated nodulosis during low dose methotrexate therapy for rheumatoid arthritis. An analysis of ten cases. J Rheumatol 1992;19:867–871.
7. Gauhar UA, Gaffo AL, Alarcon GS. Pulmonary manifestations of rheumatoid arthritis. Semin Respir Crit Care Med 2007;28:430–440.
8. Coppo P, Clauvel JP, Bengoufa D, Oksenhendler E, Lacroix C, Lassoued K. Inflammatory myositis associated with anti-U1-small nuclear ribonucleoprotein antibodies: a subset of myositis associated with a favourable outcome. Rheumatology (Oxford) 2002;41:1040–1046.
9. Khadadah ME, Jayakrishnan B, Al-Gorair S, Al-Mutairi M, Al-Maradni N, Onadeko B, Malaviya AN. Effect of methotrexate on pulmonary function in patients with rheumatoid arthritis—a prospective study. Rheumatol Int 2002;22:204–207.
10. Chang HK, Park W, Ryu DS. Successful treatment of progressive rheumatoid interstitial lung disease with cyclosporine: a case report. J Korean Med Sci 2002;17:270–273.
11. Arnett FC, Cho M, Chatterjee S, Aguilar MB, Reveille JD, Mayes MD. Familial occurrence frequencies and relative risks for systemic sclerosis (scleroderma) in three United States cohorts. Arthritis Rheum 2001;44:1359–1362.
12. Catoggio LJ, Bernstein RM, Black CM, Hughes GR, Maddison PJ. Serological markers in progressive systemic sclerosis: clinical correlations. Ann Rheum Dis 1983;42:23–27.
13. Ferri C, Valentini G, Cozzi F, Sebastiani M, Michelassi C, La Montagna G, Bullo A, Cazzato M, Tirri E, Storino F, Giuggioli D, Cuomo G, Rosada M, Bombardieri S, Todesco S, Tirri G; Systemic Sclerosis Study Group of the Italian Society of Rheumatology (SIR-GSSSc). Systemic sclerosis: demographic, clinical, and serologic features and survival in 1,012 Italian patients. Medicine (Baltimore) 2002;81 (2:139–153).
14. Bouros D, Wells AU, Nicholson AG, Colby TV, Polychronopoulos V, Pantelidis P, Haslam PL, Vassilakis DA, Black CM, du Bois RM. Histopathologic subsets of fibrosing alveolitis in patients with systemic sclerosis and their relationship to outcome. Am J Respir Crit Care Med 2002;165:1581–1586.
15. Tashkin DP, Elashoff R, Clements PJ, Goldin J, Roth MD, Furst DE, Arriola E, Silver R, Strange C, Bolster M, Seibold JR, Riley DJ, Hsu VM, Varga J, Schraufnagel DE, Theodore A, Simms R, Wise R, Wigley F, White B, Steen V, Read C, Mayes M, Parsley E, Mubarak K, Connolly MK, Golden J, Olman M, Fessler B, Rothfield N, Metersky M; Scleroderma Lung Study Research Group. Cyclophosphamide versus placebo in scleroderma lung disease. N Engl J Med 2006;354:2655–2666.
16. Goh NS, Wells AU. Scleroderma ILD stratification by computed tomography. Am J Respir Crit Care Med, in press.
17. Lomeo RM, Cornella RJ, Schabel SI, Schabel SI, Silver RM. Progressive systemic sclerosis sine scleroderma presenting as pulmonary interstitial fibrosis. Am J Med 1989;87:525–527.
18. Wells AU, Hansell DM, Rubens MB, King AD, Cramer D, Black CM, du Bois RM. Fibrosing alveolitis in systemic sclerosis: indices of lung function in relation to extent of disease on computed tomography. Arthritis Rheum 1997;40:1229–1236.
19. Silver RM, Miller KS, Kinsella MB, Smith EA, Schabel SI. Evaluation and management of scleroderma lung disease using bronchoalveolar lavage. Am J Med 1990;88:470–476.
20. Strange C, Bolster MB, Roth MD, Silver RM, Theodore A, Goldin J, Clements P, Chung J, Elashoff RM, Suh R, Smith EA, Furst DE, Tashkin DP; Scleroderma Lung Study Research

Group. Bronchoalveolar lavage and response to cyclophosphamide in scleroderma interstitial lung disease. Am J Respir Crit Care Med 2008;177:91–98.

21. Tashkin DP, Elashoff R, Clements PJ, Roth MD, Furst DE, Silver RM, Goldin J, Arriola E, Strange C, Bolster MB, Seibold JR, Riley DJ, Hsu VM, Varga J, Schraufnagel D, Theodore A, Simms R, Wise R, Wigley F, White B, Steen V, Read C, Mayes M, Parsley E, Mubarak K, Connolly MK, Golden J, Olman M, Fessler B, Rothfield N, Metersky M, Khanna D, Li N, Li G; Scleroderma Lung Study Research Group. Effects of 1-year treatment with cyclophosphamide on outcomes at 2 years in scleroderma lung disease. Am J Respir Crit Care Med 2007; 176:1026–1034.

22. Hoyles RK, Ellis RW, Wellsbury J, Lees B, Newlands P, Goh NS, Roberts C, Desai S, Herrick AL, McHugh NJ, Foley NM, Pearson SB, Emery P, Veale DJ, Denton CP, Wells AU, Black CM, du Bois RM. A multicenter, prospective, randomized, double-blind, placebo-controlled trial of corticosteroids and intravenous cyclophosphamide followed by oral azathioprine for the treatment of pulmonary fibrosis in scleroderma. Arthritis Rheum 2006;54: 3962–3970.

23. Liossis SN, Bounas A, Andonopoulos AP. Mycophenolate mofetil as first-line treatment improves clinically evident early scleroderma lung disease. Rheumatology (Oxford) 2006; 45:1005–1008.

24. Swigris JJ, Olson AL, Fischer A, Lynch DA, Cosgrove GP, Frankel SK, Meehan RT, Brown KK. Mycophenolate mofetil is safe, well tolerated, and preserves lung function in patients with connective tissue disease-related interstitial lung disease. Chest 2006;130:30–36.

25. Troshinsky MB, Kane GC, Varga J, Cater JR, Fish JE, Jimenez SA, Castell DO. Pulmonary function and gastroesophageal reflux in systemic sclerosis. Ann Intern Med 1994;121:6–10.

26. Cool CD, Kennedy D, Voelkel NF, Tuder RM. Pathogenesis and evolution of plexiform lesions in pulmonary hypertension associated with scleroderma and human immunodeficiency virus infection. Hum Pathol 1997;28:434–442.

27. Strange C, Bolster M, Mazur J, Taylor M, Gossage JR, Silver R. Hemodynamic effects of epoprostenol in patients with systemic sclerosis and pulmonary hypertension. Chest 2000; 118:1077–1082.

28. Gugnani MK, Pierson C, Vanderheide R, Girgis RE. Pulmonary edema complicating prostacyclin therapy in pulmonary hypertension associated with scleroderma: a case of pulmonary capillary hemangiomatosis. Arthritis Rheum 2000;43:699–703.

29. Ferri C, Giuggioli D, Sebastiani M, Colaci M, Emdin M. Heart involvement and systemic sclerosis. Lupus 2005;14:702–707.

30. Thompson AE, Pope JE. A study of the frequency of pericardial and pleural effusions in scleroderma. Br J Rheumatol 1998;37:1320–1323.

31. Ropes M. Systemic lupus erythematosus. Cambridge, MA: Harvard University Press, 1976.

32. Joseph J, Sahn SA. Connective tissue diseases and the pleura. Chest 1993;104:262–270.

33. Porcel JM, Ordi-Ros J, Esquerda A, Vives M, Madroñero AB, Bielsa S, Vilardell-Tarrés M, Light RW. Antinuclear antibody testing in pleural fluid for the diagnosis of lupus pleuritis. Lupus 2007;16:25–27.

34. Cheema GS, Quismorio FP, Jr. Interstitial lung disease in systemic lupus erythematosus. Curr Opin Pulm Med 2000;6:424–429.

35. Strange C, Highland KB. Interstitial lung disease in the patient who has connective tissue disease. Clin Chest Med 2004;25:549–559;vii.

36. Matthay RA, Schwarz MI, Petty TL, Stanford RE, Gupta RC, Sahn SA, Steigerwald JC. Pulmonary manifestations of systemic lupus erythematosus: review of twelve cases of acute lupus pneumonitis. Medicine (Baltimore) 1975;54:397–409.

37. Eiser AR, Shanies HM. Treatment of lupus interstitial lung disease with intravenous cyclophosphamide. Arthritis Rheum 1994;37:428–431.

38. Warrington KJ, Moder KG, Brutinel WM. The shrinking lungs syndrome in systemic lupus erythematosus. Mayo Clin Proc 2000;75:467–472.

39. Gibson CJ, Edmonds JP, Hughes GR. Diaphragm function and lung involvement in systemic lupus erythematosus. Am J Med 1977;63:926–932.

40. Karim MY, Miranda LC, Tench CM, Gordon PA, D'cruz DP, Khamashta MA, Hughes GR. Presentation and prognosis of the shrinking lung syndrome in systemic lupus erythematosus. Semin Arthritis Rheum 2002;31:289–298.

41. Zamora MR, Warner ML, Tuder R, Schwartz MI. Diffuse alveolar hemorrhage and systemic lupus erythematosus. Clinical presentation, histology, survival, and outcome. Medicine (Baltimore) 1997;76:192–202.

42. Lee CK, Koh JH, Cha HS, Kim J, Huh W, Chung MP, Koh EM. Pulmonary alveolar hemorrhage in patients with rheumatic diseases in Korea. Scand J Rheumatol 2000;29:288–294.

43. Chung SM, Lee CK, Lee EY, Yoo B, Lee SD, Moon HB. Clinical aspects of pulmonary hypertension in patients with systemic lupus erythematosus and in patients with idiopathic pulmonary arterial hypertension. Clin Rheumatol 2006;25:866–872.

44. Parambil JG, Myers JL, Lindell RM, Matteson EL, Ryu JH. Interstitial lung disease in primary Sjogren syndrome. Chest 2006;130:1489–1495.

45. Wells AU, du Bois RM. Bronchiolitis in association with connective tissue disorders. Clin Chest Med 1993;14:655–666.

46. Alkhayer M, McCann BG, Harrison BD. Lymphocytic interstitial pneumonitis in association with Sjogren's syndrome. Br J Dis Chest 1988;82:305–309.

47. Ichikawa Y, Kinoshita M, Koga T, Oizumi K, Fujimoto K, Hayabuchi N. Lung cyst formation in lymphocytic interstitial pneumonia: CT features. J Comput Assist Tomogr 1994;18:745–748.

48. Johkoh T, Muller NL, Pickford HA, Hartman TE, Ichikado K, Akira M, Honda O, Nakamura H. Lymphocytic interstitial pneumonia: thin-section CT findings in 22 patients. Radiology 1999;212:567–572.

49. Ito I, Nagai S, Kitaichi M, Nicholson AG, Johkoh T, Noma S, Kim DS, Handa T, Izumi T, Mishima M. Pulmonary manifestations of primary Sjogren's syndrome: a clinical, radiologic, and pathologic study. Am J Respir Crit Care Med 2005;171:632–638.

50. Tonami H, Matoba M, Kuginuki Y, Yokota H, Higashi K, Yamamoto I, Sugai S. Clinical and imaging findings of lymphoma in patients with Sjogren syndrome. J Comput Assist Tomogr 2003;27:517–524.

51. Hoffman GS, Kerr GS, Leavitt RY, Hallahan CW, Lebovics RS, Travis WD, Rottem M, Fauci AS. Wegener granulomatosis: an analysis of 158 patients. Ann Intern Med 1992;116:488–498.

52. Battista G, Zompatori M, Poletti V, Canini R. Thoracic manifestations of the less common collagen diseases. A pictorial essay. Radiol Med (Torino) 2003;106:445–451; quiz 452–443.

53. Seo P, Stone JH. The antineutrophil cytoplasmic antibody-associated vasculitides. Am J Med 2004;117:39–50.

54. Frankel SK, Sullivan EJ, Brown KK. Vasculitis: Wegener granulomatosis, Churg-Strauss syndrome, microscopic polyangiitis, polyarteritis nodosa, and Takayasu arteritis. Crit Care Clin 2002;18:855–879.

55. Stone JH. Limited versus severe Wegener's granulomatosis: baseline data on patients in the Wegener's granulomatosis etanercept trial. Arthritis Rheum 2003;48:2299–2309.

56. Sullivan EJ, Hoffman GS. Pulmonary vasculitis. Clin Chest Med 1998;19:759–776;ix.

57. Cordier JF, Valeyre D, Guillevin L, Loire R, Brechot JM. Pulmonary Wegener's granulomatosis. A clinical and imaging study of 77 cases. Chest 1990;97:906–912.

58. Finkielman JD, Lee AS, Hummel AM, Viss MA, Jacob GL, Homburger HA, Peikert T, Hoffman GS, Merkel PA, Spiera R, St Clair EW, Davis JC Jr, McCune WJ, Tibbs AK, Ytterberg SR, Stone JH, Specks U; WGET Research Group. ANCA are detectable in nearly all patients with active severe Wegener's granulomatosis. Am J Med 2007;120:643 e649–e614.

59. Finkielman JD, Merkel PA, Schroeder D, Hoffman GS, Spiera R, St Clair EW, Davis JC Jr, McCune WJ, Lears AK, Ytterberg SR, Hummel AM, Viss MA, Peikert T, Stone JH, Specks U; WGET Research Group. Antiproteinase 3 antineutrophil cytoplasmic antibodies and disease activity in Wegener granulomatosis. Ann Intern Med 2007;147:611–619.

60. Jayne D, Rasmussen N, Andrassy K, Bacon P, Tervaert JW, Dadonienè J, Ekstrand A, Gaskin G, Gregorini G, de Groot K, Gross W, Hagen EC, Mirapeix E, Pettersson E, Siegert C, Sinico A, Tesar V, Westman K, Pusey C; European Vasculitis Study Group. A randomized trial of

maintenance therapy for vasculitis associated with antineutrophil cytoplasmic autoantibodies. N Engl J Med 2003;349:36–44.

61. Etanercept plus standard therapy for Wegener's granulomatosis. N Engl J Med 2005;352: 351–361.

62. Keogh KA, Ytterberg SR, Fervenza FC, Carlson KA, Schroeder DR, Specks U. Rituximab for refractory Wegener's granulomatosis: report of a prospective, open-label pilot trial. Am J Respir Crit Care Med 2006;173:180–187.

63. White ES, Lynch JP. Pharmacological therapy for Wegener's granulomatosis. Drugs 2006; 66:1209–1228.

64. Guillevin L, Durand-Gasselin B, Cevallos R, Gayraud M, Lhote F, Callard P, Amouroux J, Casassus P, Jarrousse B. Microscopic polyangiitis: clinical and laboratory findings in eighty-five patients. Arthritis Rheum 1999;42:421–430.

65. Schonermarck U, Lamprecht P, Csernok E, Gross WL. Prevalence and spectrum of rheumatic diseases associated with proteinase 3-antineutrophil cytoplasmic antibodies (ANCA) and myeloperoxidase-ANCA. Rheumatology (Oxford) 2001;40:178–184.

66. Xiao H, Heeringa P, Hu P, Liu Z, Zhao M, Aratani Y, Maeda N, Falk RJ, Jennette JC. Antineutrophil cytoplasmic autoantibodies specific for myeloperoxidase cause glomerulonephritis and vasculitis in mice. J Clin Invest 2002;110:955–963.

67. Jayne D. Challenges in the management of microscopic polyangiitis: past, present and future. Curr Opin Rheumatol 2008;20:3–9.

68. Bohan A, Peter JB. Polymyositis and dermatomyositis (first of two parts). N Engl J Med 1975;292:344–347.

69. Bohan A, Peter JB. Polymyositis and dermatomyositis (second of two parts). N Engl J Med 1975;292:403–407.

70. Tan EM, Cohen AS, Fries JF, Masi AT, McShane DJ, Rothfield NF, Schaller JG, Talal N, Winchester RJ. The 1982 revised criteria for the classification of systemic lupus erythematosus. Arthritis Rheum 1982;25:1271–1277.

Chapter 9
Pulmonary Hypertension in Idiopathic Pulmonary Fibrosis

Fernando J. Martinez

Introduction

Idiopathic pulmonary fibrosis (IPF) is one of the most common of the idiopathic interstitial pneumonias [1]. It is associated with a variable prognosis that is partially predicted by baseline physiological [2] and radiological features [3,4] as well as longitudinal changes in physiology [2,5–7]. Unfortunately, recent studies have confirmed that a significant proportion of IPF patients die with accelerated disease [8]. In the placebo arm of a large randomized therapeutic trial, 21.4% of patients with IPF died during a 72-week observation period [8]; progression of IPF was thought to be causative in 89%, with 47% of these thought by the primary investigator to have occurred within 4 weeks.

A subsequent analysis from this dataset confirmed that a decrease of 10% in forced vital capacity (FVC) was the most predictive measurement of survival, although the operating characteristics of this parameter are modest [9]. A subsequent analysis of these results suggests that a decrease in FVC >10% predicted exhibited a sensitivity of 60%, specificity of 75%, positive predictive value of 31%, and negative predictive value of 91% in predicting mortality [10]. The appreciation that pulmonary hypertension (PH) may impact survival in IPF has been increasingly noted [11–13]. As such, this area is one that is worthy of review.

Prevalence/Incidence of PH in IPF

The exact incidence and prevalence of PH remains unclear. Numerous studies have shed light on this topic as enumerated in (Table 9.1). In one of the earlier studies, investigators retrospectively addressed the prevalence of right ventricular function abnormality and tricuspid regurgitation in patients evaluated for lung transplantation [14]. Of the 77 IPF patients, 50 (65%) had right ventricular dysfunction (right ventricular ejection fraction <45%), whereas almost 38% had abnormal tricuspid regurgitation on echocardiography. In a study of 27 patients followed serially in a chest clinic, echocardiography suggested PH (defined as estimated pulmonary

R.P. Baughman et al. (eds.), *Pulmonary Arterial Hypertension and Interstitial Lung Diseases,*
© Humana Press, a part of Springer Science + Business Media, LLC 2009

Table 9.1 Prevalence of PH in Selected Series of IPF Patients

Reference	n	Patient population	Study format	Assessment modality	Prevalence
Vizza et al. [14]	77	Prelung transplant evaluation	Retrospective	RVG; TTE; RHC	Decreased RVEF in 65%; Abnormal TR in 37.7%
Leuchte et al. [24]	39*	Consecutive cases	Prospective	RHC	Resting mean PAP >35 mmHg in 21.4% IPF patients
Nadrous et al. [12]	88/487	Convenience sample	Retrospective	TTE	Resting SPAP >35 mmHg in 84%
Agarwal et al. [15]	27	Consecutive cases	Prospective	TTE	Resting SPAP ≥40 mmHg or tricuspid acceleration time ≤100 ms or RV hyper-trophy/over-load in 36%
Cottin et al. [16]	43 baseline[†] 49 at follow-up	Convenience sample	Retrospective	TTE	Resting SPAP ≥45 mmHg in 47% at diagnosis 55% during follow-up
Grubstein et al. [17]	8[†]	Convenience sample	Retrospective	TTE	7/8 with SPAP >44 mmHg
Lettieri et al. [11]	79	Pre-lung transplant evaluation	Retrospective	RHC	Resting mean PAP >25 mmHg in 31.6%
Hamada et al. [13]	70	Initial evaluation of unselected population	Prospective	RHC	Resting mean PAP >25 mmHg in 8.1%
Zisman et al. [19]	61/298	Convenience sample	Retrospective	RHC	Resting mean PAP >25 mmHg in 39.3%
Shorr et al. [20]	2525/3457	US lung transplant registry	Retrospective	RHC	Resting mean PAP ≥25 mmHg in 46.1%; >40 mmHg in 9%

(continued)

Table 9.1 (continued)

Reference	n	Patient population	Study format	Assessment modality	Prevalence
Zisman et al. [26]	65	Prelung transplant evaluation (74%) or in clinical trial (26%)	Retrospective/ prospective	RHC	Resting mean PAP >25 mmHg in 41.5%
Zisman et al. [25]	60	Pre-lung transplant evaluation	Retrospective	RHC	Resting mean PAP >25 mmHg in 30%

* Twenty-eight with IPF.
† Concomitant emphysema PF.
RVG, radionuclide ventriculography; RHC, right heart catheterization; TTE, transthoracic echocardiography; RVEF, right ventricular ejection fraction; TR, tricuspid regurgitation; PAP, systolic pulmonary artery pressure; SPAP, estimated PAP; RV, right ventricle.

artery systolic pressure ≥40 mmHg or pulmonary acceleration time ≤100 ms or right ventricular hypertrophy/overload) in 36% of cases [15].

A separate group retrospectively reviewed 487 patients with IPF who were evaluated from January 1, 1994, to December 31, 1996, and they identified 136 patients who underwent echocardiography at the discretion of the managing physician [12]. After exclusion of left ventricular dysfunction, valvular heart disease, incomplete follow-up or inadequate echocardiographic images for systolic pulmonary artery pressure (SPAP) estimation, they determined that 88 patients were available for study. An estimated SPAP >35 mmHg was noted in 84% of the patients and >50 mmHg in 16%. The combination of emphysema in the upper lung zones and pulmonary fibrosis in the lower lobes on high-resolution computed tomography of the chest has been reported to be associated with a greater prevalence of PH. An estimated SPAP ≥45 mmHg was present in 47% at diagnosis and 55% during follow-up in one series [16]. A second group has reported remarkably similar data [17].

Echocardiographic data are difficult to interpret because the operating characteristics of echocardiography to estimate SPAP in patients with advanced lung disease have been reported to be quite poor [18]. In a large group of patients with interstitial lung disease evaluated for lung transplantation, the sensitivity, specificity, positive predictive value, and negative predictive value were reported as 85%, 17%, 60%, and 44%, respectively [18]. Although echo was able to estimate pressures in 44%, 52% of these measures were inaccurate by 10 mmHg or more and 48% of patients were misclassified. In a smaller sample of IPF patients a separate group (prevalence of PH of 39.3%) suggested values of 76%, 38%, 56%, and 60% for echocardiography in assessing PH [19]. It is apparent that echocardiographic assessment in IPF patients may be of limited utility.

More recent studies have used right heart catheterization (RHC) to accurately measure pulmonary pressures in patients with IPF. One investigative group reported a retrospective analysis of 79 IPF patients undergoing pretransplant RHC; PH (defined as mean pulmonary artery systolic pressure of ≥25 mmHg) was noted in 31.6% [11]. The data of Hamada et al. [13] are particularly important because they reflect the results of a prospective evaluation of 70 patients undergoing a RCH at first evaluation. Interestingly, PH (resting mean pulmonary artery systolic pressure of ≥25 mmHg) was detected in only six patients (8.1%).

Zisman et al. [19] retrospectively identified 61 of 298 patients evaluated at a single center who had undergone RHC and pulmonary function testing within 1 month of each other. Twenty-four (39.3%) of the patients exhibited a measured, resting PAP >25 mmHg. The nature of the patient population was not clearly defined. Shorr and colleagues [20] examined the United Network for Organ Sharing and the Organ Procurement and Transplant Network registry for IPF patients listed for lung transplantation between January 1995 and June 2004. Of the 3,457 patients listed, 2,525 had RHC results available; of those, 933 (37.0%) had a mean PAP > 25, whereas 231 (9.1%) had a mean PAP >40 mmHg.

These data suggest a wide prevalence of PH in patients with IPF. The differing study populations and methodologies used to define PH limits interpretation. In general, it appears that the prevalence of moderate PH in a general population of IPF patients is less than 10%. In patients with more severe disease, including those listed for lung transplantation, the prevalence increases to approximately 40%. Severe PH is unusual, even in patients listed for lung transplantation.

Few longitudinal data to clearly define incidence are available. One group reported in abstract form a baseline prevalence of 41% increasing to 90% at follow-up [21]. A second group reported a retrospective series of patients who had undergone RHC as part of lung transplant evaluation and a repeat catheterization at the time of lung transplantation; the prevalence of PH increased from 38.6% to 86.4% [22]. Because these case series have not been published in a peer-reviewed setting, it is difficult to assess methodology and, therefore, the clinical implications. Further prospective data collection is required in this arena.

Prognostic Influence of PH in IPF

The prognostic importance of PH complicating IPF has also been suggested by several groups (Table 9.2). In echocardiographically defined PH, one investigative group has noted that a SPAP >50 mmHg is associated with impaired survival (Fig. 9.1A) [12]. A separate group has demonstrated that echocardiographically defined PH in IPF patients with superimposed emphysema negatively influenced survival [16]. In a group of 79 patients undergoing RHC before listing for lung transplantation, the presence of PH predicted mortality with a sensitivity, specificity, positive predictive, and negative predictive value of 57%, 79%, 50%, and 83.6%, respectively [11]. In fact, there was a linear correlation between measured mean PAP and

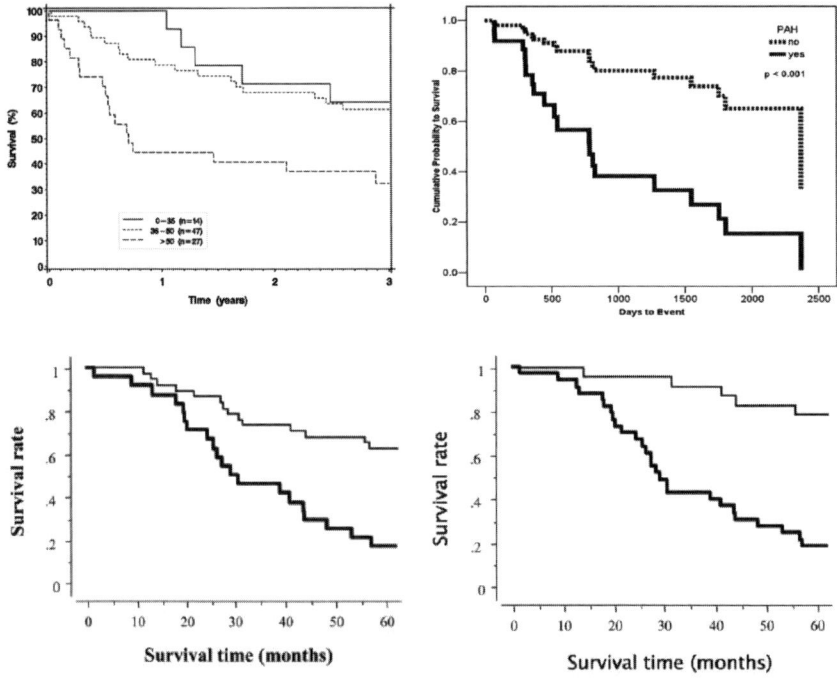

Fig. 9.1 A Kaplan-Meier survival curves for 88 patients with IPF who were stratified by echocardiographically defined systolic pulmonary artery pressure [12]. **B** Kaplan-Meier survival curves for 79 patients with IPF who were stratified by the presence of right heart catheterization-confirmed PH [11]. **C** Survival rates in patients with IPF who were segregated by right heart catheterization-confirmed mean PAP <17 mmHg (thin line). mean PAP ≥17 mmHg (bold line) [13]. **D** Survival rates of patients grouped by mean PAP <17 mmHg; a $DL_{CO} \geq 40\%$ predicted versus those with a mean PAP ≥17 mmHg /or a DL_{CO} <40% predicted [13]

greater mortality (hazard ratio 1.09; 95% confidence interval 1.02–1.16), which persisted after adjustment for FVC and diffusion capacity (of the lung) for carbon monoxide (DL_{CO}). Figure 9.1B illustrates mortality in patients with and without PH. It is notable that similar results persisted after the data were reanalyzed with those patients who underwent lung transplantation excluded.

One group has examined the influence of brain natriuretic peptide (BNP) and physiological features on survival in a large cohort (176 consecutive patients, 55 with IPF) of patients with chronic lung disease [23]. In patients with interstitial lung disease, 31 of 88 had increased levels of BNP; 11 (35.5%) of these died compared with 10 of 57 (17.5%) with normal levels of BNP. Similarly, 28 of 88 interstitial lung disease patients had a mean PAP >35 mmHg, with 12 of these patients (42.9%) dying compared with 9 of 60 (15%) without moderate-to-severe PH. When using ROC analysis in the entire cohort of 176 patients, the authors found that BNP level (area under the curve [AUC] 67.3%) and mean PAP (AUC 72.9%) predicted mortality better than total lung capacity (AUC 38.5%) and PO_2 (AUC 29.2%).

The data of Hamada et al. [13] are the most enlightening as this group prospectively studied a cohort of IPF patients who were evaluated from initial presentation with a RHC. Receiver operating characteristic analysis identified a mean PAP threshold of 17 mmHg as most predictive of long-term survival. Figure 9.1C contrasts survival for the patients with a mean PAP <17 mmHg versus those with a mean PAP ≥17 mmHg. Additional analyses suggested that grouping patients by mean PAP (< or ≥17 mmHg and DL_{CO} %predicted <40% or ≥40% predicted) was particularly predictive of long term survival (Fig. 9.1D). It is evident that complications of PH in patients with IPF are associated with a worse outcome.

Prediction of PH in IPF Patients

Given the clinical implications of complications of PH in patients with, it is important to approach diagnosis in a rigorous fashion (Table 9.3). In general, echocardiographically suggested PH has been associated with longer duration of illness, lower PaO_2, and lower FVC [15]. Another similar series using echocardiography reported that SPAP correlated inversely with DL_{CO}, PaO_2, and oxygen saturation [12]. No other measure of resting pulmonary function, including spirometry and lung volume, correlated with SPAP.

In a series of patients who underwent RHC, the presence of PH correlated with lower DL_{CO} (<40% predicted) and with a requirement for supplemental oxygen (resting SpO_2 < 88% or PaO_2 <55 mmHg) [11]. The group of patients that met both of these criteria (15.2% of the cohort) had a 10.2 greater likelihood of having PH. In fact, the combination of both of these criteria identified the presence of PH with a sensitivity of 65.0%, specificity of 94.1%, positive predictive value of 86.7%, and a negative predictive value of 92.1%. In a limited number of patients (prevalence of PH 29.4%), 6-minute walk testing while breathing room air was available. The distance walked (143.5 ± 65.5 versus 365.9 ± 81.8 meters, $p < 0.001$) and the lowest SpO_2 during the walk test ($80.1 \pm 3.7\%$ versus $88.0 \pm 3.5\%$, $p < 0.001$) were lower in those patients with PH compared with those without.

In a consecutive group of 39 patients with fibrotic lung disease (28 with IPF), the results of a 6-minute walk distance was significantly lower in those with moderate-to-severe PH (mean PAP >35 mmHg) compared with those with no-to-mild PH (185.45 ± 41.12 meters versus 303.93 ± 21.92 meters, $p < 0.05$); lung function parameters were not different between the groups [24]. These findings were generally confirmed in a subsequent larger study with a broader range of subjects (176 patients, 55 with IPF) [23].

In the dataset from the United Network for Organ Sharing and the Organ Procurement and Transplant Network registry, subjects with PH were more likely to have COPD (odds ratio [OR] 1.31; 95% confidence interval [CI] 1.03–1.67) and, in multivariate modeling, more likely to require supplemental oxygen (OR 1.22; 95% CI 1.14–1.30), have a greater pulmonary capillary wedge pressure (per 1-mmHg increase above mean cohort value: OR 1.19; 95% CI 1.16–1.21), and less likely to have a greater FEV1 (per 1% increase from mean value for cohort: OR 0.99; 95% CI 0.99–1.00) [20].

Table 9.2 Prognostic Implication of PH Complications in Patients With IPF in Selected Series

Reference	n	Prognostic implication
Nadrous et al. [12]	88	Impaired survival if estimated SPAP >50 mmHg (univariate analysis)
Cottin et al. [16]	49	Survival associated with SPAP ≥45 mmHg
Lettieri et al. [11]	79	Linear association between measured mean PAP mortality; Presence of PH was associated with worse survival
Leuchte et al. [23]	176*	Within fibrotic lung disease subgroup greater mortality in those with mean PAP >35 mmHg
Hamada et al. [13]	70	Resting mean PAP >17 mmHg was associated with worse survival; Combination of a resting mean PAP >17 mmHg DL_{CO} <40% predicted was associated with particularly poor survival

*IPF in 55 patients.
SPAP, systolic pulmonary artery pressure; PAP, pulmonary artery pressure.

Table 9.3 Prediction of Pulmonary Artery Pressures With Physiological or Clinical Measurements in Various Series of IPF Patients

Reference	Time of pulmonary artery pressure measurement pulmonary function testing or imaging	Finding
Leuchte et al. [24]	Not stated	Plasma BNP concentration directly correlated with mean PAP; a threshold of 33.3 pg/ml predicted mean PAP >35 mmHg
Nadrous et al. [12]	90 days before 14 days after	Inverse correlation between SPAP DL_{CO}, resting paO_2, resting O_2 saturation
Agarwal et al. [15]	Not stated	Longer duration of symptoms, lower FVC PaO_2 were associated with PH
Lettieri et al. [11]	Within 1 month (mean, 24.2 days)	DL_{CO} < 40% predicted requirement for oxygen supplementation (resting SpO_2 < 88% or PaO_2 < 55 mmHg) predictive of PH
Zisman et al. [19]	Within 1 month	PH predicted by SpO_2, %FVC/%DL_{CO}
Shorr et al. [20]	Not available	PH more likely with need for supplemental oxygen, higher PCWP, lower FEV_1
Zisman et al. [26]	HRCT within 1 month	Correlation was noted between mean PAP DL_{CO}, DLCO/VA%, FVC%/DL_{CO}% but not with HRCT findings

BNP, brain natriuretic peptide; PAP, pulmonary artery pressure; SPAP, estimated systolic pulmonary artery pressure; PH, pulmonary hypertension; PCWP, pulmonary capillary wedge pressure; HRCT, high-resolution computed tomography of the chest; VA, alveolar volume.

The most detailed analysis is that of Zisman et al. [19], who examined the predictive value of spirometry and DL_{CO} in identifying PH (prevalence of 39%). The mean PAP was regressed against SpO_2 and %FVC/%DL_{CO} with a resulting equation, based on multivariate modeling:

$$MPAP = -11.9 + 0.272 \times SpO_2 + 0.0659 \times (100 - SpO_2)2 + 3.06 \times (\%FVC/\%DL_{CO})$$

There was no correlation between mean PAP and individual spirometric parameters or lung volumes. When echocardiographically estimated right ventricular systolic pressure, six minute walk test distance and %DL$_{CO}$/%alveolar volume were added to the model little change occurred. Similarly replacement of SpO$_2$ with PaO$_2$ or %FVC/%DL$_{CO}$ with DL$_{CO}$ resulted in little change in the overall model. The operating characteristics of the modeling equation included a sensitivity of 71%, specificity of 81%, positive predictive value of 71%, and a negative predictive value of 81%.

In a subsequent two-center study, the use of the equation exhibited similar operating characteristics [25]. A formula-predicted MPAP >21 mmHg was associated with a sensitivity, specificity, positive predictive value, and negative predictive value of 95%, 58%, 51%, and 96%, respectively. This same group reported that semiquantitative features from computed tomography, including measures of parenchymal abnormality and pulmonary artery size, did not prove predictive of PH in IPF patients [26].

BNP may be particularly useful in identifying PH complicating IPF. In the previously mentioned study of 39 consecutive patients with fibrotic lung disease, including 28 with pulmonary fibrosis, plasma BNP level directly correlated with mean PAP [24]. In the IPF patients those with normal BNP levels (<18 pg/ml, $n = 16$) were less likely to exhibit PH compared with those with increased levels of BNP

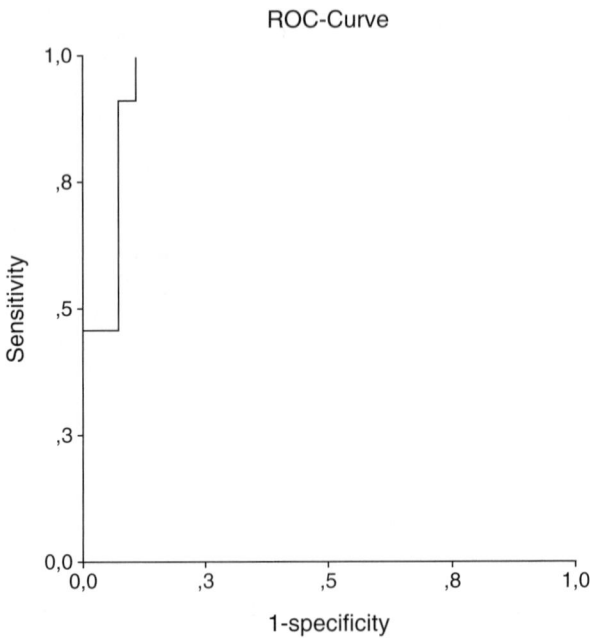

Fig. 9.2 Receiver operating characteristic analysis for BNP in 39 patients with fibrotic lung disease (including 28 with IPF). A threshold value of 33.3 pg/ml indicated severe PH (mean PAP >35 mmHg) with a sensitivity of 1.0, specificity of 0.89, and area under the curve of 95.8% ($p < 0.001$) [24]

(>18 pg/ml, $n = 12$). Furthermore, plasma BNP levels directly correlated with mean PAP and negatively correlated with cardiac index. Receiver operating characteristic analysis in the entire cohort (including 11 with secondary pulmonary fibrotic disease) suggested that a threshold level of 33.3 pg/ml exhibited a high sensitivity (100%) and specificity (89%) with an area under the curve of 95.8% ($p < 0.001$) (Fig. 9.2).

Pathogenesis of PH in IPF

A detailed discussion of the pathobiology of PH complicating IPF is beyond the scope of this chapter but a recent review has highlighted the major issues [27]. Overall there are likely multiple, global biological processes underlying the development of PH in IPF, including pulmonary artery vasoconstriction and pulmonary artery remodeling. Supporting the former is the extensive body of literature, which supports a role for hypoxia driven-vasoconstriction in the genesis of secondary PH [28]. This mechanism is particularly well acknowledged in chronic obstructive pulmonary disease, kyphoscoliosis, and the obesity-hypoventilation syndrome, where intermittent hypoxic episodes have been associated with abnormalities in right heart function [29]. Support for this mechanism in IPF includes the previously noted work suggesting an increased prevalence of PH in IPF patients with lower resting oxygen saturation or PaO_2 [12,15] or a requirement for supplemental oxygen therapy [11,20].

A mechanistic link to hypoxia has been recently supported by tissue microarray analyses from the bleomycin model of fibrosis in rodents and human IPF tissue [30]. These investigators make a cogent argument for the early role or hypoxia inducible factor 1a in the tissue remodeling of IPF, particularly in its potential association with alveolar cell and myofibroblast aberrant apoptosis. A direct link to abnormal vascular responsiveness was not reported.

Pulmonary vascular remodeling has been increasingly accepted as an important pathobiological process in PH [27]. Global, macroscopic vascular remodeling has been clearly reported in IPF, both with areas of vascular ablation and areas of neovascularization [31–33]. One investigative group has demonstrated reduced vascular density in patients with IPF, particularly within fibroblastic foci and in areas of honeycombing [34]. Interestingly, neovascularization near the fibroblastic foci was also demonstrated, suggesting vascular redistribution in this disorder. An examination of lung explants from 26 patients with IPF (19 with PH) confirmed weak positive correlations between the extent of histological fibrosis and PAP [35]. Importantly, occlusive venopathy was noted in 65% of patients, a finding that did not correlate with PAP and was noted in nonfibrotic areas.

Additional data suggesting such local vascular remodeling has been supported by preliminary data suggesting that patients with IPF and PH (defined predominantly echo-cardiographically) exhibit down-regulation of certain endothelial cell genes and up-regulation of phospholipase A2 and other factors that may be implicated in local vascular remodeling [36]. It is notable that a large number of mediators have been implicated in IPF pathogenesis that conceivably could potentiate vascular remodeling. Overproduction of profibrogenic eicosanoids has been well demonstrated in lungs of patients with IPF; some of these leukotrienes upregulate numerous potential mediators that have been implicated in pulmonary vascular remodeling [37] Endothelin-1 (ET-1) promotes pulmonary arterial vasoconstriction and induces pulmonary arterial smooth muscle growth [38]. Importantly, IPF lung has been shown to exhibit increased expression of ET-1 [39,40], whereas this expression is inversely correlated with arterial oxygen and directly with PAP [41]. Other important profibrotic cytokines that overlap between IPF and PH include platelet-derived growth factor and tumor growth factor-β [27]. Clearly, additional work is required to address the fundamental biological processes underlying fibroproliferation and pulmonary vascular remodeling as they may provide insight into novel therapeutic avenues.

Therapeutic Approach to PH Complications in IPF

The clear negative implication that PH complications in patients with IPF has on functional status (e.g., 6-minute walk distance) and survival suggests that this is an arena fruitful for therapeutic intervention. Interestingly, very little specific information has been published in this regard. Table 9.4 enumerates the limited available data with a series of therapeutic approaches. Whether agents targeting the remodeling process will have the same success remains unexplored.

Given the potential role of hypoxia in the genesis of PH complicating IPF, some have suggested the potential value of oxygen supplementation [27]. The limited available data suggest little benefit with regards to survival with oxygen supplementation in IPF [42]. There are very limited controlled data regarding oxygen therapy in interstitial lung diseases [43]. Importantly, in healthy subjects and patients with chronic obstructive pulmonary disease, short-term oxygen exposure has been demonstrated to increase oxidative stress and pulmonary inflammation [44,45]. In patients with IPF, oxidative stress has been suggested to be a key biological process perpetuating disease [46].

In contrast, one small study suggested that the combination of oxygen supplementation and low-dose inhaled nitric oxide reduced mean PAP and improved PaO_2 in 10 patients with IPF (six with PH) [47]. Interestingly, this latter approach has been used in IPF patients with severe PH as a bridge to transplantation [48]. Additional data are required to better define these therapeutic approaches in IPF patients with PH.

Two groups established the groundwork for the use of vasodilators in IPF patients with PH. Olchewski and colleagues [49] studied eight patients with fibrosing lung disease (one with IPF) and PH (estimated peak systolic pulmonary artery pressure of >50 mmHg or mean PAP >30 mmHg by RHC). A series of therapeutic interventions were administered in a randomized fashion: inhaled nitric oxide

Table 9.4 Therapeutic Intervention Studies Targeting PH in IPF

Reference	n	Therapeutic agent	Study format	Primary endpoint	Results
Yoshida et al. [47]	10 (6 with PH)	Inhaled NO O_2	Open label	Pulmonary hemodynamics	Combination of NO O_2 reduced PAP increased PaO_2
Olschewski et al. [49]	8 (1 IPF)	Inhaled NO Inhaled epoprostenol IV epoprostenol PO nifedipine or diltiazem	Romized, open label	Pulmonary hemodynamics	IV epoprostenol decreased PAP but increased pulmonary shunt decrease PaO_2; Inhaled epoprostenol decreased PAP with no effect on pulmonary shunt
Ghofrani et al. [50]	8* 8*	IV epoprostenol[†] PO sildenafil single dose[†]	Romized, open label	Pulmonary vascular resistance index	Epoprostenol decreased PVRI, systemic arterial pressure but increased pulmonary shunt decrease PaO_2 Sildenafil decreased PVRI with little change in pulmonary shunt slight rise in PaO_2
Madden et al. [51]	3	PO sildenafil 50 mg tid	Open label	Hemodynamics	Mean PAP decreased 6MWT distance increased with 8 weeks of therapy
Madden et al. [52]	2	PO sildenafil 50 mg tid	Open label	Hemodynamics	Mean PAP decreased after 8 weeks of therapy at long term follow-up (approximately 22 months)
Collard et al. [53]	14	PO sildenafil 20–50 mg tid	Open label	6MWT	9 of 11 patients improved 6MWT distance

*Pulmonary fibrosis (IPF in 7) with mean pulmonary artery pressure >35 mmHg.
[†]After nitric oxide inhalation (10–20 ppm);
PH, pulmonary hypertension; NO, nitric oxide; PAP, pulmonary artery pressure; IV, intravenous; PO, oral; PVRI, pulmonary vascular resistance index; 6MWT, 6-minute walk test.

(15–80 ppm; mean 40 ppm), intravenous epoprostenol (increasing increments of 2 ng/kg/min until discomfort was reported; mean 8 ng/kg/min), and aerosolized epoprostenol; after each dosing, 1 h was allowed for the subject to return to baseline. After these test periods, nifedipine or diltiazem was administered and hemodynamic measurement completed 30 min later.

Inhaled NO decreased mean PAP and slightly increased right ventricular ejection fraction (RVEF). Intravenous epoprostenol decreased mean PAP but at the expense of an increased in pulmonary shunt flow and a moderate decrease in SaO_2. Aerosolized epoprostenol decreased mean PAP and increased RVEF without much change in pulmonary shunt flow. Similarly, short-term challenge with a calcium channel blocker resulted in increased PAP, RVEF, and cardiac output with little change in shunt flow and arterial oxygenation.

Ghofrani and colleagues [50] studied 16 patients with pulmonary fibrosis (7 with IPF) and documented severe PH (mean PAP >35 mmHg). In the protocol, the authors used initial inhalation of nitric oxide (10–20 ppm) with subsequent randomization to intravenous infusion of epoprostenol with increasing dose in increments of 2 ng/kg every 15 min or to a single oral dose of sildenafil (50 mg). The primary endpoint was change in pulmonary vascular resistance index (PVRI), although a series of important secondary endpoints (including ventilation:perfusion matching) were also measured.

Inhalation of nitric oxide led to a rapid decrease in mean pulmonary arterial pressure and an increase in cardiac index resulting in a reduction in PVRI (Fig. 9.3). Little change in ventilation:perfusion matching was noted. Epoprostenol infusion led to an increase in cardiac index and decreased both mean pulmonary arterial pressure and PVRI (Fig. 9.3). Interestingly, major increase in pulmonary shunt flow occurred with resulting decrease in PaO_2 (Fig. 9.4). Oral sildenafil led to a vasodilatory response within 15 min, which plateaued after 45–60 min. Mean arterial pressure decreased, as did PVRI; pulmonary shunt flow decreased slightly with an increase in PaO_2 (Fig. 9.4). No major adverse events were noted with sildenafil therapy. These two studies suggest that intravenous epoprostenol is unlikely to be tolerated in this patient population but raises hope for other vasodilators.

Madden et al. [51] studied the effects of eight weeks of sildenafil (50 mg tid) in four patients with chronic obstructive pulmonary disease and three with IPF, all of whom had a mean PAP >25 mmHg. Dosing was administered for 4 days in the hospital to ensure tolerable side effect profile. In all three IPF patients, mean PAP decreased (mean 41 to 32 mmHg) whereas the 6-minute walk test distance increased (mean, 106.7–142 meters).

No adverse events were reported during a median 20 weeks of follow-up. The same group treated 16 patients with chronic lung or cardiac disease (twice with IPF) with sildenafil during a median of 22 months [52]. Both IPF patients exhibited an improvement in mean PAP during 8 weeks of therapy, which was maintained during longer-term follow-up. Overall, for the entire group, the distance on the 6-minute walk test improved in the short term, a benefit that was preserved during long-term follow-up in 13 of 15 patients.

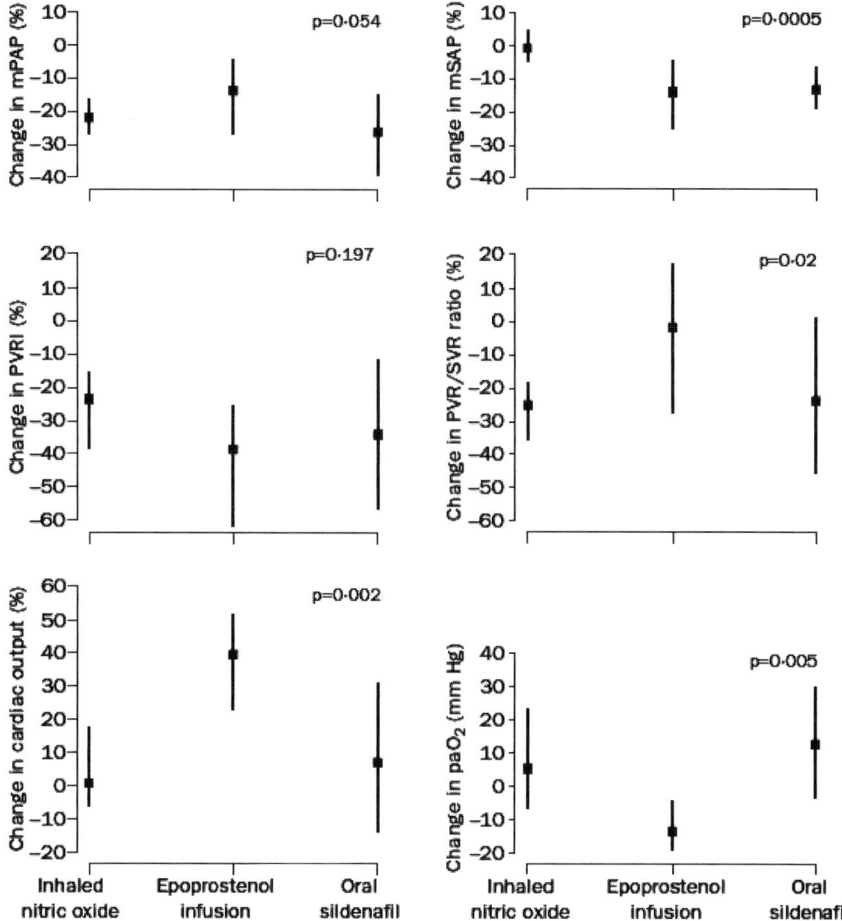

Fig. 9.3 Hemodynamic gas exchange response to inhaled nitric oxide, infused epoprostenol, and single-dose oral sildenafil (50 mg) in 16 patients with fibrotic lung disease (7 with IPF). Data are point estimates of median difference (95% CI). mPAP, mean pulmonary arterial pressure; mSAP, mean systemic arterial pressure; PVRI, pulmonary vascular resistance index; PVR/SVR ratio, ratio of pulmonary to systemic vascular resistance; paO$_2$, partial pressure of arterial oxygen. p value for difference between treatment effects. From Ghofrani et al. [50]

It was not stated if these patients included those with IPF. Most recently, Collard and colleagues [53] administered sildenafil (20–50 mg tid) to 14 patients with IPF and PH (mean PAP ≥25 mmHg on RHC or estimated peak systolic ≥35 mmHg by echocardiography). Eleven patients finished at least 3 months of therapy (median follow-up, 91 days); three patients did not complete testing (two patients discontinued sildenafil as the result of side effects attributed to the drug and in one follow-up 6-minute walk test was terminated because of chest discomfort in the patient). The mean improvement for all 11 patients was 49 meters (90% CI 17.5–84.0 meters). Six-minute walk distance improved in nine patients, with more than half improving

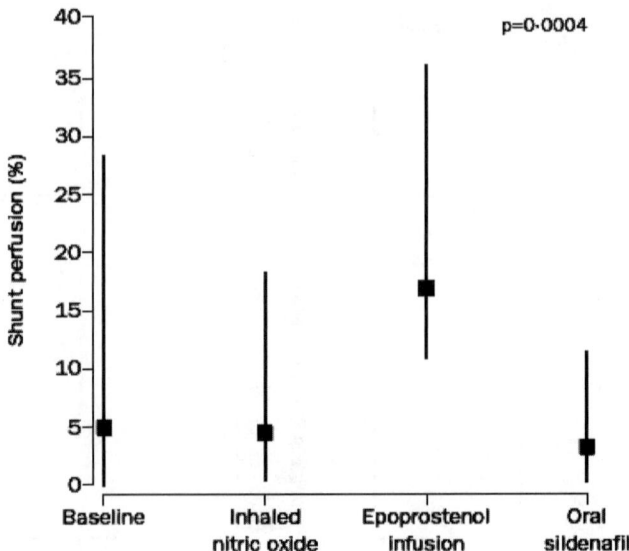

Fig. 9.4 Pulmonary shunt flow at baseline in response to vasodilator challenge with inhaled nitric oxide, infused epoprostenol, and single-dose oral sildenafil (50 mg) in 16 patients with fibrotic lung disease (7 with IPF). Data are median (range) of shunt perfusion of total pulmonary blood flow. p value for difference between treatment effects. From Ghofrani et al. [50]

by more than 20%. The totality of these preliminary data, albeit in small numbers of IPF patients, suggested a benefit of this form of vasodilator therapy.

Lung transplantation is the only therapeutic option that has been suggested to improve survival in patients with IPF (54–56). The impact of lung transplantation on IPF patients with PH has not been specifically addressed. Interestingly, Whelan et al. [57] noted that preoperative PH is a poor prognostic indicator of post transplant survivorship in IPF patients. Patients with a mean PAP >35 mmHg exhibited a 1.5-fold increased risk of mortality. This finding was not supported by a smaller, single center study [58].

Some of this may reflect the type of transplant procedure as a bilateral procedure has been suggested to offer improved survival in the setting of PH [59]. Interestingly, the new organ allocation system in the USA is based on a severity stratification with the calculation of a lung allocation score [60]. Key factors that impact the medical urgency include diagnosis with IPF strongly impacting the score as does the inclusion of pulmonary artery systolic pressure. Interestingly, preliminary data suggest that this new system preferentially places IPF patients higher on the transplant wait list [61].

Conclusions

PH can complicate IPF and appears to be associated with impaired functional status and increased mortality. The prevalence varies but is likely worse in patients with more severe disease. Patients with impaired gas exchange and worse exercise capacity are at greater risk for suffering from PH, although predictive models based on physiological parameters display only modest diagnostic accuracy. BNP levels may be quite accurate, although available data in IPF patients are limited. The pathobiology is complex but likely includes pulmonary vasoconstriction and remodeling. Current therapeutic options are limited and include vasodilator therapy and lung transplantation. Unfortunately, little controlled data exist to suggest specific treatment regimens and duration of therapy. Additional prospective investigation in this arena is sorely needed.

References

1. Noth I, Martinez F. Recent advances in idiopathic pulmonary fibrosis. Chest 2007;132:637–650.
2. Flaherty K, Rei A, Murray S, Fraley C, Colby T, Travis W, Lama V, Kazerooni E, Gross B, Toews G, Martinez F. Idiopathic pulmonary fibrosis: prognostic value of changes in physiology six-minute-walk test. Am J Respir Crit Care Med 2006;174:803–809.
3. Gay S, Kazerooni E, Toews G, Lynch J III, Gross B, Cascade P, Spizarny D, Flint A, Schork M, Whyte R, Popovich J, Hyzy R, Martinez F. Idiopathic pulmonary fibrosis. Predicting response to therapy survival. Am J Respir Crit Care Med 1998;157:1063–1072.
4. Lynch D, Godwin J, Safrin S, Starko K, Hormel P, Brown K, Raghu G, King T Jr, Bradford W, Schwartz D, Webb W, for the Idiopathic Pulmonary Fibrosis Study Group. High-resolution computed tomography in idiopathic pulmonary fibrosis. Diagnosis prognosis. Am J Respir Crit Care Med 2005;172:488–493.
5. Collard H, King T, Jr, Bartelson B, Vourlekis J, Schwarz M, Brown K. Changes in clinical physiologic variables predict survival in idiopathic pulmonary fibrosis. Am J Respir Crit Care Med 2003;168:538–542.
6. Latsi P, Du Bois R, Nicholson A, Colby T, Bisirtzoglou D, Nikolapoulou A, Veeraraghavan S, Hansell D, Wells A. Fibrotic idiopathic interstitial pneumonia. The prognostic value of longitudinal functional trends. Am J Respir Crit Care Med 2003;168:531–537.
7. Jegal Y, Kim D, Shim T, Lim C, Lee S, Koh Y, Kim WS, Kim WD, Lee J, Travis W, Kitaichi M, Colby T. Physiology is a stronger predictor of survival than pathology in fibrotic interstitial pneumonia. Am J Respir Crit Care Med 2003;171:639–644.
8. Martinez F, Safrin S, Weycker D, Starko K, Bradford W, King T Jr, Flaherty K, Schwartz D, Noble P, Raghu G, Brown K, for the IPF Study Group. The clinical course of patients with idiopathic pulmonary fibrosis. Ann Int Med 2005;142:963–967.
9. King T Jr., Safrin S, Starko K, Brown K, Noble P, Raghu G, Schwartz D. Analyses of efficacy end points in a controlled trial of interferon-γ1b for idiopathic pulmonary fibrosis. Chest 2005;127:171–177.
10. Martinez F. Idiopathic interstitial pneumonias. Usual interstitial pneumonia versus nonspecific interstitial pneumonia. Proc Am Thorac Soc 2006;3:81–95.
11. Lettieri C, Nathan S, Barnett S, Ahmad S, Shorr A. Prevalence outcomes of pulmonary arterial hypertension in advanced idiopathic pulmonary fibrosis. Chest 2006;129:746–752.
12. Nadrous H, Pellikka P, Krowka M, Swanson K, Chaowalit N, Decker P, Ryu J. Pulmonary hypertension in patients with idiopathic pulmonary fibrosis. Chest 2005;128:2393–2399.
13. Hamada K, Nagai S, Tanaka S, Ha T, Mishima M, Kitaichi M, Izumi T. Significance of pulmonary arterial pressure diffusing capacity of the lung as prognosticator in patients with idiopathic pulmonary fibrosis. Chest 2007;131:650–656.
14. Vizza C, Lynch J, Ochoa L, Richardson G, Trulock E. Right left ventricular dysfunction in patients with severe pulmonary disease. Chest 1998;113:576–583.

15. Agarwal R, Gupta D, Verma J, Aggarwal A, Jindal S. Noninvasive estimation of clinically asymptomatic pulmonary hypertension in idiopathic pulmonary fibrosis. Indian J Chest Dis Allied Sci 2005;47:267–271.

16. Cottin V, Nunes H, Brillet P, Delaval P, Devouassaoux G, Tillie-Leblond I, Israel-Biet D, Court-Fortune I, Valeyre D, Cordier J, Groupe d'Etude et de Recherche sur les Maladies Orphelines Pulmonaires (GERM O P). Combined pulmonary fibrosis emphysema: a distinct underrecognized entity. Eur Respir J 2005;26:586–593.

17. Grubstein A, Bendeyan D, Schactman I, Cohen M, Shitrit D, Kramer M. Concomitant upper-lobe bullous emphysema, lower-lobe interstitial fibrosis pulmonary hypertension in heavy smokers: report of eight cases review of the literature. Respir Med 2005;99:948–954.

18. Arcasoy S, Christie J, Ferrari V, Sutton M, Zisman D, Blumenthal N, Pochettino A, Kotloff R. Echocardiographic assessment of pulmonary hypertension in patients with advanced lung disease. Am J Respir Crit Care Med 2003;167:735–740.

19. Zisman D, Ross D, Belperio J, Saggar R, Lynch J III, Ardehali A, Karlamangia A. Prediction of pulmonary hypertension in idiopathic pulmonary fibrosis. Respir Med 2007;101: 2153–2159

20. Shorr A, Wainright J, Cors C, Lettieri C, Nathan S. Pulmonary hypertension in patients with pulmonary fibrosis awaiting lung transplantation. Eur Respir J 2007;30:715–721.

21. Yang Y, Johnson C, Hoffman K, Mulligan M, Spada C, Raghu G. Pulmonary arterial hypertension in patients with idiopathic pulmonary fibrosis when listed for lung transplantation (LT) at LT. Proc Am Thorac Soc 2006;3:A369.

22. Nathan S, Shlobin O, Ahmad S, Koch J, Barnett S, Ad N, Burton N, Leslie K. Serial development of pulmonary hypertension in patients with idiopathic pulmonary fibrosis. Respiration 2008; 76:288–94.

23. Leuchte H, Baumgartner R, Nounou M, Vogeser M, Neurohr C, Trautniz M, Behr J. Brain natriuretic is a prognostic parameter in chronic lung disease. Am J Respir Crit Care Med 2006; 173:744–750.

24. Leuchte H, Neurohr C, Baumgartner R, Holzapfel M, Gierhl W, Vogeser M, Behr J. Brain natriuretic peptide exercise capacity in lung fibrosis pulmonary hypertension. Am J Respir Crit Care Med 2004;170:360–365.

25. Zisman D, Karlamangia A, Kawut S, Shlobin O, Saggar R, Ross D, Schwarz M, Belperio J, Ardehali A, Lynch J III, Nathan S. Validation of a method to screen for pulmonary hypertension in advanced idiopathic pulmonary fibrosis. Chest 2008;133:640–645.

26. Zisman D, Karlamangia A, Ross D, Keane M, Belperio J, Saggar R, Lynch J III, Ardehali A, Goldin J. High-resolution chest computed tomography findings do not predict the presence of pulmonary hypertension in advanced idiopathic pulmonary fibrosis. Chest 2007;132:773–779.

27. Nathan S, Noble P, Tuder R. Idiopathic pulmonary fibrosis pulmonary hypertension. Connecting the dots. Am J Respir Crit Care Med 207;175:875–880.

28. Weitzenblum E, Chaouat A. Hypoxic pulmonary hypertension in man: what minimum daily duration of hypoxaemia is required? Eur Respir J 2001;18:251–253.

29. Weitzenblum E. Chronic cor pulmonale. Heart 2003;89:225–230.

30. Tzouvelekis A, Harokopos V, Paparountas T, Oikonomou N, Chatziioannou A, Vilaras G, Tsiambas E, Karameris A, Bouros D, Aidinis V. Pulmonary fibrosis comparative expression profiling suggests key role of hypoxia inducible factor 1a. Am J Respir Crit Care Med 2007; 176:1108–1119.

31. Ebina M, Shimizukawa M, Shibata N, Kimura Y, Suzuki T, Endo M, Sasano H, Kondo T, Nukiwa T. Heterogenous increase in CD34-positive alveolar capillaries in idiopathic pulmonary fibrosis. Am J Respir Crit Care Med 2004;169:1203–1208.

32. Cosgrove G, Brown K, Schiemann W, Serls A, Parr J, M Geraci, Schwarz M, Cool C, Worthen G. Pigment epithelial-derived factor in idiopathic pulmonary fibrosis. Am J Respir Crit Care Med 2004;170:242–251.

33. Simler N, Brenchley P, Horrocks A, Greaves S, Hasleton P, Egan J. Angiogenic cytokines in patients with idiopathic interstitial pneumonia. Thorax 2004;59:581–585.

34. Renzoni E, Walsh D, Salmon M, Wells A, Sestini P, Nicholson A, Veeraraghavan S, Bishop A, Romanksa H, Pantelidis P, Black C, du Bois R. Interstitial vascularity in fibrosing alveolitis. Am J Respir Crit Care Med 2003;167:438–443.
35. Colombat M, Mal H, Groussard O, Capron F, Thabut G, Jebrak G, Brugiere O, Dauriat G, Castier Y, Leseche G, Fournier M. Pulmonary vascular lesions in end-stage idiopathic pulmonary fibrosis: histopathologic study on lung explant specimens correlations with pulmonary hemodynamics. Human Pathol 2007;38:60–65.
36. Gagermeier J, Dauber J, Yousem S, Gibson K, Kaminski N. Abnormal vascular phenotypes in patients with idiopathic pulmonary fibrosis secondary pulmonary hypertension. Chest 2005;128:601S.
37. Charbeneau R, Peters-Golden M. Eicosanoids: mediators therapeutic targets in fibrotic lung disease. Clin Sci (Lond) 2005;108:479–491.
38. Budhiraja R, Tuder R, Hassoun P. Endothelial dysfunction in pulmonary hypertension. Circulation 2004;109:159–65.
39. Giaid A, Michel R, Stewart D, Sheppard M, Corrin B, Hamid Q. Expression of endothelin-1 in lungs of patients with cryptogenic fibrosing alveolitis. Lancet 1993;341:1550–1554.
40. Saleh D, Furukawa K, Tsao M, Maghazachi A, Corrin B, Yanagisawa M, Barnes P, Giaid A. Elevated expression of endothelin-1 endothelin-converting enzyme-1 in idiopathic pulmonary fibrosis: possible involvement of proinflammatory cytokines. Am J Respir Cell Mol Biol 1997;16:187–193.
41. Trakada G, Spiropoulos K. Arterial endothelin-1 in interstitial lung disease patients with pulmonary hypertension. Monaldi Arch Chest Dis 2001;56:379–383.
42. Douglas W, Ryu J, Schroeder D. Idiopathic pulmonary fibrosis. Impact of oxygen colchicine, prednisone, or no therapy on survival. Am J Respir Crit Care Med 2000;161:1172–1178.
43. Crockett A, Cranston J, Antic N. Domiciliary oxygen for interstitial lung disease. Cochrane Database of Syst Rev 2001;(3):CD002883. .
44. Carpagnano G, Kharitonov S, Foschino-Barbaro M, Resta O, Gramiccioni E, Barnes P. Supplementary oxygen in healthy subjects those with COPD increases oxidative stress airway inflammation. Thorax 2004;59:1016–1019.
45. Barbaro M, Serviddio G, Resta O, Rollo T, Tamborra R, Carpagnano G, Vendemiale G, Altomare E. Oxygen therapy at low flow rates causes oxidative stress in chronic obstructive pulmonary disease: Prevention by N-acetyl cysteine. Free Radical Res 2005;39:1111–1118.
46. Kinnula V, Fattman C, Tan R, Oury T. Oxidative stress in pulmonary fibrosis. A possible role for redox modulatory therapy. Am J Respir Crit Care Med 2005;172:417–422.
47. Yoshida M, Taguchi O, Gabazza E, Yasui H, Kobayashi T, Kobayashi H, Maruyama K, Adachi Y. The effect of low-dose inhalation of nitric oxide in patients with pulmonary fibrosis. Eur Respir J 1997;10:2051–2054.
48. Yung G, Kriett J, Jamieson S, Johnson F, Newhart J, Kinninger K, Channick R. Outpatient inhaled nitric oxide in a patient with idiopathic pulmonary fibrosis: a bridge to lung transplantation. J Heart Lung Transplant 2001;20:1224–1227.
49. Olschewski H, Ghofrani H, Walmrath D, Schermuly R, Temmesfeld-Wollbrück B, Grimminger F, Seeger W. Inhaled prostacyclin iloprost in severe pulmonary hypertension secondary to lung fibrosis [in German]. Am J Respir Crit Care Med 1999;160:600–607.
50. Ghofrani H, Wiedemann R, Rose F, Schermuly R, Olschewski H, Weissman N, Gunther A, Walmrath D, Seeger W, Grimminger F. Sildenafil for treatment of lung fibrosis pulmonary hypertension: a randomised controlled trial. Lancet 2002;360:895–900.
51. Madden B, Allenby M, Loke T, Sheth A. A potential role for sildenafil in the management of pulmonary hypertension in patients with parenchymal lung disease. Vasc Pharmacol 2006;44:372–376.
52. Madden B, Sheth A, Wilde M, Ong Y. Does sildenafil produce a sustained benefit in patients with pulmonary hypertension associated with parenchymal lung cardiac disease? Vasc Pharmacol 2007;47:184–188.
53. Collard H, Anstrom K, Schwarz M, Zisman D. Sildenafil improves walk distance in idiopathic pulmonary fibrosis. Chest 2007;131:897–899.

54. Charman S, Sharples L, McNeil K, Wallwork J. Assessment of survival benefit after lung transplantation by patient diagnosis. J Heart Lung Transplant 2002;21:226–232.
55. De Meester J, Smits JM, Persijn GG, Haverich A. Listing for lung transplantation: life expectancy transplant effect, stratified by type of end-stage lung disease, the Eurotransplant experience. J Heart Lung Transplant 2001;20:518–524.
56. Thabut G, Mal H, Castier Y, Groussard O, Brugiere O, Marrash-Chahla R, Leseche G, Fournier M. Survival benefit of lung transplantation for patients with idiopathic pulmonary fibrosis. J Thorac Cardiovasc Surg 2003;126:469–475.
57. Whelan T, Dunitz J, Kelly R, Edwards L, Herrington C, Hertz M, Dahlberg P. Effect of preoperative pulmonary artery pressure on early survival after lung transplantation for idiopathic pulmonary fibrosis. J Heart Lung Transplant 2005;24:1269–1274.
58. Huerd S, Hodges T, Grover F, Mault J, Mitchell M, Campbell D, Aziz S, Chetham P, Torres F, Zamora M. Secondary pulmonary hypertension does not adversely affect outcome after single lung transplantation. J Thorac Cardiovasc Surg 2000;119:458–465.
59. Conte J, Borja M, Patel C, Yang S, Jhaveri R, Orens J. Lung transplantation for primary secondary pulmonary hypertension. Ann Thorac Surg 2001;72:1673–1680.
60. Egan T, Kotloff R. Pro/Con debate: lung allocation should be based on medical urgency transplant survival not on waiting time. Chest 2005;128:407–415.
61. Lingaraju R, Blumenthal N, Kotloff R, Christie J, Ahya V, Sager J, Pochettino A, Hadjiliadis D. Effects of lung allocation score on waiting list rankings transplant procedures. J Heart Lung Transplant 2006;25:1167–1170.

Chapter 10
Occupational Interstitial Lung Disease Update

Lee S. Newman

Overview

Occupational exposures produce a wide range of interstitial lung disorders. Occupational etiologies account for a significant portion of all interstitial lung disease (ILD), and new causes continue to be described. All of these disorders are preventable with the reduction or elimination of workplace exposure. This chapter highlights the common, persistent diseases that continue to plague workers globally, as well as recent developments in ILD caused by exposure to metal dust and fumes, inorganic fibers, and nonfibrous inorganic dust.

ILDs caused by exposure to agents encountered in the workplace (occupational ILD) are an important and preventable group of illnesses. A large number of different agents cause occupational ILD, some well described and others poorly characterised. The list of causative agents continues to expand. The clinical, radiological, and pathological presentations of occupational ILD are very similar to nonoccupational variants because of the lung's limited patterns of response to injury [1]. The clinician must therefore maintain a high degree of suspicion and perform a thorough occupational history when confronted with a new patient presenting with ILD. The recognition of occupational ILD is especially important because of the implications with regard to primary and secondary disease prevention in exposed coworkers. This chapter will review occupational interstitial lung diseases caused by exposure to metals, inorganic fibrous dust, and inorganic nonfibrous dusts and chemicals. Hypersensitivity pneumonitis caused by organic dust exposure is discussed elsewhere in this volume.

Epidemiology

The epidemiology of occupational ILD remains poorly understood. Limitations to the epidemiologic data include nonstandardised diagnostic criteria, varied physician awareness, limitations inherent to the various data sources (death certificates, hospital discharge data, surveillance or reporting systems, etc.), and the long latency period of many agents. Occupational exposures can both cause ILD directly and

R.P. Baughman et al. (eds.), *Pulmonary Arterial Hypertension*
and Interstitial Lung Diseases,
© Humana Press, a part of Springer Science + Business Media, LLC 2009

also influence the risk of developing idiopathic forms of pulmonary fibrosis (IPF) [2]. A number of authors have investigated patients with IPF and the association of previous exposure to a variety of occupational agents [3–9]. All exposures have methodological limitations; however, metal dust exposure consistently emerges as a risk factor for IPF development. Wood dust exposure has also been shown to be a significant risk factor in some studies.

Other authors investigated what proportion of ILD is occupational, including hypersensitivity pneumonitis. In a population-based study, Coultas et al. [4] found 14% of prevalent and 12% of incident cases of ILD were occupational in origin. In data from European Registries, occupational ILD accounts for 4–18% of prevalent and 13–19% of incident cases of ILD [9]. Thus, it is important for the clinician caring for these patients to understand the approach to the diagnosis and treatment of occupational ILD and to appreciate the spectrum of causative agents.

The importance of obtaining a comprehensive occupational history from the patient cannot be overemphasized [10,11]. In one pathological series, occupational ILD was missed in 25% of the biopsies referred for "IPF" and only discovered after detailed mineralogical analysis indicated the diagnosis and further history was obtained [12]. In addition to occupational history, consideration should be given to bystander exposures, both in the home and the workplace, as illustrated by the occurrence of chronic beryllium disease in housewives and development of asbestosis in areas of significant environmental contamination as was seen in Libby, Montana, near a vermiculite mine that was laden with tremolite asbestos [13,14].

Exposure factors vary by the type of agent. Some exposures trigger an immune response, acting as antigens or haptens and lead to immune sensitization. Once sensitized, individuals are susceptible for progression to immune-mediated inflammation and subsequent fibrosis. Beryllium is the best understood example of this group of agents and is discussed in more detail in the section "Chronic Beryllium Disease." Hypersensitivity pneumonitis is discussed elsewhere in this volume. For other exposures (e.g., asbestos, coal, and silica) the cumulative exposure dose is the most important disease determinant [15]. The size, solubility, durability, and oxidative properties of inhaled agent are also important [16]. For fibers, pathogenic potential is also related to the fiber dimensions (length:diameter) as longer thinner fibers are more fibrogenic [17].

In addition to exposure, host-related factors affect pathogenesis and should be considered, including anatomic and physiologic characteristics that influence the deposition and clearance of inhaled particles (e.g., efficiency of nasal filtering and the mucociliary blanket, overall length of the respiratory tree, respiratory pattern, etc.) and genetic factors [15].

Fibrous Dust

Asbestosis

Asbestosis is the best-characterized occupational ILD caused by inorganic fibers. Asbestosis is defined as interstitial fibrosis caused by asbestos fibers [18]. There are several different types of asbestos fibers, including both serpentine (chrysotile) and amphibole (e.g., crocidolite, amosite, tremolite). In addition to interstitial fibrosis, asbestos exposure causes a variety of pleural diseases, including benign pleural effusions, pleural and diaphragmatic plaques, and diffuse pleural thickening. All fiber types have the potential to cause asbestosis, given sufficient exposure [18]. The latency between exposure onset and disease is long, ranging from 15 to greater than 40 years.

The primary symptom of asbestosis is dyspnea on exertion. Patients may also note a dry cough. Physical examination reveals bibasilar dry crackles. Clubbing also occurs. Cor pulmonale may complicate advanced disease. Pulmonary function abnormalities include reduced lung volumes and/or a reduced diffusion capacity (of the lung) for carbon monoxide (DL_{CO}). Large airway function as shown by the forced expiratory volume in 1 second/ forced vital capacity ratio is usually preserved, but the obstruction of small airways is an early finding [18,19].

The radiographic features of asbestosis are well-described. The chest radiograph typically reveals bilateral basilar predominant irregular or reticular opacities. Honeycomb change occurs in advanced cases. The high-resolution computed tomography (HRCT) is more sensitive than plain film for the detection of asbestosis [18,20]. HRCT findings include thickened interlobular septal lines and intralobular core structures (with the later being the initial or earliest CT abnormality), curvilinear lines that persist in the prone position, subpleural ground glass, and honeycombing (Fig. 10.1) [21]. These changes correlate with pathologic findings [22]. Parenchymal fibrous bands are also found but correlate better with diffuse pleural thickening [23]. The CT changes are located primarily in the basilar and subpleural regions [24]. The presence of concomitant pleural disease is an important clue. Pleural disease is rare in IPF, but more than 90% of patients with asbestosis show some pleural abnormality (either plaques, diffuse thickening, or both) on HRCT scans [24].

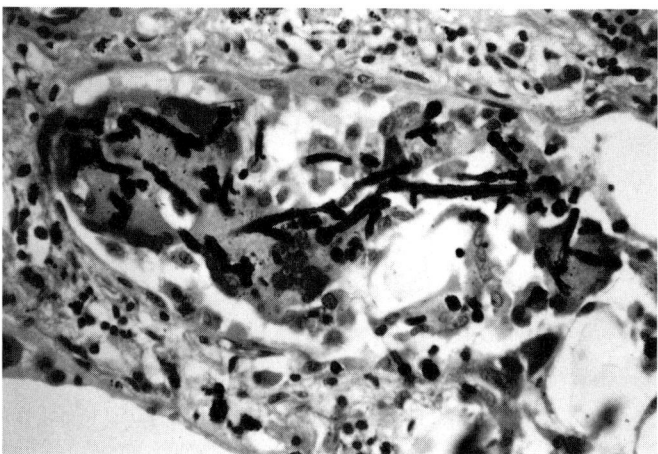

Fig. 10.1 Asbestosis. Photomicrograph demonstrates asbestos bodies ("ferruginous bodies") and adjacent macrophages in lung biopsy from a patient with asbestosis (*See Color Plates*)

However, the percentage of patients with concomitant pleural disease visible on chest x-ray is significantly lower [18,25].

Asbestosis is diagnosed according to the principles discussed previously in this chapter. When biopsies are performed, the presence of asbestos bodies (Fig. 10.2) or fiber counts can assist the clinician in a diagnosis. There are published standards for interpretation but there is significant variability between laboratories [18]. The pathologic lesion of asbestosis begins with a peribronchiolar fibrosis that then extends into surrounding alveolar walls. As the disease progresses, the pathology is similar to that encountered in usual interstitial pneumonia (UIP), and the severity can be graded according to published schemata [26].

Unfortunately, the disease is progressive in a significant proportion of patients (20–40%). Progression is typically slower than it is for idiopathic forms of pulmonary fibrosis. Risk factors for progression include cumulative exposure, severity of disease at diagnosis and, possibly, fiber type [26,27]. Therapy focuses on removal from exposure and supportive care, including Pneumovax (Merck and Co.., Whitehouse Station, NJ) and influenza vaccinations, prompt treatment of respiratory infections, supplemental oxygen to treat resting or exercise-induced hypoxemia, and diuretics for cor pulmonale. There is no known pharmacologic treatment for asbestosis. No studies have demonstrated efficacy for corticosteroids or immuno-suppressant medications.

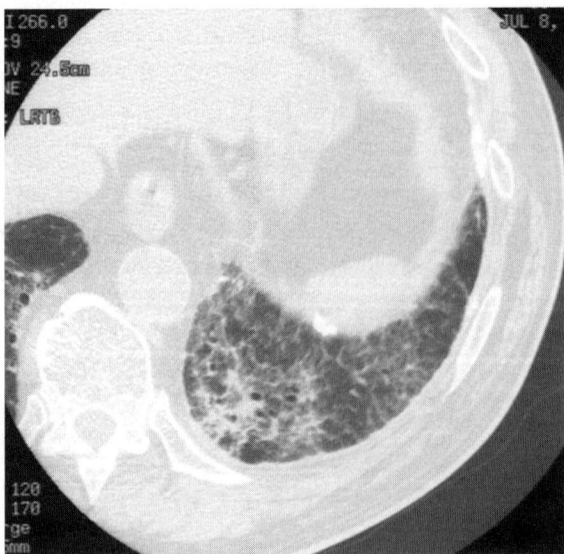

Fig. 10.2 Asbestosis. Thin-section CT at the left lung base shows typical features of asbestosis, including basilar septal thickening, linear opacities. Note also the presence of diaphragmatic pleural plaques with calcification. The combination of these pleural changes plus the interstitial changes are virtually pathognomonic for asbestosis

Flock Workers' Lung

Exposure to other types of fibers can, in some instances, cause occupational ILD. Nylon flock workers' lung was first described in 1998 [28]. It is an ILD that occurs in workers exposed to random cut nylon flock, which is a material that imparts a velvety surface when applied to adhesive fabrics or objects [29]. More recently, this condition has been described in a greeting card manufacturing facility in which the cards were coated with rayon flock in a process that included creating of peak airborne levels of exposure when compressed air was used to blow away excess [30].

With a variable latency period that ranges from 1 to 30 years, patients develop symptoms that include persistent dry cough and dyspnea. Physical examination may discover bilateral crackles. The chest radiograph shows reticulonodular infiltrates and the main CT findings from nylon flock exposure include patchy ground glass and micronodules [31]. Reticular abnormalities, consolidation, and traction bronchiectasis also occur in a minority of patients. Lung biopsies demonstrate a lymphocytic bronchiolitis and peribronchiolitis with associated lymphoid aggregates [32]. The only known effective treatment is removal from exposure.

Nonfibrous Dust

The best-characterized occupational ILD secondary to nonfibrous inorganic dust exposure is silicosis. Silicosis occurs after extensive exposure to crystalline silica (quartz, cristobalite, tridymite, etc.) [33]. Silica-related ILD presents in three ways. The most common, chronic simple silicosis, occurs after a latency period of at least 10 and as long as 40 years. The second presentation, accelerated silicosis, occurs with greater exposures. The clinical phenotype of accelerated silicosis is similar to chronic simple silicosis but the latency period is only 5 to 10 years, and the disease is usually more severe. Progressive massive fibrosis can complicate both chronic simple and accelerated silicosis (see discussion further in this section). Finally, extremely high exposures over a period of months to 2 years can cause acute silicoproteinosis, a disease that is very similar clinically and pathologically to alveolar proteinosis [34,35].

In addition to ILD, silica exposure increases one's risk for developing a variety of pulmonary and nonpulmonary illnesses. Silica exposure markedly increases one's risk of developing active tuberculosis and other mycobacterial disease. The risk increases with exposure and severity of disease on chest x-ray [36]. The incidence of both chronic bronchitis and chronic obstructive pulmonary disease is also increased in workers with silica exposure independent of tobacco abuse and even in the absence of radiographically detectable silicosis [37,38]. In addition, the risk of emphysema is increased in silica-exposed smokers (compared with smokers without silica exposure) and those with progressive massive fibrosis [39]. Silica exposure also increases the risk for developing chronic renal insufficiency and autoimmune diseases, particularly scleroderma, rheumatoid arthritis, and Wegener's granulomatosis [40]. Finally, the International Agency for Research on Cancer lists silica as a known human carcinogen, and both the American Thoracic Society and the National Institute for Occupational Safety and Health concur [37,41,42].

Patients with chronic simple silicosis are frequently asymptomatic, unless COPD is present. Symptoms develop as the disease progresses and particularly when complicated by progressive massive fibrosis [37]. Symptoms include dyspnea on exertion and productive cough. Both are of gradual onset and progress slowly. Pulmonary function tests typically reveal a mixed pattern of obstruction and restriction with a reduced diffusion capacity. Symptoms often correlate best with the obstructive abnormalities [43,44]. When complicated by severe progressive massive fibrosis, restriction predominates.

The typical radiographic finding in silicosis is upper lobe predominant nodular opacities. Hilar adenopathy is also seen and in approximately 10% of cases a characteristic pattern of "eggshell" or peripheral calcification occurs. The nodules of silicosis are typically less than 5 mm in diameter and are well-circumscribed. The nodules may coalesce to form masses, known as progressive massive fibrosis (PMF). The International Labor Organization defines a PMF lesion as a mass greater than 1 cm in diameter, whereas the Silicosis and Silicate Disease committee uses a size parameter of 2 cm [35]. As with asbestosis, CT scans demonstrate greater sensitivity than the chest radiograph [45]. CT scans also show well-circumscribed upper lobe predominant nodules, as illustrated in Fig. 10.3. The nodules are primarily posterior and central in distribution. Subpleural nodules are also common, but centrilobular

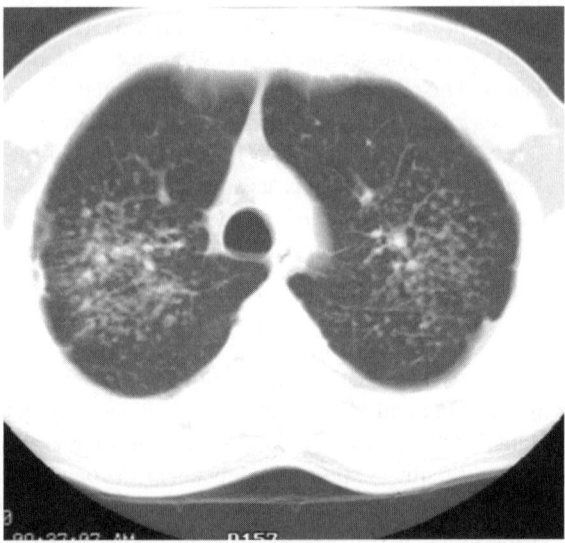

Fig. 10.3 Silicosis. Conventional CT sections in the upper lung zone illustrate the typical findings of complicated silicosis, including multiple solitary rounded nodules and coalescence of nodules. These abnormalities are most commonly found bilaterally in the mid- and upper-lung zones

nodules are unusual [46,47]. PMF lesions usually are posterior and bilateral in appearance. Unilateral lesions are a rare occurrence and appear predominantly on the right side. Rapid changes in the size of masses or the presence of cavitation should prompt a search for alternative diagnoses, particularly mycobacterial disease and lung cancer.

The diagnosis of silicosis usually does not require a lung biopsy (see previous discussion in this section). When a biopsy is performed, the pathognomonic finding is a round, hyalinized nodule known as a silicotic nodule [26,37]. Silicotic nodules are found in both the lung parenchyma and hilar lymph nodes. Diffuse interstitial fibrosis also occurs in a significant minority of patients [26,48].

Several therapies have been tried, including corticosteroids and whole lung lavage, but none are of proven benefit. Therapy thus focuses on removal from exposure and supportive care. In addition, one should screen patients with silicosis for tuberculosis with purified protein derivative skin tests. All patients with a positive test should receive treatment.

Coal Workers' Pneumoconiosis (CWP)

Also called "black lung disease," this form of occupational ILD remains a major health condition worldwide, despite our longstanding knowledge of the hazards and the ways of controlling exposure. It is caused by the chronic inhalation of coal dust, especially from anthracite and bituminous coal high in carbon content and when workers have had more than 10 years of cumulative exposure, depending upon the concentration of dust. Where quartz and coal are found together in mines, the resultant disease displays qualities of both silicosis and CWP. Typical latency is greater than 20 years.

Pathophysiologically, alveolar macrophages engulf coal dust, inducing cytokine and growth factor production, stimulating inflammation, collagen deposition, and the accretion of coal particles, resulting in formation of coal macules along bronchioles and the interstitium. These nodules are commonly associated with development of focal emphysema and varying degrees of fibrosis. Significant distortion of the lung architecture ensues, with associated airflow obstruction and varying degrees of impairment. Like silicosis, CWP is categorized as simple CWP, when the macules are individual, or as "complicated" CWP, when they coalesce or form PMF (Fig. 10.4). These large, black, parenchymal masses usually develop in the posterior of the upper lung fields. The masses may compress vascular supply and airways, or may form cavities [49].

CWP is associated with an increased risk for the development of rheumatoid arthritis. Multiple rounded nodules appearing over a relatively short time are called Caplan's syndrome and represent an immunologic response related to rheumatoid arthritis. Histologically, these nodules are similar to rheumatoid nodules, except that they show a more acute inflammatory response in their periphery.

Simple CWP is often asymptomatic; however, symptoms such as cough and shortness of breath are common in coal miners because of the bronchitis that they

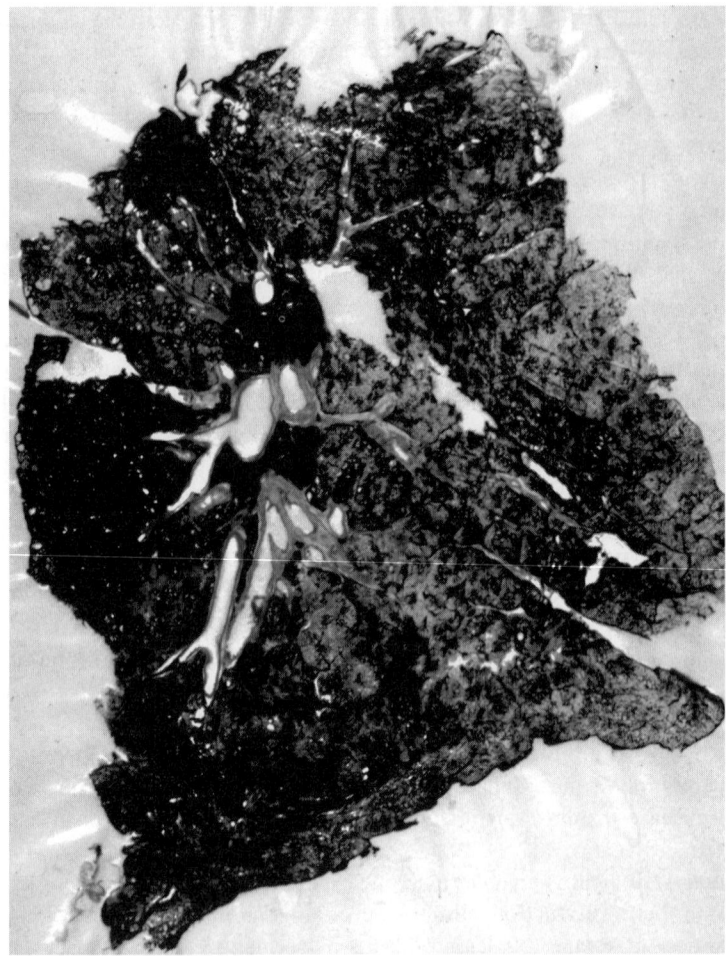

Fig. 10.4 Coal workers' pneumoconiosis. This Goff section through the entire lung of a deceased coalminer demonstrates the advanced stages of coal workers' pneumoconiosis. Note the extensive pigmentation, presence of coal macules, coalescence of these macules into conglomerate masses, and PMF in the upper lobe. Adjacent to the macules are areas of emphysema and bronchiectasis (*See Color Plates*)

develop from daily coal dust exposure. When patients develop complicated CWP, especially with PMF, progressive dyspnea is commonly reported. Pulmonary hypertension with right ventricular and respiratory failure develops in these more severe cases. Black sputum (melanoptysis) is rare and caused by rupture of PMF lesions into the airways.

Diagnosis depends on a history of exposure and the chest x-ray or CT scan appearance of diffuse small rounded opacities, with or without the presence of PMF. Chest CT is more useful for identifying CWP and for distinguishing PMF from other medical conditions, such as malignancy. Although spirometry, lung volumes, and DL_{CO} are nondiagnostic, they are important for characterizing lung impairment, as obstructive, restrictive, or mixed defects may develop [50]. Direct measures of gas exchange, such as resting arterial blood gas analysis and oximetry during exercise testing, provide additional important data for treatment and assessment of disability.

Treatment is usually unnecessary, unless patients develop complicated CWP, or show evidence of pulmonary hypertension and/or gas exchange abnormalities. Appropriate treatment with supplemental oxygen is advised for hypoxemic CWP patients. Bronchodilators, corticosteroids, and other mainstays of pulmonary pharmacotherapy are generally unhelpful.

Occupational Dust and Sarcoidosis-Like Granulomatous Pulmonary Disease

On September 11, 2001, the attack and collapse of the World Trade Center (WTC) in New York City created a massive plume of respirable airborne particulate matter [51]. In addition to high reported rates of bronchitis (so-called "WTC cough") and new-onset asthma [52], interesting data have emerged suggesting a relationship between this complex dust and combustion product mixture and the occurrence of sarcoidosis-like granulomatous pulmonary disease [53,54]. In particular, a recent study by Izbicki et al. [53] contributes evidence that occupational and environmental exposures may cause or trigger granulomatous pneumonitis and possibly some cases that have extrathoracic granulomatous inflammation as well.

Firefighting is one of a number of occupations in which environmental exposures have been implicated in sarcoidosis etiology [55–59]. Because firefighters in New York City had been the subject of a previous surveillance study that had examined sarcoidosis point prevalence and incidence in the 15 years leading up to the WTC collapse [59], Izbicki et al. [53] were able to compare rates of this disease in the pre- and post-9/11 periods by continuing a prospective surveillance study. In the 5 years after 9/11, using similar surveillance methods to the pre-9/11 period, the authors found 26 new cases [53]. Thirteen were identified during the first year after WTC dust exposure and 13 more during the next 4 years.

Calculated as incidence rates, this translated to an incidence rate of 86/100,000 in the first year after 9/11 and 22/100,000 average annual rate in the next 4 years, as compared with 15/100,000 during the 15 years before the WTC collapse. All 26 cases had intrathoracic adenopathy with biopsy-proven intrathoracic granulomatous disease, and 6 had evidence of extrathoracic disease. Notably, 16 of 18 had clinical findings consistent with asthma and a high rate of airway hyperreactivity. These data, taken in context with the body of previous literature, suggest that intense exposures to inorganic dust may contribute to sarcoidosis risk.

Metals

Chronic Beryllium Disease (CBD)

Although many metals can cause lung disease [58], the best-characterized occupational ILD secondary to metal dust and fume exposure is CBD. CBD is a granulomatous disease similar to sarcoidosis that occurs after exposure and subsequent sensitization to beryllium. Like sarcoidosis, the lung is the primary organ involved, but the skin, liver, spleen, myocardium, skeletal muscle, salivary glands, and bones may also be affected. Exposure to pure beryllium metal, beryllium alloys (with copper, nickel, magnesium, or aluminum), or beryllium oxides used in high technology ceramics can all cause CBD. Current data based on workforce screenings indicate that beryllium sensitization or CBD develops in 2–15% of those exposed [60,61]. Beryllium exposure also can cause tracheobronchitis, acute toxic pneumonitis (when inhaled at high levels), and increases the risk of lung cancer.

Unlike asbestosis and silicosis, the pathogenesis of chronic beryllium disease involves activation of the adaptive immune response. This has several important implications. First, the latency period is highly variable ranging from 2 months to more than 40 years [62,63]. Second, even seemingly small exposures can be clinically significant, as illustrated by reported cases in security guards, secretaries, and residents living near beryllium production facilities [63,64]. In addition, activation of the adaptive immune response can be detected with the beryllium lymphocyte proliferation test (BeLPT). This test is performed on either blood or bronchoalveolar lavage cells and quantifies the beryllium-specific T-cell response based on cell uptake of radiolabeled DNA precursors by T cells that have been exposed to beryllium salts in vitro [65]. In addition to its use as a clinical diagnostic tool, the BeLPT is used to screen exposed workforces.

When detected in workplace-screening programs, patients who present CBD often are asymptomatic. When symptoms occur, they may include insidious onset of dyspnea on exertion and dry cough. Constitutional symptoms, including fatigue, weight loss, fever, night sweats, arthralgias, and myalgias also occur. Physical examination reveals bilateral crackles. In advanced cases, cyanosis, digital clubbing and signs of cor pulmonale may appear. Pulmonary function tests may be normal in early disease or show airflow obstruction. As disease progresses, obstructive, restrictive, mixed patterns, and impaired DL_{CO} may all occur. Cardiopulmonary exercise testing abnormalities of ventilation or gas exchange are the most sensitive physiologic changes [66].

Radiographic changes are similar to sarcoidosis and include diffuse bilateral small opacities that are typically rounded nodules, predominantly in the middle and upper lung fields. Bilateral adenopathy is also seen but less frequently than in sarcoidosis (15–20%), and stage I radiographs (isolated hilar adenopathy) are extremely rare. CT has greater sensitivity than plain film but also may be negative in up to 25% of biopsy-proven CBD cases [58]. CT findings include bilateral small nodules (usually distributed along bronchovascular bundles), septal lines and ground glass attenuation (Fig. 10.5a and 10.5b). Enlarged hilar nodes are detected

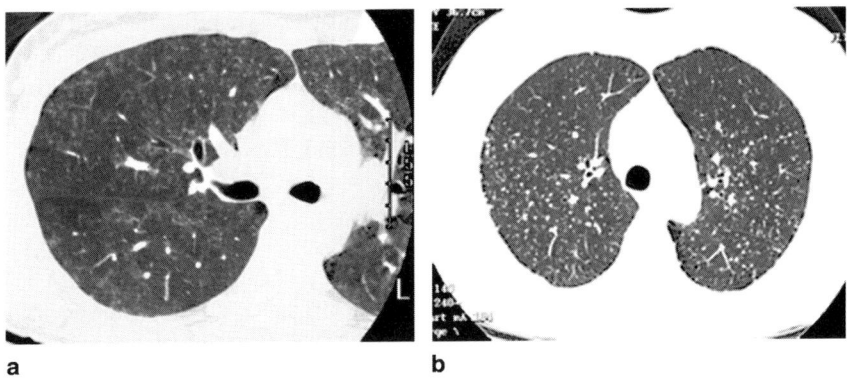

Fig. 10.5 Thin-section CT demonstrates the most common features of CBD, including hazy opacification and peripheral nodules seen in earlier stage disease (**a**) and, more prominently, diffuse nodular infiltrates characteristic of more-advanced stage CBD (**b**)

by CT in approximately one-third of cases. In patients with advanced disease, honeycombing may occur.

Published diagnostic algorithms center on the BeLPT because of its high sensitivity and specificity. Diagnosis requires a history of exposure, demonstration of a beryllium-specific immune response in blood or bronchoalveolar lavage, and evidence for lung inflammation (granulomas, mononuclear cell interstitial infiltrates, or a lymphocytic alveolitis) at bronchoscopy. When bronchoscopy with biopsy cannot be safely performed, one can make the diagnosis based on a positive blood BeLPT plus evidence of diffuse lung disease, i.e., typical x-ray or CT abnormalities, abnormal physiology, lavage lymphocytosis [67–69].

The natural history of CBD is quite variable [70]. Most patients demonstrate a slow progression of symptoms and functional abnormalities. However, some patients have a more rapid progression, whereas others remain stable for extended periods. Minimization of exposure is recommended for all patients with beryllium sensitivity or CBD. Pharmacologic treatment with corticosteroids is generally initiated in the setting of symptoms with severe or progressive functional abnormalities. There are no randomized trials documenting corticosteroid effectiveness, but its use is supported by multiple published case series. Supportive care (as described above) is also important.

Other Granuloma-Forming Metals

Hard Metal Disease

It is noteworthy that other metals can produce granulomatous occupational ILD [70]. Although less well studied than beryllium, cases of granulomatous disease have been observed in people exposed to barium, cobalt, copper, gold, lanthanides, aluminum, titanium, and zirconium.

Hard metal (also called "cemented carbides") usually comprises 80% tungsten carbide and between 10% and 25% cobalt to create a product that has 90% of the hardness of diamond. This material is used widely in manufacturing hard metal-tipped tools, such as saws, cutters, drill bits, grinding wheels, tunneling tools, as well as in defense industry applications such as armor plating and munitions.

Although there remains controversy as to whether cobalt alone can produce the clinical picture of hard metal pneumoconiosis or whether cobalt plus tungsten carbide is required, the evidence from published case series, case reports, and five population-based workplace studies provide ample evidence for the etiologic link [71]). The ILD produced by hard metal is characterized by a very wide spectrum of pathology, including desquamative pneumonitis, diffuse fibrosis, perivascular and peribronchial fibrosis, and varying degrees of more acute appearing alveolitis. In some cases, mixed-dust pneumoconiosis with nodular lesions has been reported, as have sarcoidosis-like granulomas and foreign body-type reactions. One significant commonality in most hard metal cases is the appearance of abundant multinucleated giant cells both in pathology specimens and in bronchoalveolar lavage. This has become a common pathologic feature of the disease, such that giant cell interstitial pneumonitis is often considered to be due to hard metal unless proven otherwise. The pathogenesis remains enigmatic but may involve both adaptive immune response to metal antigen as well as an effect of the metal on oxidative stress pathways.

Patients with this condition often report recent or ongoing employment in industries in which hard metal dust is generated. Symptoms may include dry cough, dyspnea, and systemic symptoms including weight loss and fever. Onset is often acute or subacute, although chronic insidious onset has also been reported. Clinical examination is nonspecific, including lung crackles and limited chest expansion, with or without wheezing. Cor pulmonale and digital clubbing can occur if the condition has not been detected early. Pulmonary physiology is nonspecific, although most typically it includes restriction, low diffusing capacity, and reduced measures of gas exchange [72]. The chest x-ray findings range from normal films, to wedge-shaped infiltrates, ground glass opacification, and a reticulonodular pattern. CT scans often show septal lines, ground glass, large peripheral cysts, and traction bronchiectasis with a mid- and upper lung zone predominance [73].

If bronchoalveolar lavage is performed, large numbers of bizarre-appearing multinucleated giant cells are a strong indication of this condition, especially if viral, bacterial, and fungal cultures are negative. Mineral analysis is advocated by some authors, using biopsy material, BAL, or, more recently, exhaled breath condensate. Such tests have yielded variability results, often showing tungsten, tantalum, and titanium. Cobalt, because of its relatively high solubility, is often absent from the mineral analyses [15].

Relatively little is known about the appropriate treatment of this condition. Removal from exposure has resulted in significant improvement and sometimes resolution of disease in some instances. Corticosteroids are commonly used, with variable results.

Chemicals That Induce Bronchiolitis Obliterans

Occupational ILD secondary to chemical agents not previously described continue to occur and clinicians need to stay alert to this possibility. Two examples include textile sprayers lung and flavoring-related bronchiolitis obliterans (also called "popcorn workers' lung"). As a generalization, when chemical exposures cause ILD, one tends to see bronchiolitis obliterans, with varying amounts of organizing pneumonia and of diffuse alveolar damage.

Textile Sprayers Lung

Textile sprayers lung or Ardystil syndrome was first reported in 1994 [74]. The initial and subsequent reports describe an epidemic of organizing pneumonia in textile printing sprayers using the chemical Acramin-FWN [75,76]. The most common symptoms are cough, epistaxis, and dyspnea. The radiography and CT reveal bilateral patchy consolidation. Small nodular infiltrates were also found on some of the CTs. Pulmonary function tests revealed restriction and/or a reduced DL_{CO}. Biopsies revealed organizing pneumonia. Many patients developed progressive disease despite removal from exposure and corticosteroids.

Flavoring-Related Bronchiolitis Obliterans

This newly described condition, first detected in workers manufacturing microwave popcorn, occurs most frequently in those individuals with heaviest short-term high exposures to a chemical called diacetyl and other components of the butter flavoring [61]. First described in 2002 [77,78], most cases have been discovered either through workplace-surveillance programs or when patients come to medical attention due to respiratory symptoms [79]. The most typical cases in the flavoring industry have developed gradually, without any obvious report of gross overexposures. Patients complain of gradual onset of dyspnea and are found to have fixed airways obstruction.

Conclusion

Occupational ILD is a diverse group of preventable pulmonary diseases that account for a significant proportion of all interstitial lung disease. There are numerous well-described and some more poorly characterized causative agents. New etiologic exposures continue to be discovered. Diagnosis requires a high degree of clinical suspicion and a thorough occupational and environmental history. Correct diagnosis is important not only for appropriate pharmaceutical treatment, but also because removal from exposure may result in clinical improvement or may slow the progression of many types of occupational ILD. In addition, any individual diagnosis of occupational ILD should prompt the clinician to work with occupational medicine specialists to investigate further. Where there is one worker with occupational lung disease, there often are coworkers with the same condition. Interventions to reduce exposure in the workplace may help reduce risk for large numbers of people.

References

1. Beckett WS. Occupational respiratory diseases. N Engl J Med 2000;342:406–413.
2. Demedts M, Wells AU, Anto JM, Costabel U, Hubbard R, Cullinan P, Slabbynck H, Rizzato G, Poletti V, Verbeken EK, et al. Interstitial lung diseases: an epidemiological overview. Eur Respir J Suppl 2001;32:2s–16s.
3. Baumgartner KB, Samet JM, Coultas DB, Stidley CA, Hunt WC, Colby TV, Waldron JA. Occupational and environmental risk factors for idiopathic pulmonary fibrosis: a multicenter case-control study. Collaborating Centers. Am J Epidemiol 2000;152:307–315.
4. Coultas DB, Zumwalt RE, Black WC, Sobonya RE. The epidemiology of interstitial lung diseases. Am J Respir Crit Care Med 1994;150:967–972.
5. Hubbard R, Cooper M, Antoniak M, Venn A, Khan S, Johnston I, Lewis S, Britton J. Risk of cryptogenic fibrosing alveolitis in metal workers. Lancet 2000;355:466–467.
6. Hubbard R, Lewis S, Richards K, Johnston I, Britton J. Occupational exposure to metal or wood dust and aetiology of cryptogenic fibrosing alveolitis. Lancet 1996;347:284–289.
7. Iwai K, Mori T, Yamada N, Yamaguchi M, Hosoda Y. Idiopathic pulmonary fibrosis. Epidemiologic approaches to occupational exposure. Am J Respir Crit Care Med 1994;150:670–675.
8. Scott J, Johnston I, Britton J. What causes cryptogenic fibrosing alveolitis? A case-control study of environmental exposure to dust. BMJ. 1990;301:1015–1017.
9. Thomeer MJ, Costabe U, Rizzato G, Poletti V, Demedts M. Comparison of registries of interstitial lung diseases in three European countries. Eur Respir J Suppl 2001;32:114s–118s.
10. Burge P. How to take an occupational exposure history relevant to lung disease. Occup Disord lung. 2002:25–32.
11. Newman LS. Occupational illness. N Engl J Med. 1995;333:1128–1134.
12. Monso E, Tura JM, Marsal M, Morell F, Pujadas J, Morera J. Mineralogical microanalysis of idiopathic pulmonary fibrosis. Arch Environ Health 1990;45:185–188.
13. Peipins LA, Lewin M, Campolucci S, Lybarger JA, Miller A, Middleton D, Weis C, Spence M, Black B, Kapil V. Radiographic abnormalities and exposure to asbestos-contaminated vermiculite in the community of Libby, Montana, USA. Environ Health Perspect 2003;111: 1753–1759.
14. Stoeckle JD, Hardy HL, Weber AL. Chronic beryllium disease. Long-term follow-up of sixty cases and selective review of the literature. Am J Med 1969;46:545–561.
15. Nemery B, Bast A, Behr J, Borm PJ, Bourke SJ, Camus PH, De Vuyst P, Jansen HM, Kinnula VL, Lison D, Pelkonen O, Saltini C. Interstitial lung disease induced by exogenous agents: factors governing susceptibility. Eur Respir J Suppl 2001;32:30s–42s.
16. Mossman BT, Churg A. Mechanisms in the pathogenesis of asbestosis and silicosis. Am J Respir Crit Care Med 1998;157:1666–1680.
17. Robledo R, Mossman B. Cellular and molecular mechanisms of asbestos-induced fibrosis. J Cell Physiol 1999;180:158–166.
18. American Thoracic Society. Diagnosis and initial management of nonmalignant diseases related to asbestos. Am J Respir Crit Care Med 2004;170:691–715.
19. Begin R, Cantin A, Berthiaume Y, Boileau R, Peloquin S, Masse S. Airway function in lifetime-nonsmoking older asbestos workers. Am J Med 1983;75:631–638.

20. Huuskonen O, Kivisaari L, Zitting A, Taskinen K, Tossavainen A, Vehmas T. High-resolution computed tomography classification of lung fibrosis for patients with asbestos-related disease. Scand J Work Environ Health 2001;27:106–112.
21. Aberle DR. High-resolution computed tomography of asbestos-related diseases. Semin Roentgenol 1991;26:118–131.
22. Akira M, Yamamoto S, Yokoyama K, Kita N, Morinaga K, Higashihara T, Kozuka T. Asbestosis: high-resolution CT-pathologic correlation. Radiology 1990;176:389–394.
23. Gevenois PA, de Maertelaer V, Madani A, Winant C, Sergent G, De Vuyst P. Asbestosis, pleural plaques and diffuse pleural thickening: three distinct benign responses to asbestos exposure. Eur Respir J 1998;11:1021–1027.
24. Copley SJ, Wells AU, Sivakumaran P, Rubens MB, Lee YC, Desai SR, MacDonald SL, Thompson RI, Colby TV, Nicholson AG, du Bois RM, Musk AW, Hansell DM. Asbestosis and idiopathic pulmonary fibrosis: comparison of thin-section CT features. Radiology 2003;229:731–736.
25. Welch LS, Michaels D, Zoloth SR. The National Sheet Metal Worker Asbestos Disease Screening Program: radiologic findings. National Sheet Metal Examination Group. Am J Ind Med 1994;25:635–648.
26. Travis W CT, Koss M, Rosado-de-Christenson M, Muller N, King T, editors. Non-neoplastic disorders of the lower respiratory tract. Am Regis of Pathol 2002:793–856.
27. Oksa P, Huuskonen MS, Jarvisalo J, Klockars M, Zitting A, Suoranta H, Tossavainen A, Vattulainen K, Laippala P. Follow-up of asbestosis patients and predictors for radiographic progression. Int Arch Occup Environ Health 1998;71:465–471.
28. Kern DG, Crausman RS, Durand KT, Nayer A, Kuhn C, 3rd. Flock worker's lung: chronic interstitial lung disease in the nylon flocking industry. Ann Intern Med 1998;129:261–272.
29. Kern DG, Kuhn C, 3rd, Ely EW, Pransky GS, Mello CJ, Fraire AE, Müller J. Flock worker's lung: broadening the spectrum of clinicopathology, narrowing the spectrum of suspected etiologies. Chest 2000;117:251–259.
30. Antao VC, Piacitelli CA, Miller WE, Pinheiro GA, Kreiss K. Rayon flock: a new cause of respiratory morbidity in a card processing plant. Am J Ind Med 2007;50:274–284.
31. Weiland DA, Lynch DA, Jensen SP, Newell JD, Miller DE, Crausman RS, Kuhn C 3rd, Kern DG. Thin-section CT findings in flock worker's lung, a work-related interstitial lung disease. Radiology 2003;227:222–231.
32. Eschenbacher WL, Kreiss K, Lougheed MD, Pransky GS, Day B, Castellan RM. Nylon flock-associated interstitial lung disease. Am J Respir Crit Care Med 1999;159:2003–2008.
33. t'Mannetje A, Steenland K, Attfield M, Boffetta P, Checkoway H, DeKlerk N, Koskela RS. Exposure-response analysis and risk assessment for silica and silicosis mortality in a pooled analysis of six cohorts. Occup Environ Med 2002;59:723–728.
34. Buechner HA, Ansari A. Acute silico-proteinosis. A new pathologic variant of acute silicosis in sandblasters, characterized by histologic features resembling alveolar proteinosis. Dis Chest 1969;55:274–278.
35. Castranova V, Vallyathan V. Silicosis and coal workers' pneumoconiosis. Environ Health Perspect 2000;108(Suppl 4):675–684.
36. Cowie RL. The epidemiology of tuberculosis in gold miners with silicosis. Am J Respir Crit Care Med 1994;150:1460–1462.
37. Adverse effects of crystalline silica exposure. American Thoracic Society Committee of the Scientific Assembly on Environmental and Occupational Health. Am J Respir Crit Care Med 1997;155:761–768.
38. Humerfelt S, Eide GE, Gulsvik A. Association of years of occupational quartz exposure with spirometric airflow limitation in Norwegian men aged 30–46 years. Thorax 1998;53:649–655.
39. Ooi GC, Tsang KW, Cheung TF, Khong PL, Ho IW, Ip MS, Tam CM, Ngan H, Lam WK, Chan FL, Chan-Yeung M. Silicosis in 76 men: qualitative and quantitative CT evaluation–clinical-radiologic correlation study. Radiology 2003;228:816–825.
40. Steenland K, Goldsmith DF. Silica exposure and autoimmune diseases. Am J Ind Med 1995; 28:603–608.

41. Department of Health and Human Services. Health effects of occupational exposure to respirable crystalline silica. 2002. Available at: http://www.cdc.gov/niosh/docs/2002-129/02-129a.html. Accessed August 12, 2008.

42. International Agency for Research on Cancer. IARC monographs on the evaluation of carcinogenic risks to humans: Silica, some silicates, coal dust and para-aramid fibrils. Lyon: IARC, 1997.

43. Kinsella M, Muller N, Vedal S, Staples C, Abboud RT, Chan-Yeung M. Emphysema in silicosis. A comparison of smokers with nonsmokers using pulmonary function testing and computed tomography. Am Rev Respir Dis 1990;141:1497–1500.

44. Wang X, Yano E. Pulmonary dysfunction in silica-exposed workers: a relationship to radiographic signs of silicosis and emphysema. Am J Ind Med 1999;36:299–306.

45. Gevenois PA, Sergent G, De Maertelaer V, Gouat F, Yernault JC, De Vuyst P. Micronodules and emphysema in coal mine dust or silica exposure: relation with lung function. Eur Respir J 1998;12:1020–1024.

46. Akira M, Higashihara T, Yokoyama K, Yamamoto S, Kita N, Morimoto S, Ikezoe J, Kozuka T. Radiographic type p pneumoconiosis: high-resolution CT. Radiology 1989;171:117–123.

47. Remy-Jardin M, Remy J, Farre I, Marquette CH. Computed tomographic evaluation of silicosis and coal workers' pneumoconiosis. Radiol Clin North Am 1992;30:1155–1176.

48. Honma K, Chiyotani K. Diffuse interstitial fibrosis in nonasbestos pneumoconiosis—a pathological study. Respiration 1993;60:120–126.

49. Hurley JF, Alexander WP, Hazledine DJ, Jacobsen M, Maclaren WM. Exposure to respirable coalmine dust and incidence of progressive massive fibrosis. Br J Ind Med. 1987;44:661–672.

50. Lyons JP, Campbell H. Relation between progressive massive fibrosis, emphysema, and pulmonary dysfunction in coalworkers' pneumoconiosis. Br J Ind Med 1981;38:125–129.

51. Lioy PJ, Weisel CP, Millette JR, Eisenreich S, Vallero D, Offenberg J, Buckley B, Turpin B, Zhong M, Cohen MD, Prophete C, Yang I, Stiles R, Chee G, Johnson W, Porcja R, Alimokhtari S, Hale RC, Weschler C, Chen LC. Characterization of the dust/smoke aerosol that settled east of the World Trade Center (WTC) in lower Manhattan after the collapse of the WTC 11 September 2001. Environ Health Perspect 2002;110:703–714.

52. Banauch GI, Dhala A, Prezant DJ. Pulmonary disease in rescue workers at the World Trade Center site. Curr Opin Pulm Med.2005;11:160–168.

53. Izbicki G, Chavko R, Banauch GI, Weiden MD, Berger KI, Aldrich TK, Hall C, Kelly KJ, Prezant DJ. World Trade Center "sarcoid-like" granulomatous pulmonary disease in New York City Fire Department rescue workers. Chest 2007;131:1414–1423.

54. Safirstein BH, Klukowicz A, Miller R, Teirstein A. Granulomatous pneumonitis following exposure to the World Trade Center collapse. Chest 2003;123:301–304.

55. Barnard J, Rose C, Newman L, Canner M, Martyny J, McCammon C, Bresnitz E, Rossman M, Thompson B, Rybicki B, Weinberger SE, Moller DR, McLennan G, Hunninghake G, DePalo L, Baughman RP, Iannuzzi MC, Judson MA, Knatterud GL, Teirstein AS, Yeager H Jr, Johns CJ, Rabin DL, Cherniack R; ACCESS Research Group. Job and industry classifications associated with sarcoidosis in A Case-Control Etiologic Study of Sarcoidosis (ACCESS). J Occup Environ Med 2005;47:226–234.

56. Kern DG, Neill MA, Wrenn DS, Varone JC. Investigation of a unique time-space cluster of sarcoidosis in firefighters. Am Rev Respir Dis 1993;148:974–980.

57. Kreider ME, Christie JD, Thompson B, Newman L, Rose C, Barnard J, Bresnitz E, Judson MA, Lackland DT, Rossman MD. Relationship of environmental exposures to the clinical phenotype of sarcoidosis. Chest 2005;128:207–215.

58. Newman LS, Rose CS, Bresnitz EA, Rossman MD, Barnard J, Frederick M, Terrin ML, Weinberger SE, Moller DR, McLennan G, Hunninghake G, DePalo L, Baughman RP, Iannuzzi MC, Judson MA, Knatterud GL, Thompson BW, Teirstein AS, Yeager H Jr, Johns CJ, Rabin DL, Rybicki BA, Cherniack R; ACCESS Research Group. A case control etiologic study of sarcoidosis: environmental and occupational risk factors. Am J Respir Crit Care Med 2004;170:1324–1330.

59. Prezant DJ, Dhala A, Goldstein A, Janus D, Ortiz F, Aldrich TK, Kelly KJ. The incidence, prevalence, and severity of sarcoidosis in New York City firefighters. Chest 1999;116:1183–1193.
60. Kelleher P, Pacheco K, Newman LS. Inorganic dust pneumonias: the metal-related parenchymal disorders. Environ Health Perspect 2000;108(Suppl 4):685–696.
61. Kreiss K, Day GA, Schuler CR. Beryllium: a modern industrial hazard. Annu Rev Public Health 2007;28:259–277.
62. Hardy HL. Beryllium poisoning—lessons in control of man-made disease. N Engl J Med 1965;273:1188–1199.
63. Kreiss K, Mroz MM, Zhen B, Martyny JW, Newman LS. Epidemiology of beryllium sensitization and disease in nuclear workers. Am Rev Respir Dis 1993;148:985–991.
64. Maier LA, Martyny JW, Liang J, Rossman MD. Recent chronic beryllium disease in residents surrounding a beryllium facility. Am J Respir Crit Care Med 2008;177:1012–1017.
65. Newman LS. Significance of the blood beryllium lymphocyte proliferation test. Environ Health Perspect 1996;104(Suppl 5):953–956.
66. Pappas GP, Newman LS. Early pulmonary physiologic abnormalities in beryllium disease. Am Rev Respir Dis 1993;148:661–666.
67. Glazer CN, L. Chronic beryllium disease: don't miss the diagnosis. J Respir Disord 2003: 357–363.
68. Newman LS, Kreiss K, King TE, Jr., Seay S, Campbell PA. Pathologic and immunologic alterations in early stages of beryllium disease. Re-examination of disease definition and natural history. Am Rev Respir Dis 1989;139:1479–1486.
69. Newman LS, Lloyd J, Daniloff E. The natural history of beryllium sensitization and chronic beryllium disease. Environ Health Perspect 1996;104(Suppl 5):937–943.
70. Newman LS. Metals that cause sarcoidosis. Semin Respir Infect 1998;13:212–220.
71. Nemery B, Abraham JL. Hard metal lung disease: still hard to understand. Am J Respir Crit Care Med 2007;176:2–3.
72. Nemery B, Verbeken EK, Demedts M. Giant cell interstitial pneumonia (hard metal lung disease, cobalt lung). Semin Respir Crit Care Med 2001;22:435–448.
73. Gotway MB, Golden JA, Warnock M, Koth LL, Webb R, Reddy GP, Balmes JR. Hard metal interstitial lung disease: high-resolution computed tomography appearance. J Thorac Imaging 2002;17:314–318.
74. Moya C, Anto JM, Taylor AJ. Outbreak of organising pneumonia in textile printing sprayers. Collaborative Group for the Study of Toxicity in Textile Aerographic Factories. Lancet 1994;344498–502.
75. Romero S, Hernandez L, Gil J, Aranda I, Martin C, Sanchez-Paya J. Organizing pneumonia in textile printing workers: a clinical description. Eur Respir J 1998;11:265–271.
76. Sole A, Cordero PJ, Morales P, Martinez ME, Vera F, Moya C. Epidemic outbreak of interstitial lung disease in aerographics textile workers—the "Ardystil syndrome": a first year follow up. Thorax 1996;51:94–95.
77. Kreiss K, Gomaa A, Kullman G, Fedan K, Simoes EJ, Enright PL. Clinical bronchiolitis obliterans in workers at a microwave-popcorn plant. N Engl J Med 2002;347:330–338.
78. Lockey J MR, Barth E, et al. Bronchiolitis obliterans in the food flavoring manufacturing industry. Am J Respir Crit Care Med 2002:A461.
79. Kanwal R, Kullman G, Piacitelli C, Boylstein R, Sahakian N, Martin S, Fedan K, Kreiss K. Evaluation of flavorings-related lung disease risk at six microwave popcorn plants. J Occup Environ Med 2006;48:149–157.

Chapter 11
Sarcoidosis

Robert P. Baughman, Elyse E. Lower, and Peter Engel

Introduction

Sarcoidosis is a granulomatous disease of unknown etiology [1]. A characteristic feature of sarcoidosis is its ability to affect multiple organs. However, the lung is the most common organ affected in sarcoidosis. In this chapter, we will focus on the pulmonary manifestations of sarcoidosis, including pulmonary hypertension, which can be a consequence of the disease.

Epidemiology and Etiology

Sarcoidosis is disease that is encountered world wide. However, it has a variable rate of incidence. Persons of Scandinavian and Irish descent in Europe and African-Americans in the USA have a greater incidence than others. The highest prevalence has been estimated to be 2–5% of these groups [2,3].

Although the disease often occurs in young adults, there is a second peak of incidence in women in their 60s [3]. In a large study of patients with newly diagnosed sarcoidosis in the USA, the median age was 40 years [4]. The disease appears to be more common in women than men, especially in African-American women and those women from Nordic populations [3,4].

Most patients with sarcoidosis have lung disease; however, the incidence of other organ involvement varies across the world. Table 11.1 demonstrates the reported incidence of various organs affected in different ethnic groups and different countries. One limitation of these data is the method of determining organ involvement. One instrument has been developed to define specific organ involvement in sarcoidosis [5]. Although it has been used in some studies, others have chosen their own definitions [6] or leave to individual institutions to determine organ involvement [7,8]. Despite these limitations, it is clear that sarcoidosis present in distinctly different ways based on ethnic background and one has to bear this in mind when assessing patients.

R.P. Baughman et al. (eds.), *Pulmonary Arterial Hypertension and Interstitial Lung Diseases,*
© Humana Press, a part of Springer Science + Business Media, LLC 2009

Table 11.1 Organ Involvement of Sarcoidosis Across the World

Organ involvement	US Caucasians	US African-Americans	Finland	Japan
Lungs	Very common*	Very common	Very common	Very common
Fibrotic lung disease	Occasional	Some	Occasional	Rare
Eye disease	Some	Common	Some	Very Common
Erythema nodosum	Some	Rare	Common	Rare
Lupus pernio	Very rare	Rare	Very rare	Very rare
Cardiac	Rare	Rare	Rare	Some
Neurologic	Rare	Rare	Rare	Rare

* Very common >50%; Common: 20–50%; Some: 10–20%; Rare: 2–10%; Very rare <2%.

The etiology of sarcoidosis remains unknown, On the basis of current evidence, sarcoidosis appears to be a specific immunologic reaction that is the result of a environmental or infectious agent in a genetically susceptible host [9]. Several antigens have been proposed as possible causes of sarcoidosis. Although each of these has support, no single agent explains all cases of sarcoidosis. It is possible that sarcoidosis is caused by multiple agents, leading to a sarcoidosis-like reaction.

An infectious agent has always been appealing as the cause of sarcoidosis. The granulomatous response looks similar to that found with tuberculosis and many fungal infections. An increased risk for sarcoidosis has been noted in health care workers [10]. Sarcoidosis has also recurred in unaffected organs transplanted into sarcoidosis patients [11–13], including patients who have developed sarcoidosis after receiving a bone marrow transplant from a sarcoidosis patient [14,15]. Chromosomal studies have indicated that the granulomas occurring in the donor lung contain cells from the host [16]. Not all donor organs from a sarcoidosis patient lead to sarcoidosis [17].

Although *Mycobacterium tuberculosis* was originally thought to be the cause of sarcoidosis, several studies failed to confirm the presence of *M. tuberculosis* in most cases. The use of polymerase chain reaction has refuted this as the cause in most cases [18]. Some authors have found evidence of mycobacteria resembling *M. tuberculosis* in tissue of sarcoidosis patients [19]. In addition, a protein specific for mycobacteria has been found not only in sarcoidosis tissue, but also in the Kveim agent [20]. Antibodies to this protein were found in the majority of patients tested [20]. In another study, Th-1 response to these proteins from peripheral blood derived lymphocytes was found in the majority of sarcoidosis patients tested [21].

Another mycobacteria that had once been proposed as the cause of sarcoidosis is a cell wall-free mycobacteria. Initial reports found that nearly all sarcoidosis cases had these organisms in their blood. However, in a subsequent double-blind study conducted by several of these same investigators, the rate of positive blood cultures was the same for the controls as for the sarcoidosis patients [22]. Similar large blinded control studies have not been done with the other potential mycobacterium markers.

Propionibacterium acnes has also been proposed as a possible infectious agent. It has been found in tissue retrieved from sarcoidosis patients [23]. This was confirmed by a multinational study of sarcoidosis patients [24]. An animal model has been developed in which granulomas can be induced by *P. acnes* antigens [25].

Other studies have suggested possible environmental agents as a cause of sarcoidosis. For example, there is an increased rate of disease among fire fighters [26]. There was also an outbreak of "sarcoidosis" among seamen on aircraft carriers [27], with a reduction in cases diagnosed after measures were instituted to minimize exposure to titanium and other metals in dust on the surface of the ships [28]. Exposure to these inorganic dusts have been proposed as a cause of sarcoidosis [29].

In a case-controlled etiologic study of sarcoidosis (ACCESS), there was an increased risk for those in a moldy environment and exposed to insecticides in the year before diagnosis [30]. This risk was greater for those with pulmonary disease as their only manifestation of their sarcoidosis. In these cases with purely thoracic sarcoidosis, one wonders if this is just a sarcoid-like reaction on patients exposed to an inhaled agent. The same question arises from the cases of sarcoid-like disease associated with the World Trade Center disaster [31].

Another aspect of the sarcoidosis is the immunologic response. It is characteristically a greater immune response characterized by the formation of granulomas. This granulomatous response seems to be the result of an antigen being presented to CD-4 T lymphocyte through the major histochemical complex [32]. This complex is through the human leukocyte antigen (HLA) interaction. Berylliosis is another granulomatous disease in which certain HLA patterns are associated with increased risk for the disease [33]. In sarcoidosis, certain HLA patterns are associated with increased risk for disease [34]. The presence of HLA-DQB1*0201 is associated with a good clinical outcome [35] and Lofgren's syndrome [36]. The presence of other HLA patterns is associated with a lower risk for sarcoidosis [37].

Diagnosis

The diagnosis of sarcoidosis requires the combination of clinical presentation and laboratory support. The hallmark of sarcoidosis is the presence of noncaseating granulomas in one or more affected organs [38]. Although the presence of granulomas is an important part of the pathologic diagnosis, most patients do not have a biopsy as part of their initial evaluation.

Although granulomas may appear in biopsies from almost any organ, the most common area in which a diagnosis is made is the thorax, either by bronchoscopy or mediastinoscopy [39]. For pulmonary sarcoidosis, the most common presenting problems are cough, dyspnea, and abnormal chest roentgenogram. For patients with symptomatic pulmonary disease, the complaints can be fairly nonspecific. In one study, more than half of sarcoidosis patients with pulmonary symptoms saw a physician at least four times before a diagnosis was made [40]. One of the causes of delay in diagnosis was the time until a chest roentgenogram was performed. The usual diagnosis made at this point was asthma or respiratory infection. However, even after a chest roentgenogram was performed, there could be a delay in diagnosis. Patients with adenopathy were diagnosed more rapidly than those without adenopathy. The authors proposed that the presence of adenopathy raised the question of malignancy and hence a greater urgency for diagnosis [40]. Interestingly, patients with skin lesions were more rapidly diagnosed than those with only pulmonary disease [40].

The clinical features which support sarcoidosis are summarized in Table 11.2 [1,38]. Although none of these features is diagnostic for sarcoidosis, they can be highly suggestive of the diagnosis. For example, the presence of symmetrical hilar and right paratracheal adenopathy (Fig. 11.1) in an asymptomatic individual is almost always sarcoidosis [41].

The presence of extrapulmonary disease is an important clinical feature of sarcoidosis. It is a useful factor in confirming the diagnosis. For example ocular, cutaneous, and hepatic involvement are common features in patients with sarcoidosis. However, they are not encountered in other conditions commonly considered in the differential diagnosis, such as idiopathic pulmonary fibrosis, hypersensitivity pneumonitis, or lymphoma. Also helpful are unusual, but relatively specific, complications of sarcoidosis such as nephrolithiasis [42], lupus pernio [43], or seventh cranial nerve paralysis [44].

As noted in Table 11.2, several laboratory tests are useful in supporting the diagnosis of sarcoidosis. Bronchoalveolar lavage (BAL) has been used widely in the study of the cause of sarcoidosis [45,46]. Its role as a diagnostic test is controversial [47]. A major limitation of BAL has been the variability of the technique in both performing the procedure and analyzing the cells retrieved. Recommendations to standardize the technique and analysis have been made [48,49].

Using a standard approach to BAL, one can make some observations about its specificity in diagnosing sarcoidosis [50]. There are two abnormalities noted in the BAL fluid of patients with sarcoidosis: increased lymphocytes and an increased CD4:CD8 ratio. In general, an increased in percentage of lymphocytes was more sensitive and increase in a CD4:CD8 ratio was more specific for sarcoidosis [51–53]. Taking a Bayesian approach to determine the value of the CD4:CD8 ratio, Welker et al. [53] found that a ratio of 3.5 markedly enhanced the post-test probability of a diagnosis of sarcoidosis in patients with a moderate pretest probability.

Table 11.2 Clinical and Laboratory Features Supporting the Diagnosis of Sarcoidosis [1,38]

Clinical Features

Skin lesions: lupus pernio, erythema nodosum, maculopapular lesions
Uveitis
Hypercalcemia or renal stones
Seventh cranial nerve paralysis
Diabetes insipidus

Laboratory features

Chest roentgenogram demonstrating symmetrical hilar adenopathy with right paratracheal enlargement
Serum angiotensin-converting enzyme level >2 times upper limit normal
BAL lymphocytosis >2 times upper limit normal
Panda/lamba sign on Gallium scan

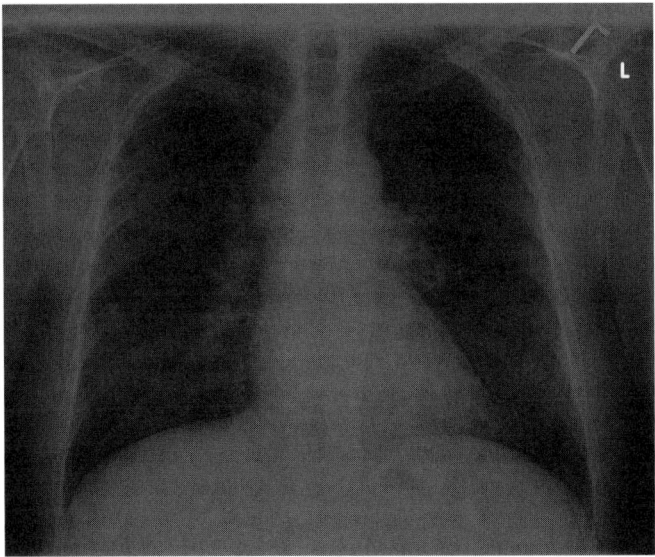

Fig. 11.1 Forty-three-year-old Caucasian man with cutaneous sarcoidosis for 5 years. Chest roentgenogram reveals prominent hilar and right paratracheal adenopathy. This is consistent with Stage 1 changes

Pulmonary Assessment

Lung involvement has been reported in more than 90% of patients in most series [3,4,54,55]. The traditional method of assessing patients has been by chest roentgenogram and pulmonary function studies. Chest roentgenogram has been classically categorized by the use of a stage system originally proposed by Scadding [56]. Stage 1 is adenopathy alone (Fig. 11.1), stage 2 adenopathy plus infiltrates, stage 3 is infiltrates alone, and stage 4 is fibrosis. Patients with normal chest roentgenogram are referred to as stage 0 [57]. The staging system has proved a useful way to stratify patients. Table 11.3 shows the proportion of patients in each of these stages at the time of diagnosis from three large series of sarcoidosis patients [4,6,55]. Each stage has been associated with a different prognosis. For example, patients with stage 1 changes have a >80% resolution of their chest roentgenogram within 2–5 years [58.59], whereas those with stage 3 changes have a less than 30% chance of resolution by that time [58].

A major limitation of the chest roentgenogram staging system is the fact that patients with stage 1 disease still have parenchymal lung disease. This can be demonstrated by bronchoscopy, with more than half of patients having a positive transbronchial biopsy [60]. BAL in stage1 disease can also show a high percentage of lymphocytes and increased CD4:CD8 ratio, indicating an active alveolitis [61]. Gallium scan has also been positive in the parenchyma of patients with stage 1 disease [61,62].

Table 11.3 Comparison of Chest X-Ray Stage at Time of Diagnosis for Different Sarcoidosis Populations

	USA [4]	Finland [208]	Japan [208]	Germany [55]*
Number studied	736	571	686	715
Chest roentgenogram stage, %				
0	8.3	1	20	0
1	39.7	48	56	35
2	36.7	40	20	51
3	9.8	11	4	14
4	5.4	0	0	0

The roentgenogram changes focus on the restrictive aspects of pulmonary sarcoidosis. The presence of interstitial lung disease by chest roentgenogram does correlate with pulmonary function and gas exchange abnormalities [63]. A normal chest roentgenogram does not predict normal lung function [4,55]. Loddenkemper et al. [55] studied new-onset disease in patients in Germany and Switzerland. They found that 12% of patients with stage 1 disease had a vital capacity between 65% and 80% of predicted, whereas 64% of patients with stage 3 disease had a normal vital capacity. In a study of 735 recently diagnosed cases of sarcoidosis in the USA, patients with more extensive lung involvement by chest roentgenogram had worse function. However, there was considerable overlap [64].

High-resolution computed tomography (HRCT) has been useful in demonstrating the fibrotic changes leading to loss of volume. The fibrotic pattern here includes not only interstitial thickening, but also honeycombing, linear nodules, and airway distortion [65] (Fig. 11.2). Figure 11.3 correlates the finding of these three main findings on CT scan and changes in pulmonary function in 68 patients studied at one institution [65]. It should be noted that obstructive disease was not a major feature of these patients, and there was no difference in the CT findings between the three groups.

Although honeycombing is the predominant cause of lung function changes, there are other reasons for restrictive disease. In patients with less advanced disease, localized air trapping has been shown to be a cause of reduced lung volume [66]. The relative importance of the reticular nodular versus the localized air trapping was studied in 45 sarcoidosis patients by Hansell et al [67]. The authors found the reticulonodular pattern was the more important in predicting lung function. They found the mosaic pattern was not associated with significant airway obstruction.

Another cause of restrictive lung disease is muscle weakness [68,69]. This can be quantitated by measurements of the maximal inspiratory and expiratory pressure. However, inspiratory and expiratory pressures also depend on lung volume, with lower volumes leading to lower pressures. Studies in sarcoidosis patients have demonstrated that muscle weakness is out of proportion to loss in lung volume [68]. This muscle weakness is associated with increasing dyspnea and worsening quality of life for the sarcoidosis patient [68,69]. Although this muscle weakness is usually due to direct muscle involvement, a neuropathy of the phrenic nerve can also lead to respiratory failure [70].

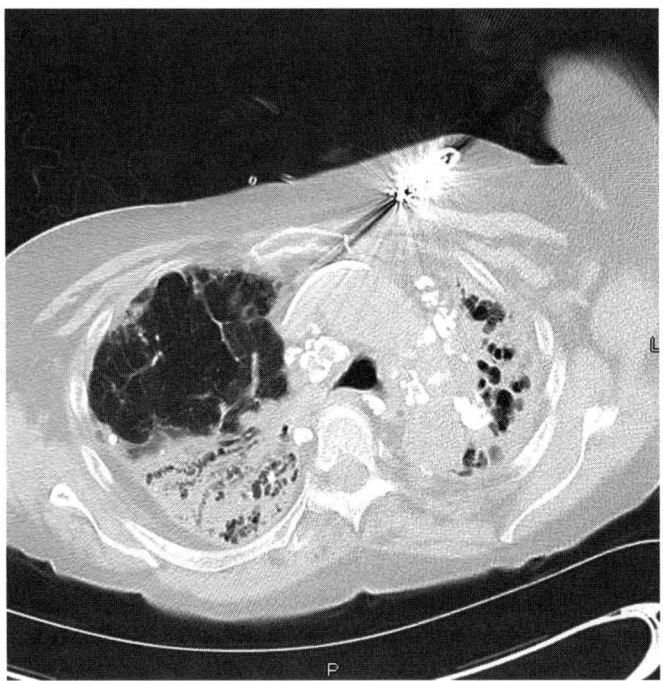

Fig. 11.2 Sixty-four year-old Caucasian woman with sarcoidosis for 3 years. HRCT scan shows bilateral honeycombing with retraction and distortion of airways. Right upper lobe also demonstrates intra-lobar thickening

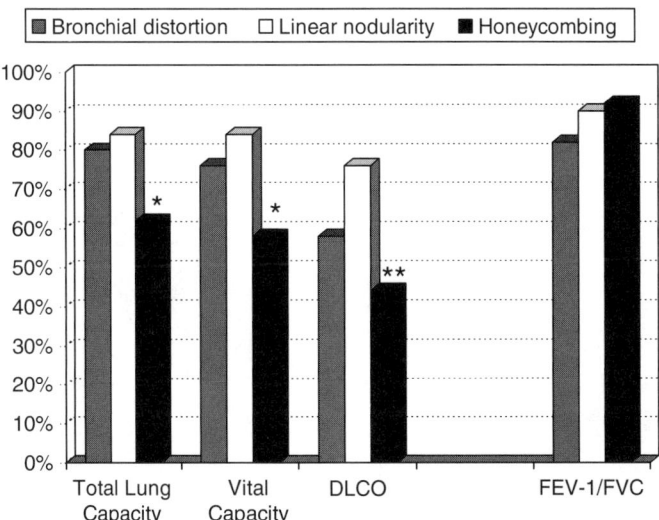

Fig. 11.3 The mean pulmonary function studies compared to HRCT patterns in 68 patients with sarcoidosis. The presence of honeycombing was associated with a significantly lower total lung capacity, forced vital capacity (FVC), and diffusion capacity (of the lung) for carbon monoxide (DL_{CO}) than the other patterns. ($^{*}p < 0.001$, $^{**}p < 0.0025$). There was no difference in forced expiratory volume in 1 second (FEV-1)/FVC between the three groups. Adapted from Abehsera et al. [65]

A co-factor here is the presence of obstructive lung disease. In some cases, the defect is combined with a restrictive defect. In one study of 715 European patients presenting with newly diagnosed sarcoidosis, 136 (19%) presented with restrictive pattern alone, 29 (4%) with obstructive pattern alone, and 22 (3%) had a combined defect [55]. In a study of African Americans, Sharma and Johnson found obstruction in 63% of the cases [71]. Cigarette smoking is another potential confounding issue, since it can cause airway obstruction [66]. However, a significant reduction in the forced expiratory volume in 1 second/forced vital capacity ratio was seen in 12% of nonsmokers in one study [64]. Sarcoidosis patients often have changes in the small airways [72]. These changes can lead to airway obstruction; however, they may not lead to significant changes in overall lung function [67].

One mechanism of obstruction is peribronchial thickening (Fig. 11.4). In addition, direct endobronchial involvement can be found in patients with sarcoidosis and can lead to significant airway narrowing. Endobronchial sarcoidosis involvement represents a distinct problem, because it can lead to irreversible bronchial stenosis [73]. In addition, a third of sarcoidosis patients appear to have airway reactivity as determined by a positive methacholine challenge [74–76]. In one study, airway hyperreactivity reactivity was associated with endobronchial disease [77].

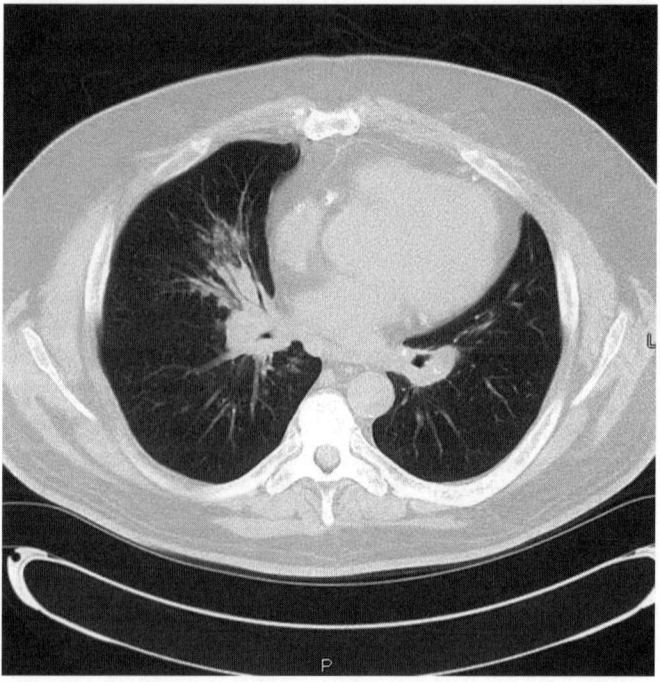

Fig. 11.4 Fifty-year-old Caucasian man with cough. CT scan showed marked peribronchial thickening of right middle lobe. On bronchoscopy, the airways were thickened. Biopsy of airways revealed numerous non caseating granulomas

Cough is a common complaint in patients with sarcoidosis [38]. In one study of acute, symptomatic pulmonary sarcoidosis patients, all patients complained of cough. Only a third of the patients had a positive methacholine challenge. Neither the duration nor severity of the cough was associated with either a positive methacholine test or presence of airway obstruction [76].

The CT scan of the chest has proved useful in characterizing the type and extent of lung involvement in many interstitial lung diseases including sarcoidosis. Figure 11.5 demonstrates the chest roentgenogram and CT scan of patient with symptomatic pulmonary sarcoidosis. When using the CT scan, one can more readily appreciate the widespread nodularity. The presence of subpleural disease and adenopathy are also more readily apparent on CT scan than can be seen on plain chest roentgenogram [78,79]. Although this increased information is useful, it has not yet been translated to prognostic information.

Another aspect of pulmonary evaluation is exercise testing. Routine cardiopulmonary exercise tests have been found to be abnormal in the majority of sarcoidosis patients [80]. In one study in which authors examined exercise alveolar-arterial gradient, with more advanced disease found by chest roentgenogram, an increase in the arterial to alveolar gradient was seen [63]. This study also examined static lung function tests and found a strong correlation between gas exchange impairment and diffusion capacity (of the lung) for carbon monoxide [63].

The changes in exercise response can be due to changes in lung function, cardiac disease, muscle strength, or pulmonary hypertension. In one study, sarcoidosis patients with normal lung function had impaired exercise studies based on increased heart rate with exercise [81]. Thus, exercise testing reveals other possible causes of dyspnea. For example, it is clear that a significant number of sarcoidosis patients have increased pulmonary artery pressures [82,83]. Although this increase occurs most frequently in patients with stage 3 and 4 disease, pulmonary hypertension can occur in patients with stage 0 or 1 disease [83].

Although the major value of exercise testing in sarcoidosis is its ability to assess the patient who is complaining of dyspnea, another indication is to potentially screen for lung disease in patients with extra pulmonary presentation, such as ocular or neurologic disease. However, the testing can be complicated and difficult to reproduce between centers. It therefore remains most commonly performed at academic centers.

Recently, there has been interest in the 6-minute walk test (6MWT) distance in various interstitial lung diseases. In idiopathic pulmonary fibrosis (IPF), walking less than 300 meters and the presence of desaturation are both associated with increased mortality [84]. The 6MWT has not been routinely evaluated in sarcoidosis. In one study of corticosteroid therapy for acute pulmonary sarcoidosis, there was some improvement in the 6MWT after 1 year of therapy, but the difference was not significant [76].

The 6MWT was prospectively studied in a group of unselected sarcoidosis patients [85]. Many factors were associated with a reduced 6MWT distance, including the percent forced vital capacity predicted (Fig. 11.6). However, the static lung function tests alone did not explain the 6MWD. The presence of pulmonary hypertension was an independent risk factor. In a multiregression analysis, it was

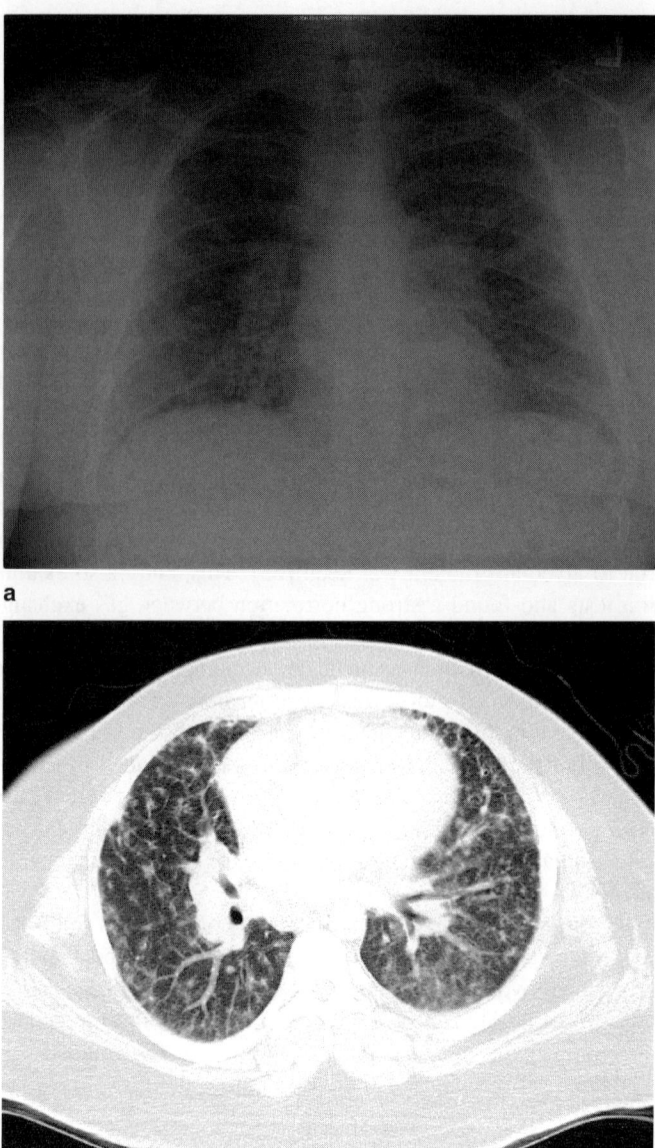

Fig. 11.5 Chest roentgenogram (5A) and CT scan (5B) or thirty-five year old African American male with adenopathy on chest roentgenogram. On CT, the diffuse, nodular ground glass areas are readily apparent

found that the patient's perceived respiratory health, as measured by the Saint George Respiratory Questionnaire (Fig. 11.7), was also a good predictor of 6MWT. Among quality of life factors affecting 6MWT, the presence of fatigue in patients with sarcoidosis predicted their 6MWT.

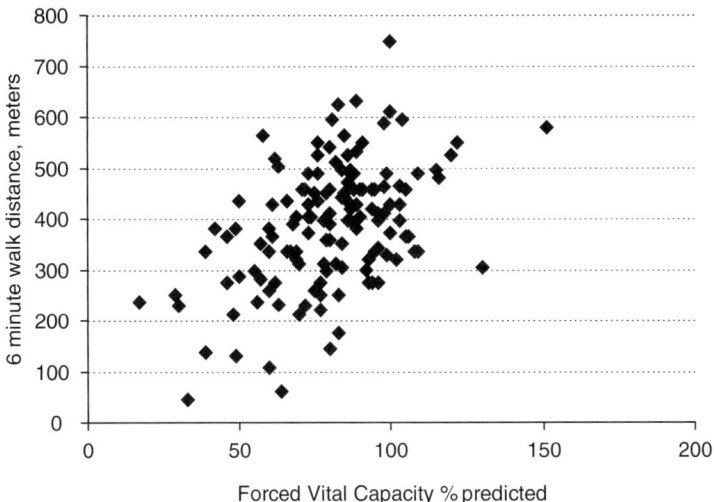

Fig. 11.6 The results of 6MWT versus pulmonary function and health assessment were determined in an unselected group of 142 sarcoidosis patients [210]. The percent predicted FVC correlated with the 6MWT (Spearman Rank rho = 0.431, $p < 0.001$). The FVC % predicted was one of several pulmonary function measures that correlated with 6MWT

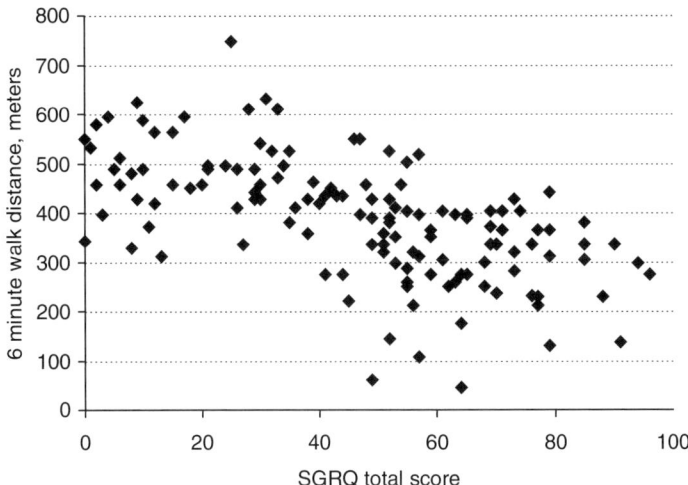

Fig. 11.7 The results of 6MWT versus pulmonary function and health assessment were determined in an unselected group of 142 sarcoidosis patients [210]. The Saint George Respiratory Questionnaire (SGRQ) total score correlated with the six minute walk distance (6MWD) (Spearman Rank rho = −0.654, $p < 0.0001$). The SGRQ ranges from 0 to 100, with the lower the score, the better a person feels about their respiratory heath. The SGRQ total was one of several health assessment instruments that correlated with 6MWD

Pulmonary Hypertension in Patients With Sarcoidosis

Pulmonary hypertension is a recognized complication of sarcoidosis [83,86]. The causes of pulmonary hypertension in this setting include direct vessel compression by adenopathy [87], arterial involvement (vasculitis) by sarcoidosis [88], pulmonary venous occlusion by granulomas [89,90], and liver disease with portopulmonary hypertension [91]. In addition, hypoxia, left ventricular disease, and pulmonary embolism may be encountered in patients with sarcoidosis.

The overall incidence of pulmonary hypertension in sarcoidosis reported by four groups is shown in Table 11.4. The greater percentage is similar to an older study, which also relied on catheterization study. The reported rate varies from 5% to 60% [82,83,92,93]. In the three studies in which the authors limited their evaluation to patients with dyspnea, the incidence of pulmonary hypertension was 50%. Handa et al. [93] conducted a prospective study of unselected sarcoidosis patients seen at a single clinic and found a lower incidence. In that study, all patients had echocardiography, but none had right heart catheterization data reported.

Pulmonary artery systolic pressure (PASP) may be estimated with the use of echocardiography and cardiac Doppler studies by applying the Bernoulli formula to tricuspid regurgitation jet velocity [94]. However, there are many limitations of this method, and echocardiography should therefore be considered a screening tool for the detection of pulmonary hypertension. In a study using echocardiography to screen for pulmonary hypertension in scleroderma [95], echocardiography was associated with both significant over- and underestimates of pulmonary artery pressure when compared with cardiac catheterization. In that study, the authors chose

Table 11.4 Rate of Pulmonary Hypertension in Sarcoidosis

City	Milan [83]	New York [82]	Kyoto [93]	Cincinnati [92]
Selection criteria	Dyspneic patients	Dyspneic patients	Prospective, unselected	Dyspneic patients
Method to confirm pulmonary hypertension	Right heart catheterization	Echocardiography	Echocardiography	Right heart Catheterization
Number studied	62	106	212	57
Number with pulmonary hypertension (%)	35 (56)*	54 (51)*	12 (5.7)*	32 (60)*†
Chest roentgenogram stage (%)				
Stage 3	No comment	6 (11)‡	No comment	9/26 (34)§
Stage 4	No comment	32 (60)‡	No comment	9/26 (34)§
Relation to DL_{CO}	No comment	Yes	No	Yes

* Number present (% total).
† Includes six patients (11% of total) with left ventricular dysfunction.
‡ Number positive and percent of those with pulmonary hypertension.
§ Number positive and percent of those with pulmonary arterial hypertension.
DL_{CO}, diffusion capacity (of the lung) for carbon monoxide.

to study dyspneic patients with estimated PASP 30–40 mmHg (within the normal range). They found pulmonary hypertension by cardiac catheterization in half of these cases.

In patients with interstitial lung disease, the predictive accuracy of echocardiography may be even more limited. Arcasoy et al. [96] studied 374 patients with advanced lung disease and found that in 52% of patients in whom correlation was possible, significant errors occurred when estimating PASP by echocardiography as compared with cardiac catheterization. In our experience, a significant number of sarcoidosis patients can have no detectable tricuspid regurgitation and still have significant pulmonary hypertension. Figure 11.8 shows the results of 91 patients studied at our institution with both echocardiogram and right heart catheterization. In 29 (32%), the PA pressure could not be estimated by the echocardiographer. Even for those in whom a PA estimate was made, there was only fair correlation between the estimated PA pressure and the directly measured number ($r = 0.56$, $p < 0.001$).

Several factors account for the predictably limited correlation between echocardiographic and catheter-derived measurements of PASP, and include (1) the time interval between noninvasive and invasive studies; (2) population studied (e.g., left heart failure patients versus patients with advanced lung disease); (3) the occurrence of marked spontaneous variation in PASP [97]; (4) the investigators' definition of pulmonary hypertension; (5) method of estimation of right atrial pressure; (6) failure to precisely capture the peak velocity of the tricuspid regurgitation jet on Doppler studies; (7) chest configuration; and (8) orientation of the heart within the chest.

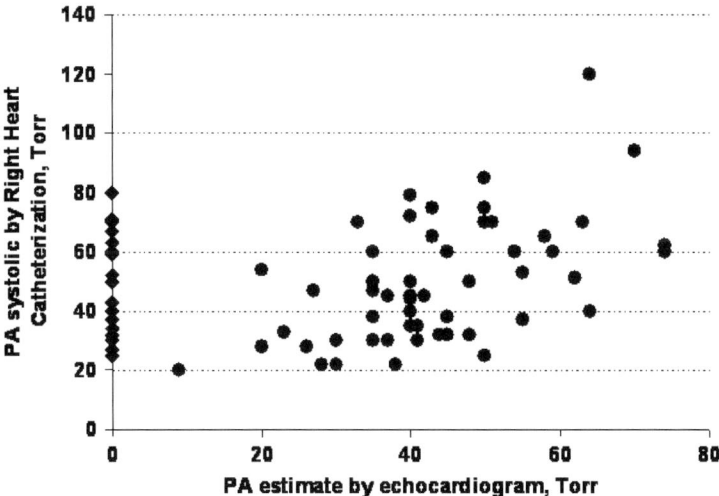

Fig. 11.8 Ninety-one patients followed at University of Cincinnati Sarcoidosis Clinic who had both right heart catheterization and echocardiogram. Of these, 29 (32%) did not have a PA pressure estimated by echocardiogram (diamonds in the above scattergram). For those with both values measured, there was a fair, but significant correlation between PA estimated by echocardiogram and measured directly by right heart catheterization ($r = 0.560$, $p < 0.0001$)

Table 11.5 Pulmonary Hypertension in Sarcoidosis Patients Seen at the University of Cincinnati Medical Center [103]

	Pulmonary arterial hypertension	Diastolic dysfunction
Number	35	12
FVC, L	1.99 (1.19–3.67)	1.81 (1.19–3.12)
Chest roentgenogram stage*		
0/1	4	7
2	7	3
3	10	0
4	14	2

*Scadding score [56].
FVC, forced vital capacity.

In patients with sarcoidosis who are awaiting lung transplantation, pulmonary hypertension has been noted in more than 70% of cases [98,99]. However, it is important to note that the presence of pulmonary hypertension (mean PAP >25 mmHg) does not necessarily imply the presence of pulmonary arterial hypertension (mean PAP >25 mmHg, mean pulmonary artery wedge pressure <15 mmHg, and pulmonary vascular resistance >3 Wood units). In a more detailed analysis of patients awaiting lung transplantation [100], it was found that the pulmonary artery wedge pressure increased as the PASP increased, suggesting that at least some cases of pulmonary hypertension are caused by left ventricular disease. Direct left ventricular involvement may be seen in sarcoidosis and may result in either systolic or diastolic left ventricular dysfunction [101,102]. In a study of 80 dyspneic sarcoidosis patients undergoing cardiac catheterization, 47 (59%) had elevated PASP; diastolic dysfunction either alone or in combination with systolic dysfunction accounted for one quarter of these cases [92]. Table 11.5 summarizes the vital capacity and chest x-ray findings of those patients with and those without left ventricular diastolic dysfunction in a study done at our institution [103]. As can be seen, these measurements do not provide sufficient information to separate the two groups. While echocardiography and cardiac Doppler studies may be helpful in suggesting the presence of left ventricular diastolic dysfunction, cardiac catheterization is often required to make a specific diagnosis.

Treatment of Patients With Sarcoidosis

Corticosteroids remain the cornerstone of systemic therapy for sarcoidosis patients. It is crucial to realize that not all patients require therapy. There remain some specific recommendations regarding who should receive therapy [38]. Certain conditions are felt to be absolute indications for therapy. These include cardiac, neurologic, ocular disease not responding to topical therapy, and hypercalcemia or hypercalciuria. Pulmonary involvement by itself does not require therapy. However, patients with dyspnea or troublesome cough should be considered for therapy. Liver involvement is rarely symptomatic, but some patients may develop irreversible cirrhosis and should be treated [104,105]. Skin involvement may respond to topical therapy. However, extensive disease or chronic problems such as lupus pernio [43] are often controlled by systemic therapy. Other organ involvement may also lead to sufficient symptoms to require therapy. Evidence-based guidelines for therapy of sarcoidosis have been established [106]. These are summarized in Table 11.6. These recommendations include the level of evidence which supports each conclusion.

Table 11.6 Evidence-Based Recommendations Regarding Therapy for Patients With Sarcoidosis

Patients with pulmonary radiographic stage I disease, with or without erythema nodosum, and with normal lung function (VC, DL_{co}) do not require treatment with corticosteroids (Grade A).

Symptomatic patients with stage II-III pulmonary lesions and an impaired lung function respond to treatment with oral corticosteroids (Grade A). Patients with newly detected disease respond better than patients who have had sarcoidosis for more than 2 years (Grade A). It is unknown for how long treatment has to be continued and what markers to be used in the decision making for tapering the dose during treatment, and when to stop treatment.

No dose–response studies have been performed. It appears that a starting dose of 30–40 mg of prednisolone per day or its equivalents is sufficient (Grade U).

Inhaled corticosteroids can be used for the treatment of bronchial sarcoidosis causing symptoms such as cough, and in patients with airway obstruction and bronchial hyperresponsiveness (Grade D).

After induction with oral corticosteroids inhaled budesonide can be used as an alternative to oral corticosteroids for long-term maintenance treatment (Grade B). Budesonide can be recommended for patients at risk of systemic side effects with oral corticosteroids, and in combination with lower doses of oral corticosteroids as an oral corticosteroid sparing treatment. These effects have been demonstrated only with budesonide.

Extrapulmonary sarcoidosis affecting vital organs with risk of organ failure development should be treated with corticosteroids on an individual patient basis (Grade D).

The use of anti malarial agent chloroquine is effective for some forms of sarcoidosis (Grade B). Hydroxychloroquine, which is less toxic, may also be effective (Grade C). Patients need to have routine eye examinations while on therapy (Grade D).

Methotrexate is steroid sparing for patients with pulmonary disease (Grade B). It is effective for pulmonary, ocular, cutaneous, and neurologic disease (Grade C). Patients on drug should undergo routine renal and hematologic monitoring (Grade D). Folic acid may reduce gastrointestinal toxicity (Grade B). Liver biopsy should be considered if the patient has received prolonged treatment to a cumulative dose of greater than 1–2 g (Grade B).

Azathioprine appears to be effective as a steroid sparing agent in sarcoidosis in some cases (Grade B). Leflunomide alone or in combination with methotrexate is effective for ocular or pulmonary sarcoidosis (Grade D). Chlorambucil is effective as other cytotoxic drugs for sarcoidosis, but is more toxic without any apparent increased efficacy compared to methotrexate or azathioprine (Grade C). Cyclophosphamide appears to be useful for refractory neurosarcoidosis (Grade B). Use of these cytotoxic drugs requires close monitor for hematologic toxicity. Cyclophosphamide is associated with bladder toxicity and monitoring urine analysis at least once a month (Grade B).

Thalidomide is effective for cutaneous sarcoidosis (Grade B). Patients need to be monitored for risk of pregnancy while taking the agent (Grade C).

(continued)

Table 11.6 (continued)

Infliximab is effective for chronic sarcoidosis (Grade C). Etanercept is not effective for most
patients with sarcoidosis (Grade C). Patients receiving drug must be carefully monitored
during infusion. The drug should be given with caution in patients with a history of heart
failure or exposure to tuberculosis (Grade C).

Tetracyclines benefit some forms of cutaneous sarcoidosis (Grade D). Cyclosporine has no
apparent benefit for pulmonary sarcoidosis (Grade B) but may help some neurosarcoidosis
(Grade D). Radiation may be useful for small, refractory sarcoidosis lesions (Grade D).
There is incomplete evidence and experience to comment on the role of pentoxifylline
or fumaric acid esters for sarcoidosis.

*Grade A: supported by at least two double-blind randomized control trials, Grade B: supported by
prospective cohort studies; Grade C: supported primarily by two or more retrospective studies; Grade
D: only one retrospective study or based on experience in other diseases; Grade U: no support.
Adapted from Baughman and Selroos [106].
DL_{CO}, diffusion capacity (of the lung) for carbon monoxide.

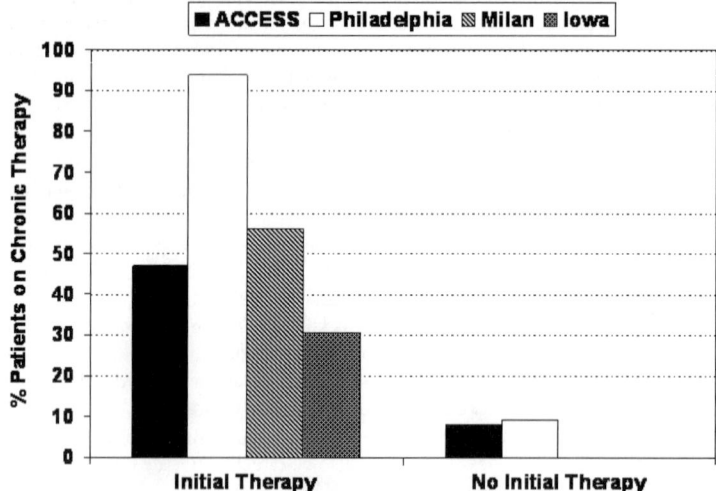

Fig. 11.9 Proportion of patients requiring chronic (at least two years) systemic therapy if they
received initial therapy [107–110]. Also shown is the proportion of patients requiring long-term
therapy if they did not receive initial systemic therapy for their sarcoidosis [108,110].

Systemic therapy is not required in all cases of sarcoidosis. In large studies, the
proportion of patients requiring initial therapy ranges from 34% to 65% [107–110].
As shown in Figure 11.9, many patients who are started on therapy will require
chronic therapy for at least 2 years 107–110. Long-term therapy is usually required
either because the patient could not be withdrawn from treatment, or symptoms
recurred when treatment was stopped. Relapses usually occurred within 6 months
of withdrawal from therapy, but could occur up to 6 years later [108]. For those
patients not requiring initial systemic therapy, there was a less than 10% chance of
needing long term therapy [108,110].

For symptomatic pulmonary disease, corticosteroid therapy has been the most widely studied [111]. Treatment with prednisone has been shown to improve the chest roentgenogram [111]. Eighteen months of corticosteroid therapy for patients with parenchymal lung disease has been shown to improve the DLCO [112], and this benefit could persist for up to 5 years after treatment [113]. A similar improvement was seen in the vital capacity [113,114]. The initial dose of corticosteroids has varied considerably among trials. In one trial demonstrating benefit for therapy, 3 months of high-dose oral corticosteroids were followed by fifteen months of high dose inhaled budesonide [112,113].

Another issue that has been poorly studied is the withdrawal of corticosteroids. It has been suggested that the sarcoidosis patient should usually be given a high dose of therapy initially and then maintained at a lower dose [115]. The trick is to give the lowest dose that does not lead to relapse. Corticosteroid dose tapering is usually done to avoid toxicity [76]. If the patient is tolerating the current dose, the regimen may be maintained longer to maximize benefit.

Alternatives to corticosteroids have been sought because of steroid toxicity. Table 11.7 lists many of these drugs, their usual doses, and recommended monitoring. As noted in Table 11.6, recommendations regarding alternatives to corticosteroids in treating sarcoidosis are often based on limited studies [116]. The two most thoroughly studied drugs are chloroquine and methotrexate.

Chloroquine and is derivative hydroxychloroquine make up the anti-malarial class of drugs. Chloroquine has been more extensively studied and found effective for cutaneous disease [117–119]. The response rate to chloroquine appears to be lower in pulmonary disease [106,118]. Chloroquine was also found to slow the progression of chronic pulmonary disease [120]. Hydroxychloroquine has also been used for cutaneous disease, but the response rate seems lower than that of chloroquine [106,121]. Since chloroquine is associated with more ocular toxicity [122–124], hydroxychloroquine is used more frequently. The antimalarials have also been reported as effected in treating hypercalcemia [125–127] and neurologic disease [128] complicating sarcoidosis.

Methotrexate is another widely studied drug in sarcoidosis [129–133]. It has been reported to be useful in treating pulmonary [132,133], cutaneous [132–134], ocular [130,132,133], and neurologic [133,135] manifestations. It has been used in treating childhood sarcoidosis, in which the clinician must try to avoid systemic corticosteroids [136]. In a randomized, double-blind placebo controlled trial, the use of methotrexate was found to be steroid sparing for patients with acute pulmonary sarcoidosis [137].

Methotrexate is a cytotoxic agent. Like all the drugs in this class, one needs to monitor the complete blood count on a regular basis when administering this agent [129]. Because bone marrow involvement can be seen in sarcoidosis [138,139], we prefer to use a relatively low dose of methotrexate. The drug is excreted by the kidney and probably should not be used in patients with significant renal dysfunction [132]. Chronic use is associated with hepatotoxicity, which can be detected by liver biopsy [140]. The use of liver function tests alone versus routine liver biopsy to screen for methotrexate hepatotoxicity is controversial [140,141]. Pulmonary toxicity is also associated with methotrexate use [142,143]. This is less frequent and

Table 11.7 Specific Drug Therapy for Sarcoidosis

Class	Drug	Dose	Suggested monitoring	Comments
Corticosteroids	Prednisone	5–40 mg	Glucose intolerance. blood pressure	Initial dose higher, reduce to minimal tolerable and effective dose
	Budesonide	800–1600 μg		Inhaled therapy
Cytotoxic	Methotrexate	5–15 mg once a week	Complete blood count (CBC), renal, hepatic every 4–8 weeks	Takes up to 6 month to be effective
	Azathioprine	50–250 mg daily	CBC, every 4–8 weeks	More leukopenic than methotrexate
	Chlorambucil	2–12 mg daily	CBC, every 4–8 weeks	Higher rate of malignancy than other agents
	Leflunomide	10–20 mg daily	CBC, renal, hepatic every 4–8 weeks	Similar to methotrexate, but less nausea
	Cyclophosphamide	50–150 mg oral daily OR 500–2000 mg intravenously every 2 weeks	CBC every 2–4 weeks, urinanalysis every month	Higher rate of side effects, but associated with greater response rate than other cytotoxic agents
Antimicrobial agents	Chloroquine		Eye exam every 6–12 months	
	Hydroxychloroquine	200–400 mg daily	Eye exam every 6–12 months	Less ocular toxicity than chloroquine
	Minocycline	100–200 mg daily		Rarely associated with immune toxicity
Cytokine modulation	Pentoxifylline	200–400 up to three times a day		High doses may be needed to block TNF-α.
	Thalidomide	50–200 mg daily	Pregnancy screening monthly	Teratogenic potential major concern
	Infliximab	5 mg/kg intravenously every 4–8 weeks after loading doses	PPD before first dose	Increase rate of infection and allergic reaction

Adapted from Baughman and Lower [209].

may only manifest itself with cough. In patients with methotrexate associated cough, discontinuation of drug seems to be adequate to control the complaint [132,144].

Azathioprine is another cytotoxic agent used to treat sarcoidosis. The response rate reported to date has been variable, from as little as 20% [145] to more than 80% [146]. In addition to pulmonary disease, the drug has been reported as effective for neurologic [147] and hepatic [148] disease. Unfortunately, the response rates of azathioprine for sarcoidosis are difficult to estimate based on the small number of treated patients reported to date [106]. Complete blood counts need to be monitored during azathioprine therapy. In particular, one must monitor for thiopurine methyltransferase-deficiency, which can lead to profound neutropenia even with small doses of the drug [149].

Other cytotoxic agents used for the treatment of patients with sarcoidosis include leflunomide, chlorambucil, and cyclophosphamide. Leflunomide has a similar mechanism of action to methotrexate and has been used in combination with that drug in treating rheumatoid arthritis [150,151]. The drug is associated with less nausea and pulmonary toxicity than methotrexate [152]. For sarcoidosis, leflunomide has been effective in more than two-thirds of patients either in place of methotrexate or in combination with the drug [144]. Chlorambucil has also been shown to be steroid sparing in sarcoidosis [153,154]. However, it is an alkylating agent and associated with a higher rate of cancer than the other cytotoxic drugs. Cyclophosphamide has been effective in over 90% of the patients reported to date [135,155]. It is usually given as intermittent, intravenous treatments to reduce toxicity. It is associated with a higher rate of nausea and bone marrow toxicity, which can be minimized with antiemetics and careful monitoring [156]. Hemorrhagic cystitis and bladder cancer are associated with prolonged use, especially if the drug is given orally [157]. Therefore, despite its greater rate of response, cyclophosphamide is usually reserved for refractory disease, including neurologic disease [135,155,158–160].

Thalidomide has been reported in several case reports to be effective for cutaneous sarcoidosis [43,161–165]. It is a serious teratogen and the drug use must be carefully monitored. The drug was originally marketed as a sleep aid, and hypersomnolence remains a dose limiting effect. Other toxicities are dose dependent and include constipation and peripheral neuropathy [43]. In a dose escalation trial, the effective dose for skin lesions was 100 mg a day in most cases [43]. That dose has limited benefit for extracutaneous manifestations [43,161,163]. In a careful study of thalidomide for pulmonary sarcoidosis, Judson et al [166] were only able to identify a modest steroid sparing effect at a dose that could be tolerated by the patients.

Excessive levels of tumour necrosis factor-alpha (TNF-α) released by alveolar macrophages have been found in patients with active sarcoidosis [167,168]. A decrease in the amount of TNF-α released has been seen after successful treatment of sarcoidosis with corticosteroids [169], methotrexate [169], and azathioprine [146]. Persistently high levels have been found in patients with refractory sarcoidosis [170]. These observations have led to the concept of targeting TNF-α as a treatment for sarcoidosis [171].

Biological agents which target TNF-α have been developed for rheumatoid arthritis and Crohn's disease. These include etanercept, a TNF-α receptor antagonist, and infliximab, a chimeric monoclonal antibody which binds TNF-α in the plasma as well as TNF-α on the cell surface [172]. Both of these drugs are effective for rheumatoid arthritis [173,174], but infliximab has proved more effective for Crohn's disease [175,176]. There is also a much greater risk for reactivation of tuberculosis associated with infliximab versus etanercept [177].

For sarcoidosis, infliximab has been reported effective in several case reports and series [178–182]. A recently completed double blind, placebo-controlled trial of chronic pulmonary sarcoidosis confirmed the effectiveness of infliximab. In that study, there was a significant increase in the forced vital capacity after 24 weeks of infliximab therapy [183]. The effect was greater for patients with more severe disease. Although the drug was well tolerated in that study and no significant side effects were encountered, others have found that infliximab is associated with allergic reactions [184], increased risk for infections [177], worsening of preexisting congestive heart failure [185], and probable increased rate of malignancy [184].

Etanercept has been shown to have a much more limited role in treating sarcoidosis. In an open label trial of pulmonary sarcoidosis, a third of patients deteriorated while on treatment and the trial was discontinued [186]. In a double-blind trial of etanercept for refractory ocular sarcoidosis, there was no difference between etanercept and placebo [187]. Etanercept shares many of the toxicities as infliximab, including possible worsening of preexisting congestive heart failure [188] and increased rate of malignancy [189]. The risk for infection and allergic reaction is smaller, but these complications still can occur.

There are several possible reasons for the difference in effectiveness of infliximab versus etanercept for sarcoidosis. These include differences in mode of action of the drug (monoclonal antibody versus receptor antagonist), peak levels of drug (intravenous versus subcutaneous administration), effect on transmembrane TNF-α (only seen with infliximab) [190], and cell lysis. Infliximab binds to TNF-α on surface of cells releasing that protein. That has been shown to lead to cell lysis and therefore reduction of the overall number of active inflammatory cells [191]. Etanercept does not bind to cells or lead to cell lysis [191].

Other drugs have been reported as possibly effective in treating sarcoidosis. Minocycline has been shown to be effective in treating cutaneous sarcoidosis [192], as have fumaric acid esters [193]. Pentoxifylline has been reported to be s useful in some cases of sarcoidosis [194]. This drug is a phosphodiesterase-3 inhibitor and has anti-TNF-α activity [195,196]. However, the drug is associated with gastrointestinal toxicity and seems to have a limited role in sarcoidosis.

Treatment of Sarcoidosis Associated Pulmonary Arterial Hypertension (SAPAH)

As noted previously, SAPAH is often encountered in sarcoidosis patients awaiting lung transplant. The presence of pulmonary hypertension is a risk factor for death while awaiting lung transplant [98,99]. Right heart failure with associated elevation of right atrial pressure is associated with an even higher risk for death [99,197]. Although lung transplantation is one approach to this condition, medical treatment of SAPAH may increase the patient's likelihood of surviving to transplant. In addition, successful medical management may avoid the need for transplant altogether.

Medical management of SAPAH is similar to that outlined for idiopathic pulmonary arterial hypertension. The guidelines for diagnosis and treatment are discussed elsewhere in this book and the principals have been adapted for SAPAH. However, the information available to date is limited regarding the outcome of treatment in these patients.

Several groups have found that sarcoidosis associated pulmonary arterial hypertension respond to epoprostenol in both the acute and chronic setting [198,199]. In one study of seven patients treated with long term epoprostenol, five of seven continued on long-term therapy. Only one of five patients given long-term therapy went on to require lung transplant, while the remaining four have done well [199]. Others have reported the usefulness of epoprostenol in the long-term management of SAPAH [92].

The use of the endothelin receptors antagonist bosentan has also been reported to be successful in treating some patients with SAPAH [92,200,201]. The use of this class of drugs is appealing, because increased levels of endothelin-1 (ET-1) levels have been detected in the blood and BAL of patients with sarcoidosis [202,203]. In one study of BAL samples, the source of the increased amounts of ET-1 were the alveolar macrophages [203]. This same group demonstrated that BAL supernatant from sarcoidosis patients stimulated fibroblast proliferation and that this could be blocked by an inhibitor which blocked both ET_A and ET_B. Thus, blockade of ET-1 receptors may not only treat SAPAH, but also treat the lung fibrosis often seen in these sarcoidosis patients. The latter hypothesis has not yet been studied.

Sildenafil has been successfully used to treat idiopathic pulmonary arterial hypertension [204]. It has also been shown to improve hemodynamics [205] and 6MWT in idiopathic pulmonary fibrosis [206]. A recent report indicated that it improved hemodynamics in sarcoidosis patients awaiting lung transplant who had significant pulmonary arterial hypertension [207]. Table 11.8 summarizes the experience of treatment with these two vasodilators studied to date for SAPAH. Although the reported experience remains small, it is clear that some patients do respond to these agents. Clinical trials looking at these and other agents are ongoing in SAPAH.

Table 11.8 Results of Therapy for SAPAH

Treatment ing	Investigator	Number started	Number treated >3 months	Number respond-
Epoprostenol	Fisher [199]	7	5	4
	Baughman [92]	2	1	1
Bosentan	Sharma [201]	1	1	1
	Foley [200]	1	1	1
	Baughman [92]	5*	5	3

*Some patients treated with more than one drug for SAPAH.

Conclusion

Sarcoidosis is one of the most common idiopathic interstitial lung diseases. Although the prognosis for patients is often good, there is a subset of chronic disease. These patients often require years of corticosteroids and steroid-sparing agents to control their disease. Pulmonary hypertension is a frequent complication of advanced pulmonary disease. Some of the treatments for idiopathic pulmonary arterial hypertension have also been successful in treating sarcoidosis associated pulmonary arterial hypertension.

References

1. Baughman RP, du Bois RM, Lower EE. Sarcoidosis. Lancet 2003;361:1111–1118.
2. Rybicki BA, Major M, Popovich J, Jr., et al. Racial differences in sarcoidosis incidence: a five year study in a health maintenance organization. Am J Epidemiol 1997;145:234–241.
3. Hillerdal G, Nou E, Osterman K, et al. Sarcoidosis: epidemiology and prognosis. A 15-year European study. Am Rev Respir Dis 1984;130:29–32.
4. Baughman RP, Teirstein AS, Judson MA, et al. Clinical characteristics of patients in a case control study of sarcoidosis. Am J Respir Crit Care Med 2001;164:1885–1889.
5. Judson MA, Baughman RP, Teirstein AS, et al. Defining organ involvement in sarcoidosis: the ACCESS proposed instrument. Sarcoidosis Vasc Diffuse Lung Dis 1999;16:75–86.
6. Pietinalho A, Ohmichi M, Hiraga Y, et al. The mode of presentation of sarcoidosis in Finland and Hokkaido, Japan. A comparative analysis of 571 Finnish and 686 Japanese patients. Sarcoidosis 1996;13:159–166.
7. Izumi T. Symposium: population differences in clinical features and prognosis of sarcoidosis throughout the world. Sarcoidosis 1992;9:S105–S118.
8. Siltzbach LE, James DG, Neville E, et al. Course and prognosis of sarcoidosis around the world. Am J Med 1974;57:847–852.
9. ACCESS Research Group. Design of a case control etiologic study of sarcoidosis (ACCESS). J Clin Epidemiol 1999;52:1173–1186.
10. Hills SE, Parkes SA, Baker SB. Epidemiology of sarcoidosis in the Isle of Man–2: Evidence for space-time clustering. Thorax 1987;42:427–430.
11. Johnson BA, Duncan SR, Ohori NP, et al. Recurrence of sarcoidosis in pulmonary allograft recipients. American Review of Respiratory Disease 1993;148:1373–137X.
12. Martinez FJ, Orens JB, Deeb M, et al. Recurrence of sarcoidosis following bilateral allogeneic lung transplantation. Chest 1994;106:1597–1599.
13. Nunley DR, Hattler B, Keenan RJ, et al. Lung transplantation for end-stage pulmonary sarcoidosis. Sarcoidosis Vasc Diffuse Lung Dis 1999;16:93–100.
14. Sundar KM, Carveth HJ, Gosselin MV, et al. Granulomatous pneumonitis following bone marrow transplantation. Bone Marrow Transplant 2001;28:627–630.
15. Heyll A, Meckenstock G, Aul C, et al. Possible transmission of sarcoidosis via allogeneic bone marrow transplantation. Bone Marrow Transplant 1994;14:161–164.
16. Milman N, Andersen CB, Burton CM, et al. Recurrent sarcoid granulomas in a transplanted lung derive from recipient immune cells. Eur Respir J 2005;26:549–552.
17. Heatly T, Sekela M, Berger R. Single lung transplantation involving a donor with documented pulmonary sarcoidosis. J Heart Lung Transplant 1994;13:720–723.
18. Hance AJ. The role of mycobacteria in the pathogenesis of sarcoidosis. Semin Respir Infect 1998;13:197–205.
19. Drake WP, Pei Z, Pride DT, et al. Molecular analysis of sarcoidosis tissues for mycobacterium species DNA. Emerg Infect Dis 2002;8:1334–1341.

20. Song Z, Marzilli L, Greenlee BM, et al. Mycobacterial catalase-peroxidase is a tissue antigen and target of the adaptive immune response in systemic sarcoidosis. J Exp Med 2005;201:755–767.
21. Drake WP, Dhason MS, Nadaf M, et al. Cellular recognition of Mycobacterium tuberculosis ESAT-6 and KatG peptides in systemic sarcoidosis. Infect Immun 2007;75:527–530.
22. Brown ST, Brett I, Almenoff PL, et al. Recovery of cell wall-deficient organisms from blood does not distinguish between patients with sarcoidosis and control subjects. Chest 2003;123: 413–417.
23. Ishige I, Usui Y, Takemura T, et al. Quantitative PCR of mycobacterial and propionibacterial DNA in lymph nodes of Japanese patients with sarcoidosis. Lancet 1999;354:120–123.
24. Eishi Y, Suga M, Ishige I, et al. Quantitative analysis of mycobacterial and propionibacterial DNA in lymph nodes of Japanese and European patients with sarcoidosis. J Clin Microbiol 2002;40:198–204.
25. Minami J, Eishi Y, Ishige Y, et al. Pulmonary granulomas caused experimentally in mice by a recombinant trigger-factor protein of Propionibacterium acnes. J Med Dent Sci 2003;50: 265–274.
26. Prezant DJ, Dhala A, Goldstein A, et al. The incidence, prevalence, and severity of sarcoidosis in New York City firefighters. Chest 1999;116:1183–1193.
27. Jajosky P. Sarcoidosis diagnoses among U.S. military personnel: trends and ship assignment associations. Am J Prev Med 1998;14(3):176–183.
28. Gorham ED, Garland CF, Garland FC, et al. Trends and occupational associations in incidence of hospitalized pulmonary sarcoidosis and other lung diseases in Navy personnel: a 27-year historical prospective study, 1975–2001. Chest 2004;126:1431–1438.
29. Drent M, Bomans PH, Van Suylen RJ, et al. Association of man-made mineral fibre exposure and sarcoidlike granulomas. Respir Med 2000;94:815–820.
30. Newman LS, et al. Etiology of sarcoidosis: environmental and occupational factors associated with sarcoidosis risk. Ann Intern Med 2002; in press.
31. Izbicki G, Chavko R, Banauch GI, et al. World Trade Center "sarcoid-like" granulomatous pulmonary disease in New York City Fire Department rescue workers. Chest 2007;131: 1414–1423.
32. Moller DR, Chen ES. Genetic basis of remitting sarcoidosis: triumph of the trimolecular complex? Am J Respir Cell Mol Biol 2002;27:391–395.
33. Richeldi L, Sorrentino R, Saltini C. HLA-DPB1 Glutamate 69: a genetic marker of beryllium disease. Science 1993;262:242–244.
34. Rossman MD, Thompson B, Frederick M, et al. HLA-DRB1*1101: a significant risk factor for sarcoidosis in blacks and whites. Am J Hum Genet 2003;73:720–735.
35. Sato H, Grutters JC, Pantelidis P, et al. HLA-DQB1*0201: a marker for good prognosis in British and Dutch patients with sarcoidosis. Am J Respir Cell Mol Biol 2002;27:406–412.
36. Grunewald J, Eklund A. Sex-specific manifestations of Lofgren's syndrome. Am J Respir Crit Care Med 2007;175(1):40–44.
37. Foley PJ, McGrath DS, Petrek M, et al. HLA-DRB1 position 11 residues are a common protective marker for sarcoidosis. Am J Respir Cell Mol Biol 2001;25:272–277.
38. Hunninghake GW, Costabel U, Ando M, et al. ATS/ERS/WASOG statement on sarcoidosis. American Thoracic Society/European Respiratory Society/World Association of Sarcoidosis and other Granulomatous Disorders. Sarcoidosis Vasc Diffuse Lung Dis 1999;16:149–173.
39. Teirstein AS, Judson MA, Baughman RP, et al. The spectrum of biopsy sites for the diagnosis of sarcoidosis. Sarcoidosis Vasc Diffuse Lung Dis 2005;22:139–146.
40. Judson MA, Thompson BW, Rabin DL, et al. The diagnostic pathway to sarcoidosis. Chest 2003;123:406–412.
41. Winterbauer RH, Belic N, Moores KD. A clinical intepretation of bilateral hilar adenopathy. Ann Intern Med 1973;78:65–71.
42. Rizzato G, Colombo P. Nephrolithiasis as a presenting feature of chronic sarcoidosis: a prospective study. Sarcoidosis 1996;13:167–172.
43. Baughman RP, Judson MA, Teirstein AS, et al. Thalidomide for chronic sarcoidosis. Chest 2002;122:227–232.

44. Winget D, O'Brien GM, Lower EE, et al. Bell's palsy as an unrecognized presentation for sarcoidosis. Sarcoidosis 1994;11:S368–S370.
45. Hunninghake GW, Crystal RG. Pulmonary sarcoidosis: a disorder mediated by excess helper T-lymphocyte activity at sites of disease activity. N Engl J Med 1981;305:429–432.
46. Semenzato G, Chilosi M, Ossi E, et al. Bronchoalveolar lavage and lung histology: comparative analysis of inflammatory and immunocompetent cells in patients with sarcoidosis and hypersensitivity pneumonitis. Am Rev Respir Dis 1985;132:400–404.
47. Kantrow SP, Meyer KC, Kidd P, et al. The CD4/CD8 ratio in BAL fluid is highly variable in sarcoidosis]. Eur Respir J 1997;10:2716–2721.
48. Klech H, Pohl W. Technical recommendations and guidelines for bronchoalveolar lavage (BAL). Eur Respir J 1989;2:561–585.
49. Haslam PL, Baughman RP. ERS task force report on measurement of acellular components in BAL. Eur Resp Rev 1999;9:25–27.
50. Baughman RP, Drent M. Role of bronchoalveolar lavage in interstitial lung disease. Clin Chest Med 2001;22:331–341.
51. Poulter LW, Rossi GA, Bjermer L, et al. The value of bronchoalveolar lavage in the diagnosis and prognosis of sarcoidosis. Eur Respir J 1990;3:943–944.
52. Drent M, Jacobs JA, Cobben NA, et al. Computer program supporting the diagnostic accuracy of cellular BALF analysis: a new release. Respir Med 2001;95:781–786.
53. Welker L, Jorres RA, Costabel U, et al. Predictive value of BAL cell differentials in the diagnosis of interstitial lung diseases. Eur Respir J 2004;24:1000–1006.
54. Sugisaki K, Yamaguchi T, Nagai S, et al. Clinical characteristics of 195 Japanese sarcoidosis patients treated with oral corticosteroids. Sarcoidosis Vasc Diffuse Lung Dis 2003;20:222–226.
55. Loddenkemper R, Kloppenborg A, Schoenfeld N, et al. Clinical findings in 715 patients with newly detected pulmonary sarcoidosis—results of a cooperative study in former West Germany and Switzerland. WATL Study Group. Wissenschaftliche Arbeitsgemeinschaft fur die Therapie von Lungenkrankheitan. Sarcoidosis Vasc Diffuse Lung Dis 1998;15:178–182.
56. Scadding JG. Prognosis of intrathoracic sarcoidosis in England. Br Med J 1961;4:1165–1172.
57. DeRemee RA. The roentgenographic staging of sarcoidosis. Historic and contemporary perspectives. Chest 1983;83:128–133.
58. Nagai S, Shigematsu M, Hamada K, et al. Clinical courses and prognoses of pulmonary sarcoidosis. Curr Opin Pulm Med 1999;5:293–298.
59. Neville E, Walker AN, James DG. Prognostic factors predicting the outcome of sarcoidosis: an analysis of 818 patients. Q J Med 1983;208:525–533.
60. Koonitz CH, Joyner LR, Nelson RA. Transbronchial lung biopsy via the fiberoptic bronchoscope in sarcoidosis. Ann Intern Med 1976;85:64–66.
61. Abe S, Munakata M, Nishimura M, et al. Gallium-67 scintigraphy, bronchoalveolar lavage, and pathologic changes in patients with pulmonary sarcoidosis. Chest 1984;85:650–655.
62. Sulavik SB, Spencer RP, Palestro CJ, et al. Specificity and sensitivity of distinctive chest radiographic and/or 67Ga images in the noninvasive diagnosis of sarcoidosis. Chest 1993; 103:403–409.
63. Medinger AE, Khouri S, Rohatgi PK. Sarcoidosis: the value of exercise testing. Chest 2001; 120:93–101.
64. Yeager H, Rossman MD, Baughman RP, et al. Pulmonary and psychosocial findings at enrollment in the ACCESS study. Sarcoidosis Vasc Diffuse Lung Dis 2005;22:147–153.
65. Abehsera M, Valeyre D, Grenier P, et al. Sarcoidosis with pulmonary fibrosis: CT patterns and correlation with pulmonary function. AJR Am J Roentgenol 2000;174:1751–1757.
66.Terasaki H, Fujimoto K, Muller NL, et al. Pulmonary sarcoidosis: comparison of findings of inspiratory and expiratory high-resolution CT and pulmonary function tests between smokers and nonsmokers. AJR Am J Roentgenol 2005;185:333–338.
67. Hansell DM, Milne DG, Wilsher ML, et al. Pulmonary sarcoidosis: morphologic associations of airflow obstruction at thin-section CT. Radiology 1998;209:697–704.
68. Baydur A, Alsalek M, Louie SG, et al. Respiratory muscle strength, lung function, and dyspnea in patients with sarcoidosis. Chest 2001;120:102–108.

69. Brancaleone P, Perez T, Robin S, et al. Clinical impact of inspiratory muscle impairment in sarcoidosis. Sarcoidosis Vasc Diffuse Lung Dis 2004;21:219–227.
70. Robinson LR, Brownsberger R, Raghu G. Respiratory failure and hypoventilation secondary to neurosarcoidosis. Am J Respir Crit Care Med 1998;157:1316–1318.
71. Sharma OP, Johnson R. Airway obstruction in sarcoidosis. A study of 123 nonsmoking black American patients with sarcoidosis. Chest 1988;94:343–346.
72. Ploysongsang Y, Roberts RD. The pathophysiology and response to steroid therapy in sarcoidosis. Respiration 1986;49:204–215.
73. Chambellan A, Turbie P, Nunes H, et al. Endoluminal stenosis of proximal bronchi in sarcoidosis: bronchoscopy, function, and evolution. Chest 2005;127:472–481.
74. Bechtel JJ, Starr TI, Dantzker DR, et al. Airway hyperreactivity in patients with sarcoidosis. Am Rev Respir Dis 1981;124:759–761.
75. Olafsson M, Simonsson BG, Hansson SB. Bronchial reactivity in patients with recent pulmonary sarcoidosis. Thorax 1985;40:51–53.
76. Baughman RP, Iannuzzi MC, Lower EE, et al. Use of fluticasone in acute symptomatic pulmonary sarcoidosis. Sarcoidosis Vasc Diffuse Lung Dis 2002;19:198–204.
77. Shorr AF, Torrington KG, Hnatiuk OW. Endobronchial involvement and airway hyperreactivity in patients with sarcoidosis. Chest 2001;120:881–886.
78. Muller NL, Mawson JB, Mathieson JR, et al. Sarcoidosis: correlation of extent of disease at CT with clinical, functional, and radiographic findings. Radiology 1989;171:613–618.
79. Remy JM, Beuscart R, Sault MC, et al. Subpleural micronodules in diffuse infiltrative lung diseases: evaluation with thin-section CT scans. Radiology 1990;177:133–139.
80. Akkoca O, Celik G, Ulger F, et al. Exercise capacity in sarcoidosis. Study of 29 patients. Med Clin (Barc) 2005;124:686–689.
81. Delobbe A, Perrault H, Maitre J, et al. Impaired exercise response in sarcoid patients with normal pulmonary functio. Sarcoidosis Vasc Diffuse Lung Dis 2002;19:148–153.
82. Sulica R, Teirstein AS, Kakarla S, et al. Distinctive clinical, radiographic, and functional characteristics of patients with sarcoidosis-related pulmonary hypertension. Chest 2005;128:1483–1489.
83. Rizzato G, Pezzano A, Sala G, et al. Right heart impairment in sarcoidosis: haemodynamic and echocardiographic study. Eur J Respir Dis 1983;64(2):121–128.
84. Lama VN, Flaherty KR, Toews GB, et al. Prognostic value of desaturation during a 6-minute walk test in idiopathic interstitial pneumonia. Am J Respir Crit Care Med 2003;168:1084–1090.
85. Baughman RP, Sparkman BK, Lower EE. Six minute walk test and health status assessment in sarcoidosis. Chest 2007;132:207–213.
86. Nunes H, Humbert M, Capron F, et al. Pulmonary hypertension associated with sarcoidosis: mechanisms, haemodynamics and prognosis. Thorax 2006;61:68–74.
87. Battesti JP, Georges R, Basset F, et al. Chronic cor pulmonale in pulmonary sarcoidosis. Thorax 1978;33:76–84.
88. Smith LJ, Lawrence JB, Katzenstein AA. Vascular sarcoidosis: a rare cause of pulmonary hypertension. Am J Med Sci 1983;285:38–44.
89. Hoffstein V, Ranganathan N, Mullen JB. Sarcoidosis simulating pulmonary veno-occlusive disease. Am Rev Respir Dis 1986;134:809–811.
90. Nunes H, Humbert M, Capron F, et al. Pulmonary hypertension associated with sarcoidosis: mechanisms, haemodynamics and prognosis. Thorax 2006;61:68–74.
91. Salazar A, Mana J, Sala J, et al. Combined portal and pulmonary hypertension in sarcoidosis. Respiration 1994;61:117–119.
92. Baughman RP, Engel PJ, Meyer CA, et al. Pulmonary hypertension in sarcoidosis. Sarcoidosis Vasc Diffuse Lung Dis 2006;23:108–116.
93. Handa T, Nagai S, Miki S, et al. Incidence of pulmonary hypertension and its clinical relevance in patients with sarcoidosis. Chest 2006;129:1246–1252.
94. Yock PG, Popp RL. Noninvasive estimation of right ventricular systolic pressure by Doppler ultrasound in patients with tricuspid regurgitation. Circulation 1984;70:657–662.

95. Hachulla E, Gressin V, Guillevin L, et al. Early detection of pulmonary arterial hypertension in systemic sclerosis: a French nationwide prospective multicenter study. Arthritis Rheum 2005;52:3792–3800.

96. Arcasoy SM, Christie JD, Ferrari VA, et al. Echocardiographic assessment of pulmonary hypertension in patients with advanced lung disease. Am J Respir Crit Care Med 2003;167: 735–740.

97. Rich S, D'Alonzo GE, Dantzker DR, et al. Magnitude and implications of spontaneous hemodynamic variability in primary pulmonary hypertension. Am J Cardiol 1985;55: 159–163.

98. Arcasoy SM, Christie JD, Pochettino A, et al. Characteristics and outcomes of patients with sarcoidosis listed for lung transplantation. Chest 2001;120:873–880.

99. Shorr AF, Davies DB, Nathan SD. Predicting mortality in patients with sarcoidosis awaiting lung transplantation. Chest 2003;124:922–928.

100. Shorr AF, Helman DL, Davies DB, et al. Pulmonary hypertension in advanced sarcoidosis: epidemiology and clinical characteristics. Eur Respir J 2005;25:783–788.

101. Fahy GJ, Marwick T, McCreery CJ, et al. Doppler echocardiographic detection of left ventricular diastolic dysfunction in patients with pulmonary sarcoidosis. Chest 1996;109: 62–66.

102. Chapelon-Abric C, de ZD, Duhaut P, et al. Cardiac sarcoidosis: a retrospective study of 41 cases. Medicine (Baltimore) 2004;83:315–334.

103. Baughman RP, Engel PJ. Not all pulmonary hypertension in sarcoidosis is due to pulmonary arterial hypertension. 2007: in press.

104. Maddrey WC, Johns CJ, Boitnott JK. et al. Sarcoidosis and chronic hepatic disease: a clinical and pathologic study of 20 patients. Medicine 1970;49:375–395.

105. Judson MA. Hepatc, splenic, and gastrointestinal involvement with sarcoidosis. Sem Resp Crit Care Med 2002;23:529–543.

106. Baughman RP, Selroos O. Evidence-based approach to the treatment of sarcoidosis. In: Gibson PG, Abramson M, Wood-Baker R, et al,, editors. Evidence-based respiratory medicine. Malden: Blackwell Publishing Ltd.; 2005. p. 491–508.

107. Hunninghake GW, Gilbert S, Pueringer R, et al. Outcome of the treatment for sarcoidosis. Am J Respir Crit Care Med 1994;149:893–898.

108. Gottlieb JE, Israel HL, Steiner RM, et al. Outcome in sarcoidosis. The relationship of relapse to corticosteroid therapy. Chest 1997;111:623–631.

109. Rizzato G, Montemurro L, Colombo P. The late follow-up of chronic sarcoid patients previously treated with corticosteroids. Sarcoidosis 1998;15:52–58.

110. Baughman RP, Judson MA, Teirstein A, et al. Presenting characteristics as predictors of duration of treatment in sarcoidosis. QJM 2006;99:307–315.

111. Paramothayan S, Jones PW. Corticosteroid therapy in pulmonary sarcoidosis: a systematic review. JAMA 2002;287:1301–1307.

112. Pietinalho A, Lindholm A, Haahtela T, et al. Inhaled budesonide for treatment of pulmonary sarcoidosis. Results of a double-blind, placebo-controlled, multicentre study. Eur Respir J 1996;9(suppl 23):406s.

113. Pietinalho A, Tukiainen P, Haahtela T, et al. Early treatment of stage II sarcoidosis improves 5-year pulmonary function. Chest 2002;121:24–31.

114. Gibson GJ, Prescott RJ, Muers MF, et al. British Thoracic Society Sarcoidosis study: effects of long term corticosteroid treatment. Thorax 1996;51:238–247.

115. Judson MA. An approach to the treatment of pulmonary sarcoidosis with corticosteroids: the six phases of treatment. Chest 1999;115:1158–1165.

116. Paramothayan S, Lasserson T, Walters EH. Immunosuppressive and cytotoxic therapy for pulmonary sarcoidosis. Cochrane Database Syst Rev 2003;(3):CD003536.

117. British Tuberculosis Association. Chloroquine in the treatment of sarcoidosis. Tubercle 1967;48:257–272.

118. Siltzbach LE, Teirstein AS. Chloroquine therapy in 43 patients with intrathoracic and cutaneous sarcoidosis. Acta Med Scand 1964;425:302S–308S.

119. Zic J, Horowitz D, Arzubiaga C, et al. Treatment of cutaneous sarcoidosis with chloroquine: review of the literature. Arch Dermatol 1991;127:1034–1040.
120. Baltzan M, Mehta S, Kirkham TH, et al. Randomized trial of prolonged chloroquine therapy in advanced pulmonary sarcoidosis. Am J Respir Crit Care Med 1999;160:192–197.
121. Jones E, Callen JP. Hydroxychloroquine is effective therapy for control of cutaneous sarcoidal granulomas. J Am Acad Dermatol 1990;23:487–489.
122. Canadian Consensus Conference on hydroxychloroquine. J Rheumatol 2000;27:2919–2921.
123. Bartel PR, Roux P, Robinson E, et al. Visual function and long-term chloroquine treatment. South African Med J 1994;84:32–34.
124. Silman A, Shipley M. Ophthalmological monitoring for hydroxychloroquine toxicity: a scientific review of available data. Br J Rheumatol 1997;36:599–601.
125. Adams JS, Diz MM, Sharma OP. Effective reduction in the serum 1,25-dihydroxyvitamin D and calcium concentration in sarcoidosis-associated hypercalcemia with short-course chloroquine therapy. Ann Intern Med 1989;111:437–438.
126. Barre PE, Gascon-Barre M, Meakins JL, et al. Hydroxychloroquine treatment of hypercalcemia in a patient with sarcoidosis undergoing hemodialysis. Am J Med 1987;82:1259–1262.
127. O'Leary TJ, Jones G, Yip A, et al. The effects of chloroquine on serum 1,25-dihydroxyvitamin D and calcium metabolism in sarcoidosis. N Engl J Med 1986;315:727–730.
128. Sharma OP. Effectiveness of chloroquine and hydroxychloroquine in treating selected patients with sarcoidosis with neurologic involvement. Arch Neurol 1998;55:1248–1254.
129. Baughman RP, Lower EE. A clinical approach to the use of methotrexate for sarcoidosis. Thorax 1999;54:742–746.
130. Dev S, McCallum RM, Jaffe GJ. Methotrexate for sarcoid-associated panuveitis. Ophthalmology 1999;106:111–118.
131. Lacher MJ. Spontaneous remission response to methotrexate in sarcoidosis. Ann Intern Med 1968;69:1247–1248.
132. Lower EE, Baughman RP. Prolonged use of methotrexate for sarcoidosis. Arch Intern Med 1995;155:846–851.
133. Vucinic VM. What is the future of methotrexate in sarcoidosis? A study and review. Curr Opin Pulm Med 2002;8:470–476.
134. Webster GF, Razsi LK, Sanchez M, et al. Weekly low-dose methotrexate therapy for cutaneous sarcoidosis. J Am Acad Dermatol 1991;24:451–454.
135. Lower EE, Broderick JP, Brott TG, et al. Diagnosis and management of neurologic sarcoidosis. Arch Intern Med 1997;157:1864–1868.
136. Gedalia A, Molina JF, Ellis GS, et al. Low-dose methotrexate therapy for childhood sarcoidosis. J Pediatr 1997;130:25–29.
137. Baughman RP, Winget DB, Lower EE. Methotrexate is steroid sparing in acute sarcoidosis: results of a double blind, randomized trial. Sarcoidosis Vasc Diffuse Lung Dis 2000;17:60–66.
138. Lower EE, Smith JT, Martelo OJ, et al. The anemia of sarcoidosis. Sarcoidosis 1988;5:51–55.
139. Browne PM, Sharma OP, Salkin D. Bone marrow sarcoidosis. JAMA 1978;240:43–50.
140. Baughman RP, Koehler A, Bejarano PA, et al. Role of liver function tests in detecting methotrexate-induced liver damage in sarcoidosis. Arch Intern Med 2003;163:615–620.
141. Kremer JM, Alarcon GS, Lightfoot RW, Jr., et al. Methotrexate for rheumatoid arthritis. Suggested guidelines for monitoring liver toxicity. American College of Rheumatology. Arthritis Rheum 1994;37:316–328.
142. Kremer JM, Alarcon GS, Weinblatt ME, et al. Clinical, laboratory, radiographic, and histopathologic features of methotrexate-associated lung injury in patients with rheumatoid arthritis: a multicenter study with literature review. Arthritis Rheum 1997;40:1829–1837.
143. Zisman DA, McCune WJ, Tino G, et al. Drug-induced pneumonitis: the role of methotrexate. Sarcoidosis Vasc Diffuse Lung Dis 2001;18:243–252.
144. Baughman RP, Lower EE. Leflunomide for chronic sarcoidosis. Sarcoidosis Vasc Diffuse Lung Dis 2004;21:43–48.

145. Lewis SJ, Ainslie GM, Bateman ED. Efficacy of azathioprine as second-line treatment in pulmonary sarcoidosis. Sarcoidosis Vasc Diffuse Lung Dis 1999;16:87–92.
146. Muller-Quernheim J, Kienast K, Held M, et al. Treatment of chronic sarcoidosis with an azathioprine/prednisolone regimen. Eur Respir J 1999;14:1117–1122.
147. Agbogu BN, Stern BJ, Sewell C, et al. Therapeutic considerations in patients with refractory neurosarcoidosis. Arch Neurol 1995;52:875–879.
148. Kennedy PT, Zakaria N, Modawi SB, et al. Natural history of hepatic sarcoidosis and its response to treatment. Eur J Gastroenterol Hepatol 2006;18:721–726.
149. Escousse A, Mousson C, Santona L, et al. Azathioprine-induced pancytopenia in homogenous thiopurine methyltransferase-deficient renal transplant recipients: a family study. Transplant Proc 1995;27:1739–1742.
150. Kremer JM, Genovese MC, Cannon GW, et al. Concomitant leflunomide therapy in patients with active rheumatoid arthritis despite stable doses of methotrexate. A randomized, double-blind, placebo-controlled trial. Ann Intern Med 2002;137:726–733.
151. Kremer JM, Caldwell JR, Cannon GW, et al. The combination of leflunomide and methotrexate in patients with active rheumatoid arthritis who are failing on methotrexate treatment alone: a double-blind placebo controlled study. 2000: S224.
152. Osiri M, Shea B, Robinson V, et al. Leflunomide for the treatment of rheumatoid arthritis: a systematic review and metaanalysis. J Rheumatol 2003;30:1182–1190.
153. Israel HL, McComb BL. Chlorambucil treatment of sarcoidosis. Sarcoidosis 1991;8:35–41.
154. Kataria YP. Chlorambucil in sarcoidosis. Chest 1980;78:36–42.
155. Doty JD, Mazur JE, Judson MA. Treatment of corticosteroid-resistant neurosarcoidosis with a short-course cyclophosphamide regimen. Chest 2003;124:2023–2026.
156. Baughman RP, Lower EE. Use of intermittent, intravenous cyclophosphamide for idiopathic pulmonary fibrosis. Chest 1992;102:1090–1094.
157. Talar-Williams C, Hijazi YM, Walther MM, et al. Cyclophosphamide-induced cystitis and bladder cancer in patients with Wegener granulomatosis. Ann Intern Med 1996;124:477–484.
158. Bradley DA, Lower EE, Baughman RP. Diagnosis and management of spinal cord sarcoidosis. Sarcoidosis Vasc Diffuse Lung Dis 2006;23(1):58–65.
159. Rosenbaum JT. Treatment of severe refractory uveitis with intravenous cyclophosphamide. J Rheumatol 1994;21:123–125.
160. Zuber M, Defer G, Cesaro P, et al. Efficacy of cyclophosphamide in sarcoid radiculomyelitis. J Neurol Neurosurg Psychiatry 1992;55:166–167.
161. Carlesimo M, Giustini S, Rossi A, et al. Treatment of cutaneous and pulmonary sarcoidosis with thalidomide. J Am Acad Dermatol 1995;32:866–869.
162. Lee JB, Koblenzer PS. Disfiguring cutaneous manifestation of sarcoidosis treated with thalidomide: a case report. J Am Acad Dermatol 1998;39:835–838.
163. Nguyen YT, Dupuy A, Cordoliani F, et al. Treatment of cutaneous sarcoidosis with thalidomide. J Am Acad Dermatol 2004;50:235–241.
164. Oliver SJ, Kikuchi T, Krueger JG, et al. Thalidomide induces granuloma differentiation in sarcoid skin lesions associated with disease improvement. Clin Immunol 2002;102:225–236.
165. Rousseau L, Beylot-Barry M, Doutre MS, et al. Cutaneous sarcoidosis successfully treated with low doses of thalidomide. Arch Dermatol 1998;134:1045–1046.
166. Judson MA, Silvestri J, Hartung C, et al. The effect of thalidomide on corticosteroid-dependent pulmonary sarcoidosis. Sarcoidosis Vasc Diffuse Lung Dis 2006;23:51–57.
167. Baughman RP, Strohofer SA, Buchsbaum J, et al. Release of tumor necrosis factor by alveolar macrophages of patients with sarcoidosis. J Lab Clin Med 1990;115:36–42.
168. Ziegenhagen MW, Benner UK, Zissel G, et al. Sarcoidosis: TNF-alpha release from alveolar macrophages and serum level of sIL-2R are prognostic markers. Am J Respir Crit Care Med 1997;156:1586–1592.
169. Baughman RP, Lower EE. The effect of corticosteroid or methotrexate therapy on lung lymphocytes and macrophages in sarcoidosis. Am Rev Respir Dis 1990;142:1268–1271.

170. Ziegenhagen MW, Rothe E, Zissel G, et al. Exagerated TNFalpha release of alveolar macrophages in corticosteroid resistant sarcoidosis. Sarcoidosis Vasc Diffuse Lung Dis 2002;19:185–190.

171. Baughman RP, Iannuzzi M. Tumour necrosis factor in sarcoidosis and its potential for targeted therapy. BioDrugs 2003;17:425–431.

172. Gartlehner G, Hansen RA, Jonas BL, et al. The comparative efficacy and safety of biologics for the treatment of rheumatoid arthritis: a systematic review and metaanalysis. J Rheumatol 2006;33:2398–2408.

173. Lovell DJ, Giannini EH, Reiff A, et al. Etanercept in children with polyarticular juvenile rheumatoid arthritis. Pediatric Rheumatology Collaborative Study Group. N Engl J Med 2000;342:763–769.

174. Kavanaugh A, Clair EW, McCune WJ, et al. Chimeric anti-tumor necrosis factor-alpha monoclonal antibody treatment of patients with rheumatoid arthritis receiving methotrexate therapy. J Rheumatol 2000;27:841–850.

175. Sands BE, Anderson FH, Bernstein CN, et al. Infliximab maintenance therapy for fistulizing Crohn's disease. N Engl J Med 2004;350:876–885.

176. Sandborn WJ, Hanauer SB, Katz S, et al. Etanercept for active Crohn's disease: a randomized, double-blind, placebo-controlled trial. Gastroenterology 2001;121:1088–1094.

177. Keane J, Gershon S, Wise RP, et al. Tuberculosis associated with infliximab, a tumor necrosis factor-alpha neutralizing agent. N Engl J Med 2001;345:1098–1104.

178. Baughman RP, Bradley DA, Lower EE. Infliximab for chronic ocular inflammation. Int J Clin Pharmacol Ther 2005;43:7–11.

179. Baughman RP, Lower EE. Infliximab for refractory sarcoidosis. Sarcoidosis Vasc Diffuse Lung Dis 2001;18:70–74.

180. Doty JD, Mazur JE, Judson MA. Treatment of sarcoidosis with infliximab. Chest 2005; 127:1064–1071.

181. Saleh S, Ghodsian S, Yakimova V, et al. Effectiveness of infliximab in treating selected patients with sarcoidosis. Respir Med 2006;100(11):2053–2059.

182. Yee AMF, Pochapin MB. Treatment of complicated sarcoidosis with infliximab anti-tumor necrosis-alpha therapy. Ann Intern Med 2001;135:27–31.

183. Baughman RP, Drent M, Kavuru M, et al. Infliximab therapy in patients with chronic sarcoidosis and pulmonary involvement. Am J Respir Crit Care Med 2006;174:795–802.

184. Hanauer SB. Review article: safety of infliximab in clinical trials. Alimentary Pharm Therapeutics 1999;13(Suppl 4):16–22.

185. Chung ES, Packer M, Lo KH, et al. Randomized, double-blind, placebo-controlled, pilot trial of infliximab, a chimeric monoclonal antibody to tumor necrosis factor-alpha, in patients with moderate-to-severe heart failure: results of the anti-TNF Therapy Against Congestive Heart Failure (ATTACH) trial. Circulation 2003;107:3133–3140.

186. Utz JP, Limper AH, Kalra S, et al. Etanercept for the treatment of stage II and III progressive pulmonary sarcoidosis. Chest 2003;124:177–185.

187. Baughman RP, Lower EE, Bradley DA, et al. Etanercept for refractory ocular sarcoidosis: results of a double-blind randomized trial. Chest 2005;128:1062–1067.

188. Mann DL, McMurray JJ, Packer M, et al. Targeted anticytokine therapy in patients with chronic heart failure: results of the Randomized Etanercept Worldwide Evaluation (RENEWAL). Circulation 2004;109:1594–1602.

189. Wegener's Granulomatosis Etanercept Trial (WGET) Research Group. Etanercept plus standard therapy for Wegener's granulomatosis. N Engl J Med 2005;352:351–361.

190. Wallis RS, Ehlers S. Tumor necrosis factor and granuloma biology: explaining the differential infection risk of etanercept and infliximab. Semin Arthritis Rheum 2005;34(5 Suppl 1): 34–38.

191. Van den Brande JM, Braat H, van den Brink GR, et al. Infliximab but not etanercept induces apoptosis in lamina propria T-lymphocytes from patients with Crohn's disease. Gastroenterology 2003;124:1774–1785.

192. Bachelez H, Senet P, Cadranel J, et al. The use of tetracyclines for the treatment of sarcoidosis. Arch Dermatol 2001;137:69–73.
193. Breuer K, Gutzmer R, Volker B, et al. Therapy of noninfectious granulomatous skin diseases with fumaric acid esters. Br J Dermatol 2005;152:1290–1295.
194. Zabel P, Entzian P, Dalhoff K, et al. Pentoxifylline in treatment of sarcoidosis. Am J Respir Crit Care Med 1997;155:1665–1669.
195. Marques LJ, Zheng L, Poulakis N, et al. Pentoxifylline inhibits TNF-alpha production from human alveolar macrophages. Am J Respir Crit Care Med 1999;159(2):508–511.
196. Strieter RM, Remick DG, Ward PA, et al. Cellular and molecular regulation of tumor necrosis factor-alpha production by pentoxifylline. Biochem Biophys Res Commun 1988;155: 1230–1236.
197. Judson MA. Lung transplantation for pulmonary sarcoidosis. Eur Respir J 1998;11:738–744.
198. Preston IR, Klinger JR, Landzberg MJ, et al. Vasoresponsiveness of sarcoidosis-associated pulmonary hypertension. Chest 2001;120:866–872.
199. Fisher KA, Serlin DM, Wilson KC, et al. Sarcoidosis-associated pulmonary hypertension: outcome with long-term epoprostenol treatment. Chest 2006;130:1481–1488.
200. Foley RJ, Metersky ML. Successful Treatment of Sarcoidosis-Associated Pulmonary Hypertension with Bosentan. Respiration 2008;75:211–214.
201. Sharma S, Kashour T, Philipp R. Secondary pulmonary arterial hypertension: treated with endothelin receptor blockade. Tex Heart Inst J 2005;32:405–410.
202. Letizia C, Danese A, Reale MG, et al. Plasma levels of endothelin-1 increase in patients with sarcoidosis and fall after disease remission. Panminerva Med 2001;43:257–261.
203. Terashita K, Kato S, Sata M, et al. Increased endothelin-1 levels of BAL fluid in patients with pulmonary sarcoidosis. Respirology 2006;11:145–151.
204. Galie N, Ghofrani HA, Torbicki A, et al. Sildenafil citrate therapy for pulmonary arterial hypertension. N Engl J Med 2005;353:2148–2157.
205. Ghofrani HA, Wiedemann R, Rose F, et al. Sildenafil for treatment of lung fibrosis and pulmonary hypertension: a randomised controlled trial. Lancet 2002;360:895–900.
206. Collard HR, Anstrom KJ, Schwarz MI, et al. Sildenafil improves walk distance in idiopathic pulmonary fibrosis. Chest 2007;131:897–899.
207. Milman N, Burton CM, Iversen M, et al. Pulmonary hypertension in end-stage pulmonary sarcoidosis: therapeutic effect of sildenafil? J Heart Lung Transplant 2008;27:329–334.
208. Pietinalho A, Ohmichi M, Lofroos AB, et al. The prognosis of sarcoidosis in Finland and Hokkaido, Japan. A comparative five-year study of biopsy-proven cases. Sarcoidosis Vasc Diffuse Lung Dis 2000;17:158–166.
209. Baughman RP, Lower EE. Therapy for sarcoidosis. Eur Respir Mon 2005;32:301–315.
210. Baughman RP, Sparkman BK, Lower EE. Six-minute walk test and health status assessment in sarcoidosis. Chest 2007;132:207–213.

Index

Printed in the United States of America